Manual of
Minor Oral Surgery
for the General Dentist

Manual of Minor Oral Surgery for the General Dentist

Edited by

Karl R. Koerner

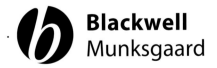

Karl R. Koerner, BS, DDS, MS, is an editor of and contributor to *Manual of Oral Surgery for General Dentists* (Blackwell Publishing) and has co-authored *Color Atlas of Minor Oral Surgery*, 2nd ed. (Mosby) and *Clinical Procedures for Third Molar Surgery*, 2nd ed. (PennWell). He also is editor of and contributor to a *Dental Clinics of North America* (Saunders) volume on basic oral surgery. Dr. Koerner has produced video programs and contributed articles to publications such as *General Dentistry, Dentistry Today, Dental Economics*, and the *Journal of Public Health Dentistry.*

Dr. Koerner is a past president of the Utah Dental Association and a former delegate to the ADA House. He has served as Utah Academy of General Dentistry (AGD) president, is a Fellow in the AGD, and has membership in the International College of Dentists. He is licensed in Utah to administer IV sedation and licensed to practice dentistry in Utah, Idaho, and California. His practice is now limited to oral surgery.

Dr. Koerner has been teaching clinical courses on oral surgery to other dentists in the United States and abroad since 1981. In 2002, he joined Clinical Research Associates (CRA) in Provo, Utah, as an evaluator and clinician and began teaching their "Update" courses throughout the country and abroad. Since 2002, he has co-presented more than 90 courses for CRA and serves on their advisory board.

© 2006 by Blackwell Munksgaard,
published by Blackwell Publishing Professional,
a Blackwell Publishing Company

Blackwell Publishing Professional
2121 State Avenue, Ames, Iowa 50014-8300, USA
Tel: +1 515 292 0140

Editorial Offices:
9600 Garsington Road, Oxford OX4 2DQ
Tel: 01865 776868

Blackwell Publishing Asia Pty Ltd,
550 Swanston Street, Carlton South,
Victoria 3053, Australia
Tel: +61 (0)3 9347 0300

Blackwell Wissenschafts Verlag,
Kurfürstendamm 57,
10707 Berlin, Germany
Tel: +49 (0)30 32 79 060

Europe and Asia
All rights reserved. No part of this publication may be reproduced, stored in a retrieval system, or transmitted, in any form or by any means, electronic, mechanical, photocopying, recording or otherwise, except as permitted by the UK Copyright, Designs and Patents Act 1988, without the prior permission of the publisher.

The right of the Author to be identified as the Author of this Work has been asserted in accordance with the Copyright, Designs and Patents Act 1988.

North America
Authorization to photocopy items for internal or personal use, or the internal or personal use of specific clients, is granted by Blackwell Publishing, provided that the base fee is paid directly to the Copyright Clearance Center, 222 Rosewood Drive, Danvers, MA 01923. For those organizations that have been granted a photocopy license by CCC, a separate system of payments has been arranged. The fee code for users of the Transactional Reporting Service is ISBN-13: 978-0-8138-0559-7/2006.

Library of Congress Cataloging-in-Publication Data

Manual of minor oral surgery for the general dentist / edited by Karl R. Koerner.
    p. ; cm.
    Includes bibliographical references and index.
    ISBN-13: 978-0-8138-0559-7 (alk. paper)
    ISBN-10: 0-8138-0559-7 (alk. paper)
    1. Dentistry, Operative. 2. Mouth—Surgery.
3. Dentistry. [DNLM: 1. Oral Surgical Procedures.
2. Surgical Procedures, Minor. WU 600 M294
2006] I. Koerner, Karl R.

    RK501.M34 2006
    617.6_05—dc22

                       2005028549

For further information on
Blackwell Publishing, visit our Dentistry Subject Site: www.dentistry.blackwellmunksgaard.com

The last digit is the print number: 9 8 7 6 5 4 3 2

Contents

Contributors   vii
Preface   ix

Chapter 1   Patient Evaluation and Medical History   3
  Dr. R. Thane Hales
Chapter 2   Surgical Extractions   19
  Dr. Hussam S. Batal and Dr. Gregg Jacob
Chapter 3   Surgical Management of Impacted Third Molar Teeth   49
  Dr. Pushkar Mehra and Dr. Shant Baran
Chapter 4   Pre-Prosthetic Oral Surgery   81
  Dr. Ruben Figueroa and Dr. Abhishek Mogre
Chapter 5   Conservative Surgical Crown Lengthening   99
  Dr. George M. Bailey
Chapter 6   Endodontic Periradicular Microsurgery   137
  Dr. Louay Abrass
Chapter 7   The Evaluation and Treatment of Oral Lesions   201
  Dr. Joseph D. Christensen and Dr. Karl R. Koerner
Chapter 8   Anxiolysis for Oral Surgery and Other Dental Procedures   221
  Dr. Fred Quarnstrom
Chapter 9   Infections and Antibiotic Administration   255
  Dr. R. Thane Hales
Chapter 10   Management of Perioperative Bleeding   277
  Dr. Karl R. Koerner, and Dr. William L. McBee
Chapter 11   Third World Volunteer Dentistry   295
  Dr. Richard C. Smith

Index   319

Contributors

Number in brackets following each name is the chapter number.

Louay M. Abrass, DMD [6]
Assistant Clinical Professor, Department of Endodontics, Boston University School of Dental Medicine
Adjunct Assistant Professor, Department of Endodontics, University of Pennsylvania School of Dental Medicine
Private Practice Limited to Endodontics in Boston and Wellesley, Massachusetts

George M. Bailey, DDS, MS [5]
Associate Professor, University of Utah Medical School and Creighton School of Dentistry
President and Lecturer CPSeminars
Private Practice Periodontics

Shant Baran, DMD [3]
Resident, Department of Oral and Maxillofacial Surgery, Boston University School of Dental Medicine and Boston Medical Center, Boston, Massachusetts

Hussam S. Batal, DMD [2]
Assistant Professor, Department of Oral and Maxillofacial Surgery, Boston University, Boston, Massachusetts

Joseph D. Christensen, DMD [7]
Private General Practice, Salt Lake City, Utah

Ruben Figueroa, DMD, MS [4]
Oral and Maxillofacial Surgeon
Assistant Professor, Director Predoctoral Oral and Maxillofacial Surgery, Director Oral Surgery Clinic, Boston University, Henry Goldman School of Dental Medicine, Boston, Massachusetts

R. Thane Hales, DMD [1, 9]
Founder and Director of the Wasatch Surgical Institute
International Lecturer and Clinician, Private Practice, Ogden, Utah

Gregg A. Jacob, DMD [2]
Private Practice, Summit Oral and Maxillofacial Surgery, P.A., Summit, New Jersey

Karl R. Koerner, DDS, MS [Editor, 7, 10]
International Lecturer and Clinician
Private General Practice Limited to Oral Surgery, Salt Lake City, Utah
Formerly Consultant and Instructor for Clinical Research Associates, Provo, Utah

William L. McBee, DDS [10]
Private Practice Limited to Oral and Maxillofacial Surgery, Provo, Utah

Pushkar Mehra, BDS, DMD [3]
Director, Department of Dentistry and Oral and Maxillofacial Surgery, Boston Medical Center
Director, Department of Oral and Maxillofacial Surgery, Boston University Medical Center
Assistant Professor, Department of Oral and Maxillofacial Surgery, Boston University School of Dental Medicine, Boston, Massachusetts

Abhishek Mogre BDS [4]
Current Advanced Standing DMD Student
Vice President Predoctoral Association of Oral and Maxillofacial Surgery, Boston University, Henry Goldman School of Dental Medicine, Boston, Massachusetts

Dr. Fred Quarnstrom, DDS [8]
Clinical Faculty of Dentistry, University of British Columbia
Affiliate Assistant Professor, University of Washington School of Dentistry
Dental Anesthesiologist also in General Dental Practice, Seattle, Washington

Richard C. Smith, DDS [11]
Chairman of Ayuda Incorporated
Private General Practice (Retired), Westlake Village, California

Preface

This handbook is a guide for the general dentist who enjoys doing oral surgery. A broad range of knowledge and expertise in this area is found among dentists. Some have had extensive experience and training through general practice residencies, military or other postgraduate programs, or a mentoring experience with a more experienced dentist; others have had only minimal instruction and training in dental school.

Dental school oral surgery training varies widely based on individual school requirements for graduation. In addition, some schools offer elective or extramural experiences, others do not. Even in the same dental school class, a few students might have the opportunity to perform extensive exodontia, but others will remove only a few teeth before moving on to private practice. This handbook is meant to diminish the discrepancy between experienced and inexperienced generalists and provide an information base for the interested clinician. This book presents a review of procedures and principles in each of several clinical surgical areas; this review will enable a dentist to perform according to established standards of care.

It is assumed that the reader possesses fundamental knowledge and skills in oral anatomy, patient/operator positioning for surgery, the care of soft and hard tissue during surgery, and basic patient management techniques. Therefore, the authors have skipped to the crux of each procedure, addressing such things as case selection, step-by-step operative procedures, and the prevention and/or management of complications. This handbook will help dentists perform procedures more quickly, smoothly, easily, and safely—thereby greatly minimizing doctor frustration and patient dissatisfaction.

The procedures covered in this book are also done by oral and maxillofacial surgeons and/or periodontists and endodontists. There are times that the patient would be better served by being referred to the specialist, such as when the patient is extremely apprehensive, medically compromised, an older patient with dense bone, or has other mitigating circumstances. This book will help readers more clearly understand the scope of each procedure and more accurately define their capabilities and comfort zones.

Procedures described are mainly dentoalveolar in nature, such as "surgical" extractions, the removal of impacted wisdom teeth (mainly in younger patients), preprosthetic surgery, apicoectomy and retrofil cases, surgical crown lengthening, and biopsy. Supportive topics include patient evaluation and case selection and the management of problems such as bleeding and infection. One chapter involves logistical considerations and the use of basic surgical principles for those volunteering services in a third-world setting.

This book is a ready reference for the surgery-minded general practioner. Within these pages, the authors share many pearls gleaned from years of experience and training to increase the readers' confidence and competence.

ix

Manual of
Minor Oral Surgery
for the General Dentist

Chapter 1

Patient Evaluation and Medical History

Dr. R. Thane Hales

Introduction

The purpose of this book is to provide the general dentist with specific information about oral surgery procedures that are performed daily in general dentists' offices. Some advanced information is also given to provide the more experienced general dentist the opportunity to further his or her skills and knowledge.

The ability of a general dentist to perform these procedures is based on a number of factors. Some dentists have a great interest in surgery, while others have very little interest. Some dentists have had a general practice residency or other postgraduate training or experience; others may not have had the opportunity. Some are in areas that have little or no support from a specialist, which makes some surgery mandatory in their practices. Currently, it is accepted that regardless of who performs dental procedures, be they a generalist or a specialist, the standards of care are the same. If a general dentist wants to include the removal of third molars in his or her practice, he or she will usually need more training than that provided in dental school.

Just having the desire to do this procedure will not, in and of itself, qualify a person. The best thing a general dentist can do is to first obtain additional training. Surgical expertise is improved by taking postgraduate courses. The clinician then learns to diagnose the less complicated procedures and does them with supervision until they are performed well. State laws do not discriminate between a general dentist and a specialist. A license gives the same perogative to a generalist that an oral surgeon has to extract teeth. Therefore, the generalist has a greater responsibility to acquire training and knowledge if he or she expects to do more complex procedures. This responsibility includes not only receiving instruction in step-by-step surgical techniques, but also the medical management of such patients and any complications that might arise.

Surgical skill is only part of the equation. The judgment of the practitioner in making appropriate decisions regarding the patient's total condition is vital when doing surgical procedures. Anxiety management should be addressed before the surgical procedure is

4   CHAPTER 1

started. Will sedation be needed to accomplish the treatment? Some patients require sedation in order to make them feel comfortable about the surgery. The dentist who doesn't fully understand the many facets of treating an extremely anxious and medically compromised patient should find an appropriate network of specialists in medicine and/or dentistry and then use a multidisciplinary team approach.

Dentists must never forget the human elements of kindness, compassion, and caring. The patient wants to be treated just like any person would want to be treated. Dentists need to have enough insight into the patients' fears and concerns to be able to calm and reassure them that they can handle any and all contingencies with competence. A little compassion and empathy go a long way in today's "rushed" society.

Humanism and compassion are the two most important factors by which a patient judges a dentist's skill. Especially in the mind of the patient, the technical aspect of surgery is secondary to the surgeon's ability to manage pain and anxiety. It is a given that a surgeon has the ability to handle tissues with great skill, care, and judgment; the proper handling of and respect for tissues will enable them to heal more quickly and without as many complications.

Medical History

The most important information that a clinician can acquire is the medical history of a patient. If any problem is expressed in the history, a skilled clinician should be able to decide whether the patient is capable of undergoing the procedure. The dentist should be fully able to predict how medical problems might interfere with the patient's ability to heal and whether they might react to the anesthetic, antibiotics, or other medications.

The doctor needs to have a detailed questionnaire that covers all major medical problems that could exist in a patient and a space

on the form for any other condition not mentioned. The questionnaire must make sure that the doctor is advised of any complications a patient may have had in the past. The doctor then must be able to fully evaluate the patient's situation relative to the procedure.

In the process of getting medical information or even biographical data, the doctor should observe the patient for any illogical statements or inconsistent responses that might need further evaluation. A bright, well-trained assistant is priceless in a private practice—especially during the filling out of patient forms and in helping to acquire accurate medical information. He/she should bring to the attention of the doctor any problem on the form that might influence the procedure. The assistant must also highlight medical problems and mark the outside of the chart with a coded warning that the patient is at medical risk.

All medical questionnaires should include a history and description of the patient's chief complaint. Patients should fill out the form in their own words and give as much information as they can about their problems. The clarity of this information, accompanied by careful and skillful questioning by the doctor, can help him or her form a reasonable diagnosis. If the patient is unable to competently give this information, then all aspects of the information should be suspect. A diagnosis can be moved to the next step only if there is a complete and reliable review of the patient's status. The form should include a statement of confidentiality reassuring patients that records will be protected. The only people having access to the records will be the doctors in the practice or the patient's physician (with permission of the patient). A signature line is also required to verify that the patient has understood the questions and that they have been answered satisfactorily.

Specifically, the medical history form should include medical problems patients might have that would compromise their safety (unless proper steps are taken by the dentist). The cardiovascular system is a main consideration. Any history of angina, myocardial infarction, murmurs, or rheumatic fever should be taken seriously, and appropriate steps should be taken to protect the patient. Other illnesses like hepatitis, asthma, diabetes, kidney disease, sexually transmitted disease, seizures, artificial joints, heart valves, and specific allergies should be noted. Allergies that should be addressed are mainly those to medications and other items used in a dental office, such as latex. The use of any anticoagulants (which now include some of the common herbal compounds), corticosteroids, hypertension medication, and other medications should be thoroughly reviewed.[1] Female patients, even young unmarried females, should be asked whether there is any possibility that they are pregnant. The medical history should be updated annually. A good hygienist or assistant should interview the patient to find out whether there has been any change since the patient's last visit. The hygienist should then record the changes on the chart and bring them to the attention of the doctor.

After the medical history form is filled out, the doctor sits with the patient and reviews the form in detail. It is crucial that the patient understands everything they are talking about. This is a good time to evaluate the patient's ability to respond and comprehend his or her condition. Any signs of nervous or psychological behavior should be noted. The interview should help determine whether the patient is responsible enough for the physician to trust the information the patient has given on the medical form. If there is any doubt, a responsible family member should be consulted, and when necessary, a call to the patient's physician should be made.

Form 1.1 shows a typical medical history form. Each provider must take responsibility for the content of his or her own forms.[2] Another important legal paper that has

proven worthwhile is the consent to proceed form (Form 1.2). It gives added protection to the office staff.[2]

HIPPA

The dentist is, of course, subject to HIPPA (Health Insurance Portability and Accountability Act of 1996) regulations. HIPAA requires that all health plans, including the Employee Retirement Income Security Act (ERISA), health care clearinghouses, and any dentist who transmits health information in an electronic transaction, use a standard format. Those plans and providers that choose not to use the electronic standards can use a clearinghouse to comply with the requirement. Providers' paper transactions are not subject to this requirement. The security regulations, which the Department of Health and Human Services released under HIPPA, were conceived to protect electronic patient health information. Protected patient health information is anything that ties a patient's identity to that person's health, health care, or payment for health care, such as X-rays, charts, or invoices. Transactions include claims and remittances, eligibility inquiries and response, and claim status and response. Self-training kits can be purchased from the American Dental Association. Electronic processing has become the standard and, in many ways, makes the provider's life much easier.[3]

Physical Examination

The clinician or a well-trained hygienist or assistant should begin the exam with the measurement of vital signs. This both serves as a screening device for unsuspected medical problems and gives a good baseline for future evaluations. The technique of measuring blood pressure and pulse rate is shown in Figure 1.1.

Despite elevated blood pressure being common, the devices to examine this critical

Medical History

Patient's Name _____ Date of Birth _____

Physician's Name _____ Phone number _____

Please answer the following questions as completely as possible

1. Do you consider yourself to be in good health?   YES   NO
2. Are you now or have you been under a physician's care within the past year?   YES   NO
   If yes, specify the condition being treated: _____
3. Do you take any medication, including birth control pills?   YES   NO
   Please specify name and purpose of medication: _____
   _____
   _____
4. Do you have or have you ever had any heart or blood problems?   YES   NO
5. Have you ever been told that you have a heart murmur?   YES   NO
6. Do you require antibiotic medication before treatment for a heart condition?   YES   NO
7. Do you now have or have you ever had high blood pressure?   YES NO
8. Have you ever been diagnosed as being HIV positive or having AIDS?   YES NO
9. Have you ever had hepatitis or liver disease?   YES   NO
10. Have you ever had rheumatic fever, ___ asthma, ___ blood disorder, ____
    diabetes ___; rhermatism ____; arthritis ____; tuberculosis ___; venereal disease ___; heart attack ___;
    kidney disease ___; immune system disorder ___; any other diseases ___
    If so, specify: _____
11. Do you bleed easily?   YES   NO
12. Have you ever had any severe or unusual reaction to, or are you allergic to, any drugs, including the following:

    Penicillin____   Ibuprofen_____
    Aspirin_____   Codeine_____
    Acetaminophen____   Barbiturates_____

    Are you taking any of the following medications?
    Antibiotics _____   Digitalis or heart medication_____
    Anticoagulants (Blood thinners)_____   Nitroglycerin_____
    Aspirin _____   Antihistamine_____
    Tranquilizers _____   Oral contraceptives_____
    Insulin_____
13. Do you faint easily?   YES   NO
14. Have you ever had a reaction to dental treatment or local anesthetic?   YES   NO
15. Are you allergic to any local anesthetic?   YES   NO
16. Do you have any other allergies?   YES   NO
    If yes, please describe: _____
    _____
    _____
17. Have you ever had a nervous breakdown or undergone psychiatric treatment?   YES   NO
18. Have you ever had an addiction problem with alcohol or drugs?   YES   NO
19. Women: Are you or could you be pregnant   YES   NO
    Are you breast feeding now?   YES   NO
20. Are you in pain now?   YES   NO
21. When did you last see a dentist?_____
22. Who was your last dentist? _____
23. Are your teeth affecting your general health?   YES   NO
24. Do you have or have you had bleeding or sensitive gums?   YES   NO
25. Have you ever taken Fen Phen or similar appetite-suppressant drugs?   YES   NO
26. Do you smoke? If yes, how many cigarettes a day   YES   NO
27. Do you drink alcohol? If yes, how often   YES   NO

I hereby certify that the answers to the forgoing questions are accurate to the best of my ability. Since a change in my medical condition or in medications I take can affect dental treatment, I understand the importance of and agree to take the responsibility for notifying the dentist of any changes at any subsequent appointment.

Signature _____ Date _____

(Patient, legal guardian, or authorized agent of patient)

Form 1–1

Consent to Proceed

I herby authorize Dr._____ and/or such associates or assistants as s/he may designate to perform those procedures as may be deemed necessary or advisable to maintain my dental health or the dental health of any minor or other individual for which I have responsibility, including arrangement and/or administration of any sedative (including nitrous oxide), analgesic, therapeutic, and/or other pharmaceutical agent(s) including those related to restorative, palliative, therapeutic, or surgical treatments.

I understand that the administration of local anesthetics may cause an untoward reaction or side effects, which may include, but are not limited to, bruising; hematoma; cardiac stimulation; muscle soreness; and temporary or, rarely, permanent numbness. I understand that occasionally needles break and may require surgical retrieval.

I understand that as part of dental treatment, including preventive procedures such as cleanings and basic dentistry including fillings of all types, teeth may remain sensitive or even possibly quite painful both during and after completion of treatment. After lengthy appointments, jaw muscles may also be sore and tender. Gums and surrounding tissues may also be sensitive or painful during and/or after treatment. Although rare, it is also possible for the tongue, cheek, or other oral tissues of the mouth to be inadvertently abraded or lacerated during routine dental procedures. In some cases sutures or additional treatment may be required.

I understand that as part of dental treatment, items including, but not limited to, crowns, small dental instruments, drill components, etc. may be aspirated (inhaled into the respiratory system) or swallowed. This unusual situation may require a series of x-rays to be taken by a physician or hospital and may, in rare cases, require a bronchoscope or other procedures to ensure safe removal.

I do voluntarily assume any and all possible risks, including the risk of substantial and serious harm, if any, that may be associated with general preventive and operative treatment procedures in hopes of obtaining the potential desired results, which may or may not be achieved, for my benefit or the benefit of my minor child or ward. I acknowledge that the nature and purpose of the forgoing procedures have been explained to me if necessary and that I have been given the opportunity to ask questions.

Patient Name_____

Signature_____
(Patient, legal guardian, or authorized agent of patient)

Witness_____

Form 1–2

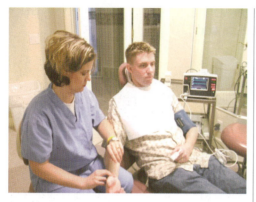

Figure 1-1. Blood pressure and pulse. Mercury sphygmomanometers are still considered a gold standard for blood pressure, but most offices now use digital equipment.

Table 1-1. Blood pressure classification

Systolic BP	Diastolic BP	Classification
<120	<80	Normal
120–139	80–89	Prehypertension
140–159	90–99	Stage 1 mild hypertension
>160	>100	Stage 2 moderate hypertension
>200	>110	Stage 3 severe hypertension

BP = blood pressure.

vital sign are frequently not accurate. The dentist must routinely calibrate blood pressure equipment against a standard mercury instrument and update the training of staff members periodically to ensure accuracy. Even when automated devices are used, those responsible for recording blood pressure must be properly trained, to reduce human error.

Of the millions of people who have hypertension, a large percentage are unaware. The dental team can be instrumental in discovering this significant and life-threatening health problem. Current studies note that nearly one-third of the U.S. population has **hypertension**—defined as a systolic blood pressure higher than 139 mm Hg or a diastolic blood pressure higher than 89 mm Hg. Another one-quarter of the U.S. population has **prehypertension**—defined by a systolic blood pressure between 120 and 139 mm Hg and a diastolic blood pressure between 80 and 89 mm Hg.[4] (Note: Recent public health trends are in the direction of advocating even more conservative values than those mentioned here and in Table 1.1.)

Normal to various high values are illustrated in Table 1.1.

Systolic and diastolic blood pressures, as opposed to pulse pressure, remain the best means to classify hypertension. The risk of stroke begins to increase steadily as blood pressure rises from 115/75 mm Hg to higher values.

About 15 to 20 percent of patients with stage I hypertension have elevated blood pressure only in the office setting of a health care provider. This type of transient hypertension is more common in older men and women, and antihypertensive treatment in these patients may reduce office blood pressure but not affect ambulatory blood pressure.

When the blood pressure reading is mild to moderately high, the patient should be referred to their primary care physician for hypertensive therapy. The patient should be monitored on each subsequent visit before treatment. If needed, the operator can use anxiety control protocol (see Table 1.2 later in this chapter).

When severe hypertension exists, defer treatment and refer the patient to a primary care or emergency room physician. These patients can be walking potential stroke victims.

A pulse rate should be taken and recorded. The most common method is to use the tips of the middle and index fingers of the right hand to palpate the radial artery at the patient's wrist. See Figure 1.1.

The heart rate is determined by counting the number of pulses for 30 seconds and then multiplying that number by two. This yields the number of beats per minute. If there is a weakened pulse or irregular rhythm, elective treatment should not be performed unless the operator has received clearance by the patient's physician.

HEAD AND NECK EXAMINATION

The physical evaluation of a dental patient will focus on the oral cavity and surrounding head and neck region, but the clinician should also carefully visually evaluate the rest of the patient for abnormalities.

The physical evaluation is usually accomplished in four primary ways: inspection, palpation, percussion, and auscultation (listening with a stethoscope to the sounds made by the heart, lungs, and blood). The dentist should also examine skin texture and look for possible skin lesions on the head, neck, and any other exposed parts of the body. Submandibular lymph nodes and those on the neck should be palpated. Include examination of the hair, facial symmetry, eye movements and conjunctiva color, and facial masses. Inspect the oral cavity thoroughly, including the oropharynx, tongue, floor of the mouth, and oral mucosa for any abnormal-looking tissue or indurated areas.

SUSPICIOUS LESIONS

All suspicious lesions should have a biopsy. According to the guidelines of the American Dental Association, any lesion that has an abnormal appearance and a duration of 14 days or more should be biopsied. The specimen should be sent to an oral pathology laboratory. Labs that specialize in the histological examination of excisional and incisional biopsies usually provide specimen jars at no charge. Dentists must take the lead in this effort. Red and white lesions or a combination of both types are particularly suspicious and must be taken seriously. See Figure 1.2. Oral cancer is usually very invasive and de-

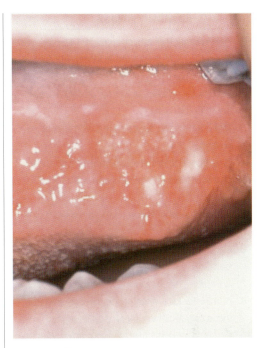

Figure 1-2. Squamous cell carcinoma on the lateral border of the tongue.

structive. It can be found in people without the characteristic risk factors of tobacco and alcohol use and even in children. A thorough exam is mandatory.

ANXIETY CONTROL

The incorporation of good anxiety-reducing methods is essential. See Table 1.2.

Common Diseases and Conditions Affecting Dental Patients

When the evaluation is completed, the clinician should have a good idea of the condition of the patient. As dental treatment poses no risk to most people, the dentist may become complacent when presented with a high-risk patient and not perform the necessary steps to completely analyze the situation. A careful and systematic approach must be used to deal with medically compromised patients. Only in this way can potential

CHAPTER 1

Table 1-2. Antianxiety protocol

1. Administration of a hypnotic agent to promote sleep the night before the appointment for surgery. (Ambien 10 mg)
2. Administer sedative agent for anxiety control 2 hours before surgery.
3. Make a morning appointment with little or no waiting.
4. Give frequent verbal reassurances with other distracting conversations not related to the surgery.
5. Warn the patient before doing anything that is uncomfortable.
6. Keep surgical instruments and needles out of sight.
7. Administer nitrous oxide oxygen.
8. Administer local anesthetics carefully and use those of sufficient duration and intensity.
9. Use epinephrine 1:100,000, but no more than 4 ml, for a total adult dose of 0.04 mg in any 30-minute period.
10. Administer intravenous sedation if available, with sufficient monitoring incorporated by licensed personnel.
11. After surgery give verbal and written instructions on postoperative care.
12. Write prescriptions for effective analgesics.
13. Give reassurance and get information about whom to call if problems arise.
14. Call the patient at home that evening to see how they are doing and whether there are any questions or problems.

complications be managed or avoided. Following are a few of the most common diseases and conditions that a clinician will encounter.

Cardiovascular Disease

The progressive narrowing of the arteries to the heart leads to a difference in myocardial oxygen demand and supply. This demand can be further increased by exertion, digestion, or anxiety during surgical procedures. When the muscle of the heart becomes ischemic, it can produce pressure in the chest with pain radiating to the arms, neck, or jaw. Other symptoms include sweating and a slowed heart rate. This condition is called **angina pectoris**. Angina is usually reversible if the proper medications and oxygen are administered quickly. Oxygen, nitroglycerin, and aspirin should be available in the office.

If, during the examination, the dentist determines that the patient has experienced obstruction of the arterial blood flow to the heart, certain precautions must be taken. The practitioner's responsibility to the patient is to have necessary medications on hand and initiate preventive measures even before treatment is begun. This will reduce the chance that a surgical procedure will precipitate an anginal episode. If the patient is easily prone to this condition, supplemental oxygen is recommended. Oral sedation or nitrous oxide can be helpful to relax these patients. If anginal pain is a problem during a dental appointment, the operator should activate the Emergency Medical System (call 911). The patient's physician should be consulted prior to subsequent appointments.

Giving a local anesthetic with epinephrine to a patient with a history of cardiac problems has always been controversial, but generally, the benefits outweigh the risks. Endogenous adrenalin surges in response to pain stimulation can be equal to or more dangerous than the small amount of vasoconstrictor. It is recommended, however, that with these patients, the dose not exceed 4 ml of local anesthetic and an epinephrine concentration of 1:100,000, for a total adult dose of .04 mg per 30-minute period.[1]

Monitoring of the vital signs should be done at regular intervals during surgery. Verbal contact should be ongoing and unforced. Always have a fresh bottle of nitroglycerin and a good supply of oxygen available.

Many scenarios should alert the dentist that the patient is having more than angina. The following symptoms could indicate a heart attack or **myocardial infarction** (MI). Among them are the following:

1. The chest pain does not go away.
2. The chest pain goes away but comes back.
3. The chest pain worsens.[5]

If these symptoms persist, the dentist must get the patient to an emergency room or call the Emergency Medical System (911).

Myocardial Infarction (MI)

Care must be taken with patients who have a history of MI. The blockage of a coronary artery must be recognized and treated immediately. The infarcted area dies, becomes nonfunctional, and eventually necrotic. The myocardium around the infarction is slightly damaged but usually heals. It may form a nidus that can precipitate abnormal rhythms.

The management of a patient with a history of MI is as follows (as recommended by the American Heart Association):

1. Consult the patient's physician.
2. Defer all elective procedures for at least six months after an infarction. After clearance from the patient's physician, implement the antianxiety protocol. Give supplemental oxygen during each dental appointment.
3. Have nitroglycerin available. If oral surgery is needed, consider referring the patient to an oral and maxillofacial surgeon.[6]

Heart Bypass Grafts

Bypass graft patients should also be scheduled for dental treatment no sooner than six months after surgery. This is the routine unless there have been complications during healing—then it could be longer. Always keep the anxious patient as relaxed as possible. Carefully monitor the vital signs throughout treatment. A pulse oximeter is a great instrument to have attached to any patient with a history of heart disease. If the office is equipped with a heart monitoring device (or EKG), it should be used to detect any arrhythmias.

Congestive Heart Failure

This disease of the heart occurs when the myocardium is unable to act as an efficient pump. The heart cannot deliver the output necessary to maintain the circulatory system, and the blood begins to pool and back up. The major effect is seen in the pulmonary system, the hepatic system, and the mesenteric vascular beds.

The symptoms of congestive heart failure are orthopnea, ankle swelling, and dyspnea. Orthopnea is a shortness of breath when the patient is lying down. The patient feels some comfort in sleeping with the upper body elevated to enhance breathing. These patients are usually on a variety of medications to reduce fluids. Diuretics and digitoxin are administered to increase cardiac output. The patient may also be taking beta blockers or calcium channel antagonists to control the work load of the heart.

Patients who are generally well controlled with their medication can undergo routine dental surgery or other treatments. The dentist should initiate anxiety control and give supplemental oxygen during surgery.

Any clinician who serves the medically compromised heart patient must be well qualified to handle emergencies. If not, he or she should refer the patient to a specialist.

Liver Dysfunction

The patient who suffers from hepatic damage, usually from some infectious disease or alcohol abuse, will need to be given special consideration. This would include a reduction in dose or total avoidance of drugs that are metabolized in the liver. This requires the prescribing dentist to be cognizant of the metabolic processes of the drug he or she prescribes. The patient may be prone to bleeding because of the fact that many coagulation factors produced in the liver are diminished. A partial prothrombin time (PTT) or a prothrombin time (PT) is useful in evaluation, especially in the severely liver-damaged patient. Many patients with liver disease are infectious but can be managed with routine universal precautions.

DIABETES

Diabetes is classified into insulin-dependent and non-insulin-dependant patients. Insulin-dependent diabetics usually have a history of diabetes from childhood or early adulthood. The underproduction of insulin is the major problem.

Elevated serum glucose short-term is not dangerous to the diabetic, but hypoglycemia from not eating after an insulin load can cause disorientation and possible diabetic or insulin shock. This state must be treated with a glucose load in order to stabilize the patient. A drink of orange juice when the patient is conscious is effective. Emergency kits should provide a safe mode of delivery for the needed glucose. To manage an insulin-dependent diabetic, do the following:

1. Make certain the diabetes is well controlled. Consult the patient's physician before treatment is initiated.
2. Place the patient on an anxiety reduction protocol if necessary but do not use deep sedation.
3. Do not schedule long procedures and make short morning appointments.
4. Ask the patient before proceeding what he or she has eaten and whether he or she has balanced it with insulin.

5. Monitor the patient's vital signs continuously.
6. Have the patient eat a normal breakfast with the normal insulin dose.
7. Make sure that the patient is advised to adjust the insulin dose to the caloric intake after the surgery. Difficulty in eating may cause some alteration in balance. Consult the patient's physician if necessary.
8. Watch for signs of hypoglycemia.
9. Keep in touch with the patient on the development of infection. Do what is necessary to prevent infection. If any is noticed, treat it aggressively.
10. Have a source of glucose available in the office (orange juice, glucose package, etc.).[1]

In a non-insulin-dependant diabetic, all dental procedures can be performed without special precautions—unless the diabetes becomes uncontrolled.[7] Table 1.3 shows the symptoms of hypoglycemia.

BLEEDING

Bleeding disorders are discussed in Chapter 10.

EPILEPSY

The most common type of seizure an epileptic patient will have is a grand mal episode. These episodes occur when an area of the brain is depolarizing (firing) spontaneously. Ask the patient the following questions before treatment:

- What type of seizures do you have?
- What is the medication you are taking?
- What is the aura you experience before the seizure?

The drugs that are taken by an epileptic are CNS depressants. The most common are Dilantin, Phenobarbital, Tegretol, and Depakote.

Table 1-3. Signs of diabetic hypoglycemia

Frequent urination	Pale
Excessive thirst	Sweating
Extreme hunger	Increased fatigue
Unusual weight loss	Disoriented
Irritability	Blurry vision

During the medical history find out the frequency, severity, and duration of the episodes from the patient and family members.[7] Usually, the seizures last one to three minutes. If one lasts five minutes or more, it can be life-threatening. After an epileptic episode of one or two minutes, the patient will be extremely tired and usually disoriented. The only thing you can do during the convulsions is protect the patient from injury. No attempt is to be made to move the patient to the floor. Insert any mouth props before the procedure (tied with floss). Do not try to insert a mouth prop during an episode, as you may damage the teeth or gingiva. These patients should be scheduled for treatment within a reasonable time after the seizure-control medicine is taken. Consult with a family member and release them to a responsible adult.

PREGNANCY

The concern for the pregnant female is not only her welfare but the care of the fetus. Potential genetic damage from drugs and radiation are serious concerns. It is always best to defer surgery for the pregnant patient until after delivery.

The patient who requires surgery and/or medication during pregnancy is at best in a high-risk situation and should be treated as such. Drugs are rated by the FDA as to their possible effect on the fetus. These classifications are A, B, C, D, and X. A classification drugs are the safest. D and X are the least safe. The most likely to have a teratogenic effect are the D and X drugs, but doses of C and even B drugs should be used with extreme caution.[8, 9]

Drugs considered the safest are acetaminophen, penicillin, codeine, erythromycin, and cephalosporin. Aspirin and ibuprofen are contraindicated because of the possibility of postpartum bleeding and prolonging of the pregnancy.[7]

Avoid keeping the near-term patient in a supine position, as that position can compress the vena cava and limit blood flow. Do not treat any pregnant patients in their first or last trimester unless absolutely necessary. Even then, it is prudent to consult the patient's physician.

BREAST-FEEDING

Obviously, the doctor must not prescribe medications that are known to enter breast milk and potentially affect infants. Only a few drugs commonly used in dentistry could harm an infant. Some of these include hydrocortisones, tetracyclines, metronidazole, and aminoglycosides.

Acceptable drugs delivered during breast-feeding can be administered according to the age and size of the baby. The older the child, the less chance of a problem with the drug. The duration of the medication is also a factor. Any drug given long-term must be avoided unless prescribed by the mother's physician. Any drug that is commonly administered to an infant should be fine to administer to a breast-feeding mother, but the duration should be shortened.[8] See Table 1.4 for a list of drugs that can be used sparingly and of those that would harm a breast-fed infant.

Basic Life Support

It is essential that all office personnel attend a training program in basic life support. A brief review of the technique is appropriate here.

The acronym for treating emergencies is

CHAPTER 1

Table 1-4. Breast-feeding mothers and drugs

Drugs that can be used sparingly	Drugs that are potentially harmful to the infant
Acetaminophen	Ampicillin
Antihistamines	Aspirin
Codiene	Atropine
Erythromycin	Barbiturates
Flouride	Chloral hydrate
Lidocaine	Diazepam
Meperidine	Metronidazol
Oxacillin	Penicillin
Clindamycin	Tetracyclines

PABC and **D**. This acronym is used in all emergencies—not just heart attacks.

P Position
A Airway
B Breathing
C Circulation
D Definitive treatment

A brief description of each letter is as follows.

P, POSITIONING THE PATIENT

Positioning the patient is the first step. The right position is the one that is most comfortable for the patient, if conscious. For cardiac arrest, the patient needs to be flat on his or her back. If asthmatic, patients probably will want to sit up, which helps their ability to breathe. If a patient is conscious, he or she can tell you what position feels the best. If the patient is unconscious, place the patient horizontally with the feet slightly elevated. The most common reason the patient loses consciousness is low blood pressure. With the feet elevated slightly, the patient can receive a larger flow of blood to the head and, thus, stimulate the brain. The patient can still breathe in the horizontal or supine position, but the head must be on the same plane as the heart, not lower.

A, AIRWAY

The second letter in the acronym is for airway. Airway management is critical in an unconscious patient. The head is tilted back, and the chin is lifted. One hand is placed on the forehead, with two fingers of the other hand on the mandible to rotate the head back. The tongue is attached to the mandible so that when you pull the mandible forward, the tongue also moves forward. This opens the airway so the patient can breathe, or so you can breathe for the patient. Make sure that no obstructions are in the mouth or throat.

B, BREATHING

The person attending must place his or her ear one inch away from the patient's nose. Watch the chest and see whether it is moving. The chest may move, indicating that the patient is trying to breathe, but it does not mean the patient is breathing. The patient might have an obstruction. It is crucial that you feel air coming through the mouth or nose. In a cardiac arrest, the patient must be supine but not have the heart higher than the head. The legs can be elevated slightly to increase the blood flow to the brain, but if the heart is higher than the head, breathing becomes more difficult.

If the patient is not breathing, it is called **apnea**. The rescuer must provide supplemental breathing to the victim to oxygenate the blood.

C, CIRCULATION

Maintain the head tilt and check for the carotid pulse. Knowing how to check the carotid pulse is critical. Studies have shown that the carotid pulse is missed 40 percent of the time by medical personnel and paramedics. To locate the carotid artery, maintain head tilt and place the fingers on the Adam's apple or thyroid cartilage. The fingers are

PATIENT EVALUATION AND MEDICAL HISTORY 15

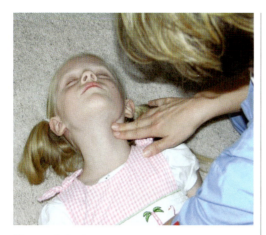

Figure 1-3. Carotid pulse. The carotid pulse is missed 40 percent of the time.

then, with moderate pressure, slid down the neck toward the rescuer, into a groove on the side of the neck formed by the sternocleidomastoid muscle. The carotid artery is located in that groove. See Figure 1.3. The pulse should be checked for 10 seconds. If a pulse is not felt, start compressions immediately. You are now circulating oxygenated blood to the victim's brain. With the 2005 American Heart Association changes, a lay rescuer does not assess signs of circulation before beginning chest compressions.

D, Definitive Treatment

The final part of the equation is the diagnosis of the problem. If the doctor can diagnose the problem, then, if trained to do so, he or she can give the patient the appropriate medication. However, remember that drugs do not save the patient; proper life support does. If the dentist is not trained in Advanced Cardiac Life Support (ACLS), then it is best to continue with basic life support until help arrives.

Clinical signs are what the doctor can see, and symptoms are what the patient tells you. Signs and symptoms of concern are as follows:

1. Altered consciousness
2. Respiratory depression
3. Allergic reaction
4. Chest pain[1, 10]

Basic Life Support, CPR

The following is a step-by-step outline of cardiopulmonary resuscitation. This list is for review but is not intended to replace formal training.

Cardiopulmonary Resuscitation (CPR)
1. **Call 911**
   Check the victim for unresponsiveness. If there is no response, call 911 and return to the victim. Ask for assistance. In most locations, the emergency dispatcher can assist you with CPR instructions. If you are not alone, have someone else call and you begin CPR.
2. **Breathe**
   Clear the mouth of any foreign objects. Tilt the head back, lift the chin up, and listen for breathing. Put your ear one inch from the victim's nose and mouth. If the patient is not breathing normally, pinch his or her nose, cover the mouth with yours, and blow until you see the chest rise. Give two breaths. All breaths should be given over 1 second with sufficient volume to achieve visible chest rise.

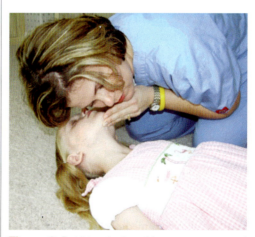

Figure 1-4. Listen for breathing.

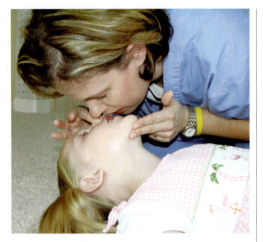

Figure 1-5. Breathe two breaths for two seconds each.

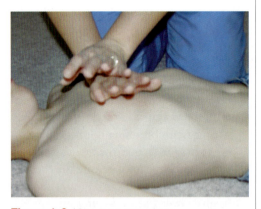

Figure 1-6. Chest compressions.

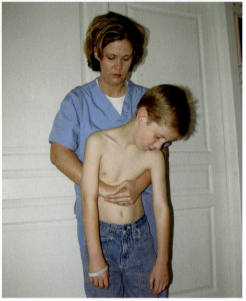

Figure 1-7. Heimlich maneuver. Repeat abdominal thrusts.

3. **Chest Compressions**

    If the victim is unconscious and unresponsive, begin chest compressions. Push down on the chest 1 1/2 to 2 inches, 30 times right between the nipples. On a small child or infant, compress the chest 1 to 1.5 inches. Compress the chest at the rate of 100/minute. The rescuer should then breathe twice for every 30 compressions.

    Continue administering CPR until help arrives. Paramedics will continue life support and transport to a medical center or emergency room.

CHOKING

When a patient has a foreign body lodged in the throat, it is important to act immediately. Most of the time the dentist is able to quickly remove the object before it gets too far into the trachea to see. If patients struggle, they will usually grab the throat. This is the universal sign for choking. The following steps are to be followed for adults as well as children.

First Aid for a Choking Conscious Adult and for Children (1–8 years old)

Determine whether the person can speak or cough. If not, proceed to the next step. Perform an abdominal thrust (Heimlich maneuver) repeatedly until the foreign body is expelled. See Figures 1.7 and 1.8. A chest thrust may be used for markedly obese persons or those in the late stages of pregnancy. If the adult or child becomes unresponsive, perform CPR; if you see an object in the throat or mouth, remove it.

PATIENT EVALUATION AND MEDICAL HISTORY

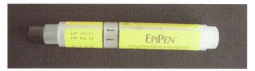

Figure 1-9. Epinephrine syringe. This is the only drug that should be preloaded in an emergency kit.

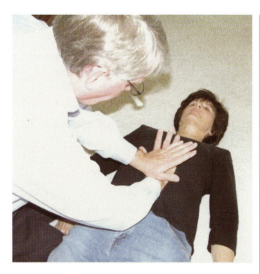

Figure 1-8. Floor position for abdominal thrusts.

Emergency Kit

Several emergency kits on the market contain the basic drugs and apparatus to help in certain emergencies.

Epinephrine is the only drug that is of immediate help with anaphylaxis but it must be given within the first few minutes of symptoms. This is the only drug you should have in a preloaded syringe. See Figure 1.9.

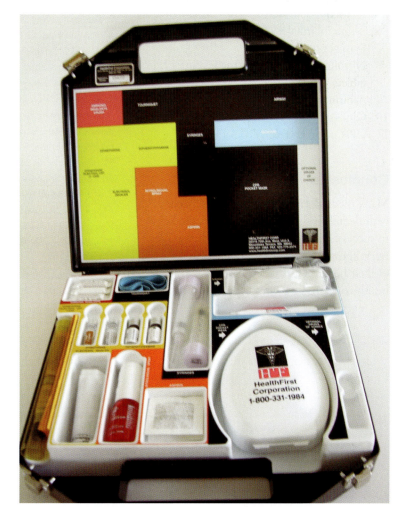

Figure 1-10. Emergency kit.

CHAPTER 1

Epinephrine can be administered into the thigh muscle right through the clothing if necessary. Each minute that passes without epinephrine when a patient is experiencing anaphylactic shock considerably lessens the chances of recovery. You can give 1 cc of 1:1000 epinephrine up to three times in intervals of five minutes. Also administer oxygen. Do not leave the patient until help arrives.

A good emergency kit should include the following:

1. Ammonia inhalants
2. Tourniquet
3. CPR pocket mask
4. Epinephrine in a preloaded syringe (1:1000)
5. Diphenhydramine
6. Albuterol inhaler
7. Syringes
8. Nitrolingual spray or nitroglycerin tablets
9. Aspirin
10. Glucose
11. CPR pocket mask

Conclusion

Many medical problems can and do occur with dental treatment. Prevention is the key to successful and uneventful procedures. We must know our patients and be clearly aware of their health status. Each patient who has health concerns in their medical history must be evaluated thoroughly. If the clinician is not aware of the effect surgery or routine dental treatments will have on the patient, then a consultation with the patient's physician is mandatory. We must be prepared for possible medical problems and have a good understanding of basic life support measures.

Bibliography

1. L. Peterson, E. Ellis, J. Hupp, M. Tucker. *Contemporary Oral and Maxillofacial Surgery*, 4th edition. St. Louis: Mosby, 2003.
2. Adapted from Professional Insurance Exchange standard consent to proceed form, March, 2005.
3. American Dental Association Health Insurance Portability and Accountability Act, HIPPA, requirements at ADA.org.
4. L. Barclay, C. Vega. The American Heart Association Updates Recommendations for Blood Pressure Measurements. *Medscape Medical News*, www.medscape.com, Dec., 2004.
5. S.F. Malamed. *Emergency Medicine.* Millennium Productions DVD, 2003.
6. *Basic Life Support for Healthcare Providers*, American Heart Association, 1997.
7. J. Little, D. Falave, C. Miller, N. Rhodus. *Dental Management of the Medically Compromised Patient*, 6th edition. St Louis: Mosby, 2002.
8. T.W. Hale, *Medications and Mother's Milk: A Manual of Lactational Pharmacology, 11th ed.* Pharmasoft Publishing L.P., Amarillo, TX, 2004.
9. *Pregnancy categories for prescription drugs*, FDA Drug Bull. 1982.
10. S. F. Malamed. *Medical Emergencies in the Dental Office*, 5th edition. St. Louis: Mosby, 1999.

Chapter 2

Surgical Extractions

Dr. Hussam S. Batal and Dr. Gregg Jacob

Introduction

The purpose of this chapter is to review the principles of surgical extractions. This chapter provides the dentist with general surgical principles and techniques that can be used for evaluation and treatment. Basic extraction techniques are discussed in the context of surgical extraction only. **Surgical extraction** is defined in this chapter as extraction of a tooth that requires the elevation of a soft tissue flap, bone removal, and/or sectioning of the tooth. Despite the fact that the majority of extractions performed in the dental office are forceps extractions, surgical extractions are frequently indicated when forceps extractions are inadequate for a variety of reasons.

In most cases, an adequate preoperative assessment will allow the dentist to predict the difficulty of the extraction. Combining good clinical and radiographic evaluations will allow the dentist to determine the best approach for the extractions. However, even with the best assessment, approximately 10 percent of forceps extractions will become complicated and require some form of surgical extraction.

Surgical extractions should not be reserved only for the most extreme situations. When used appropriately, surgical extractions may actually be more conservative and cause less morbidity than forceps extractions. For example, in some cases, excessive force might be required to extract a tooth, resulting in the fracture of roots, adjacent bone, or both. In general, surgical extractions should be considered when strong force might be needed to remove a tooth. Using surgical extraction techniques instead will allow for the **controlled** removal of bone or the sectioning of tooth, leading to a more predictable outcome.

General Principles

Dentists performing surgical extractions should have a clear understanding of anatomical structures in the surgical site. When considering the surgical extractions of teeth, several principles should be followed. These principles include proper preoperative evaluation, proper development of a soft tissue flap so that adequate access and visualization are obtained, creation of an adequate path of removal, use of controlled force to decrease the risk of root or bone fracture, and proper reapproximation of the soft tissue

Table 2-1. Indications for the extraction of teeth

1—Dental caries
2—Periodontal disease
3—Orthodontic reasons
4—Prosthetic reasons
5—Teeth associated with pathology
6—Radiation therapy
7—Chemotherapy
8—Malpositioned teeth compromising periodontal health of adjacent teeth
9—Teeth with serious infection
10—Economics
11—Teeth in line of a jaw fracture
12—Unrestorable fractured teeth

Table 2-2. Clinical factors predicting the difficulty of extractions

1—Extensive loss of coronal tooth structure
2—Thickness of the buccal plate
3—Limited access to the area of extraction
4—Limited access to the tooth in the dental arch
5—Increased age of the patient
6—History of past root canal therapy

flap. An understanding of these principles and adherence to sound surgical techniques will ensure the successful surgical extraction of teeth and uneventful healing of the surgical site.

PREOPERATIVE EVALUATION

The extraction of teeth is one of the most commonly performed surgical procedures. Table 2.1 presents the main indications for tooth removal.

A thorough review of the patient's medical history, social history, medications, and allergies is mandatory prior to any surgical procedure. The dentist should perform thorough preoperative clinical and radiographic evaluations of the tooth to be extracted. A careful preoperative evaluation allows the dentist to predict the difficulty of the extraction and minimizes the incidence of complications. Good clinical and radiographic evaluations will allow the dentist to anticipate any potential problems and modify the surgical approach accordingly for a more favorable outcome.

CLINICAL EXAM

When a clinical evaluation of the tooth to be extracted is performed, many factors need to

be taken into consideration. Some of them present a "red flag" or predictor of difficulty. See Table 2.2.

ACCESS TO THE SURGICAL SITE

Access to the tooth might be impeded, causing the dentist to have difficulty with the instrumentation needed for extraction. Difficult access can result from a limited mouth opening that minimizes access and visibility in general, but especially to the posterior teeth. Depending on the degree of access limitation, even a simple forcep extraction might need to be surgically removed because of the inability to apply forceps. The most common causes for restricted mouth opening are odontogenic infections affecting the masticator spaces and temporomandibular joint disorders. Other less common reasons include microstomia and muscle fibrosis due to radiation therapy or burns.

Difficult access can also result from the location of the tooth in the dental arch. Access to the maxillary third molar might be difficult even in a patient with no restriction to the mouth opening. This is because when the patient fully opens, the coronoid process moves into the area of the maxillary third and second molars, limiting instrumentation access. Access into this area can be improved by having the patient close slightly and move the mandible laterally to the side of the tooth to be extracted. This will move the coronoid process away from the surgical site and improve access.

SURGICAL EXTRACTIONS   21

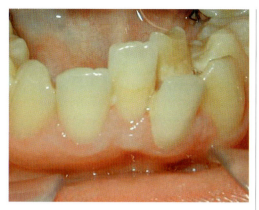

Figure 2-1. Severe crowding in the dental arch can limit access to the application of a forcep.

Another cause of difficult access is severe crowding in the dental arch limiting availability of the clinical crown of the tooth. This type of limited access is most commonly seen in the mandibular anterior and premolar teeth. Attempts at forceps extractions in such cases can result in damage to adjacent teeth. See Figure 2.1.

Condition of the Tooth

The presence of extensive caries or large restorations weakens the tooth and often results in crown fracture during forceps extractions. See Figure 2.2. In addition, the presence of extensive caries can make adapting the beaks of the forceps difficult, especially if the caries is on the buccal or palatal/lingual aspect of the tooth. In such cases, a surgical extraction should be performed so that the beaks of the forceps can be seated as apically as possible, beyond the area of the caries on sound tooth structure.

Condition of the Bone Surrounding the Tooth

The extractions of most teeth depend on the expansion of the buccal bone. If the buccal bone is especially thick or dense, adequate expansion is less likely, increasing the risk of tooth fracture at the time of extraction. The bone in older patients tends to be more dense compared to the bone in younger patients. Patients with a grinding habit often have thick, dense bone. The presence of obvious buccal exostoses also makes expansion of the buccal bone difficult. See Figure 2.3. Consideration should be given to surgical extraction if a tooth is surrounded by thick, dense bone to decrease the risk of tooth fracture during extraction and to ensure a more predictable outcome.

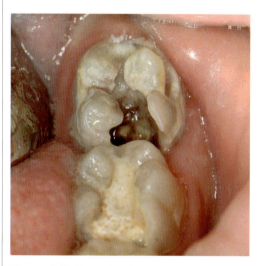

Figure 2-2. Extensive dental caries weakens the coronal tooth structure. Since this can result in crown fracture during the extraction, these teeth are better approached surgically.

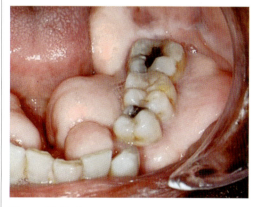

Figure 2-3. Significant exostoses can limit the amount of buccal bone expansion. These teeth are best approached by a surgical extraction.

Radiographic Evaluation

Radiographic evaluation of the tooth to be extracted is critical. A radiograph of diagnostic quality provides important information that cannot be obtained from a clinical evaluation. Periapical and panoramic radiographs are the most commonly used radiographs. A good-quality panoramic radiograph provides information about the general condition and anatomy of the teeth and their relationship to adjacent anatomic structures. However, it lacks the detail that can be provided by a good-quality periapical radiograph. The panoramic radiograph is the most commonly used radiograph for the evaluation of third molars. Occasionally, an occlusal radiograph can be used to assess the buccolingual or buccopalatal location of an impacted tooth, such as an impacted cuspid.

The dentist performing radiographic evaluation of the tooth to be extracted should consider several factors including the relationship of the tooth to adjacent anatomical structures, the tooth anatomy, and the condition of the surrounding bone. See Table 2.3.

Anatomy of the Tooth

The number of roots on the tooth should be evaluated, and any variation from normal should be noted. See Figure 2.4. The length and shape of the roots should be evaluated. The shorter and more conical the roots, the easier the extraction. The longer, thinner, and more curved the roots, the more difficult the extraction and the higher the risk of root fracture. See Figures 2.5 and 2.6. Teeth with dilacerated roots can be extremely difficult to extract, and a surgical extraction should be performed for such teeth.

For multirooted teeth, the degree of root divergence should also be evaluated. The greater the degree of divergence, the greater the difficulty of extraction. See Figure 2.7. Compare the dimension at the point of maximum divergence of the roots to the di-

Table 2-3. Radiographic factors predicting the difficulty of extraction

1—Severely divergent roots
2—Root dilacerations
3—Endodontically treated teeth with or without post and core
4—Increased number of roots present
5—Evidence of external or internal resorption
6—Presence of hypercementosis/bulbous roots
7—Long roots
8—Dense bone
9—Horizontal root fracture

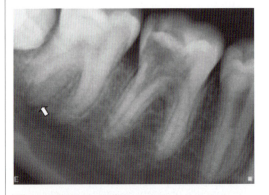

Figure 2-4. A lower second molar with anomalous roots (white arrow). Careful evaluation of a periapical radiograph will allow the operator to note any variation in anatomy and thereby determine the correct surgical plan.

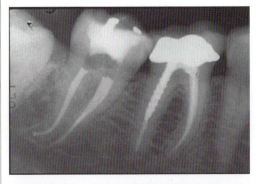

Figure 2-5. Teeth with thin long roots or dilacerations of the root are best approached surgically to decrease the chances of root fracture.

SURGICAL EXTRACTIONS 23

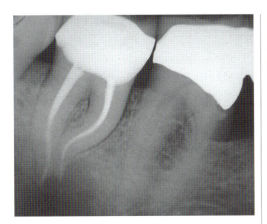

Figure 2-6. Another example of teeth with thin long roots.

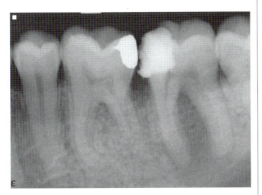

Figure 2-7. The greater the degree of divergence of the roots, the greater the difficulty of the extraction. These molars should be sectioned to develop a path of withdrawal for each root separately.

mension of the tooth at the crest of bone. If the dimension at the point of maximum divergence of the roots is greater than the dimension of the tooth at the crest of bone, then the extraction can be expected to be more difficult. Sectioning of the tooth will probably be required to create an adequate path of withdrawal. See Figure 2.8A,B.

Relationship of the Tooth to Anatomic Structures

The relationship of the tooth to be extracted to anatomic structures such as the maxillary

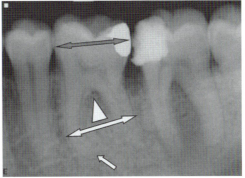

Figure 2-8A. When evaluating this periapical radiograph, a measurement is made at the widest portion of the root (double-headed white arrow) and compared to a measurement at the contact points of the crown (double-headed dark arrow). If the root measurement is greater than at the contact points, this indicates an inadequate path of withdrawal. Also note the curvature on the mesial root (single white arrow). This tooth is best approached by sectioning the tooth between mesial and distal roots. Some bone should be removed from the buccal in the furcation area (white triangle) before tooth sectioning.

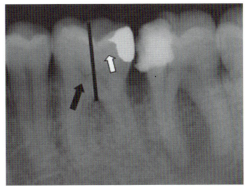

Figure 2-8B. On the lower first molar, the distal root should be removed first (white arrow), and then the mesial root (black arrow). This sequence will prove easier because of the curvature on the mesial root.

sinus or inferior alveolar nerve should be evaluated.

Maxillary Sinus

Great variation exists in the relationship of the maxillary posterior teeth to the maxillary

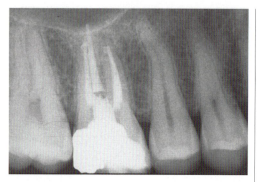

Figure 2-9. A first molar with a minimal relationship to the maxillary sinus. The tooth is totally surrounded by bone.

Table 2-4. Teeth at risk for sinus exposure

1—Lone standing maxillary molar with pneumatized maxillary sinus
2—Roots projecting into a severely pneumatized maxillary sinus and minimal coronal bone visible radiographically
3—Long divergent bulbous roots with a pneumatized sinus into the trifurcation area
4—Teeth with advanced periodontal disease but with no mobility; also teeth with the maxillary sinus extending into the trifurcation area

sinus: The roots might be completely encased by bone with minimal relationship to the maxillary sinus (see Figure 2.9), or the maxillary sinus might extend into the furcation area of the roots with paper-thin bone separating the roots from the maxillary sinus. See Figure 2.10. In general, the degree of maxillary sinus pneumatization increases with advancing age and with loss of maxillary posterior teeth. Various degrees of maxillary sinus involvement can result from the removal of maxillary posterior teeth. This can vary from the displacement of a root tip into the maxillary sinus to the development of an oroantral communication or fistula.

Teeth at the greatest risk for sinus exposure or communication (see Table 2.4) are best approached by surgical extraction. Flap reflection with sectioning of teeth along with possible buccal bone removal can minimize the chance of sinus exposure or root displacement into the sinus.

Inferior Alveolar Neurovascular Bundle

Evaluation of the proximity of the inferior alveolar neurovascular bundle is especially critical prior to extractions of mandibular third molars. Extractions of mandibular third molars are associated with the highest risk of injury to the inferior alveolar nerve. Appropriate evaluation of the relationship of the mandibular third molars to this nerve, and an altered surgical approach, decreases the risk of complications. See Figure 2.11.

CONDITION OF THE TOOTH

Evaluate the tooth for the presence of internal or external resorption. If extensive resorption is present, fracture of the root can be expected at the level of the resorption. Surgical extraction is usually needed for the removal of such teeth. See Figure 2.12.

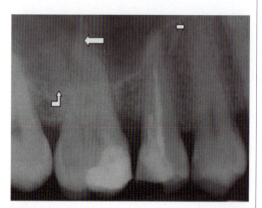

Figure 2-10. A first molar with a pneumatized sinus into the furcation area (angled white arrow). Also note the curvature of the mesiobuccal root (white straight arrow). There is also close proximity of the premolar roots to the sinus (small double-ended arrow). This tooth is best approached surgically by sectioning off the palatal root and then dividing the mesiobuccal and distobuccal roots to decrease the chance of sinus communication and improve the path of removal.

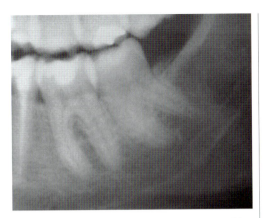

Figure 2-11. This tooth has a close relationship between the mandibular molars and the mandibular canal. As long as the operator does not instrument apical to the sockets, there should be no injury to the inferior alveolar nerve.

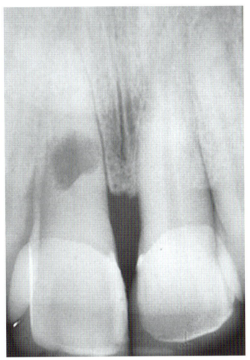

Figure 2-12. Internal resorption of tooth #9. Depending on the extent of the internal resorption, the tooth can fracture at the level of the resorption during extraction, requiring surgical removal of the root tip.

A tooth that has been endodontically treated can be difficult to extract for several reasons. See Figure 2.13. Unless the tooth was endodontically treated recently, it tends to be very brittle and fractures easily. Furthermore, an endodontically treated tooth often has a large restoration or a crown, further complicating the extraction. Therefore, a tooth that has been endodontically treated is often best managed with a surgical extraction.

The tooth should also be evaluated for the possibility of ankylosis. The periodontal ligament space around the tooth should be visible. Otherwise, the tooth might be ankylosed. An ankylosed tooth should be approached as a surgical extraction.

A tooth with hypercementosis (see Figure 2.14) can be difficult to extract due to an inadequate path of withdrawal. A surgical extraction should be performed so that an adequate path of withdrawal can be created to facilitate the extraction.

CONDITION OF THE BONE

The bone surrounding the tooth to be extracted should be carefully evaluated. A radiograph of good quality should allow an as-

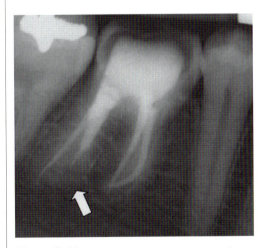

Figure 2-13. Endodontic treatment can make teeth brittle and prone to fracture during removal—requiring surgical extraction.

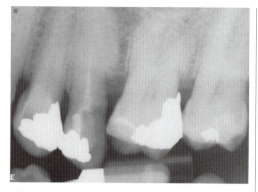

Figure 2-14. Hypercementosis on a maxillary second premolar with a bulbous root.

sessment of the relative density of the bone. Bone that appears relatively radiolucent is less dense and is more likely to expand, making the extraction easier. However, bone that is relatively radiopaque is more dense and less likely to expand, making the extraction more difficult.

Flap Design, Development, and Management

Before beginning any surgical extraction we should review the appropriate design and execution of that procedure. A well-designed treatment plan will enable potentially difficult surgery to be performed efficiently and painlessly for both the patient and the treating dentist. Paramount to any surgical treatment plan is the development of an appropriate surgical flap. Adequate flap design plays a vital role in exposure and access for the surgical extraction of teeth. Good surgical principles and techniques will help to avoid tissue trauma and subsequent delayed healing.

The dentist must consider a number of factors simultaneously in preparing for a surgical extraction. First and foremost are the indications for flap development, as the inappropriate decision to lay a flap might lead to unnecessary trauma, swelling, and discomfort for the patient. Conversely, not laying a flap when needed might also complicate the surgery and lead to a more difficult procedure for the patient. The general indications for flap reflection include the following:

- To allow for complete access and visualization of the surgical field.
- To allow for bone removal and tooth sectioning.
- To prevent unnecessary trauma to soft tissue and bony structures.

After the decision to raise a flap has been made, the treating dentist must decide on the type and design of the flap. In the design process, several factors should be taken into consideration, including vascular supply to the flap, regional anatomy, underlying bony anatomy, health of the tissues to be incised, and the ability to place an incision in a discrete and cosmetic location that can be repositioned postoperatively in a tension-free fashion.

Generally, most surgical extractions will require the elevation of a full-thickness mucoperiosteal flap. This flap includes the overlying gingiva, mucosa, submucosa, and underlying periosteum in one piece. In order to properly develop this type of flap, one must create sharp, discrete, full-thickness incisions that extend completely to the underlying bone. See Figure 2.15. Sharp incisions made in this fashion will allow the effective elevation of a full-thickness flap without tearing the periosteum or gingival tissue—thus avoiding unnecessary bleeding into the surgical field or delayed healing of the flap.

When considering flap design, the surgeon must decide which flap will allow the most effective visualization and execution of the surgical procedure while maintaining minimal invasiveness. A few basic surgical principles must be kept in mind. First, when outlining the flap, the base must be broader than the apex to allow for maintenance of an adequate, independent blood supply. See

SURGICAL EXTRACTIONS   27

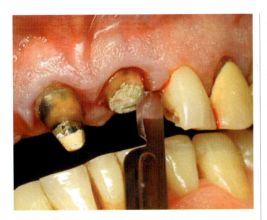

Figure 2-15. When making an incision, the #15 blade should be carried down to the bone in a full-thickness fashion.

Figure 2.16. If this basic principle is violated, the flap risks devascularization and necrosis with delayed healing. Second, the margin of the flap should never be placed over a bony prominence, as this may prohibit tension-free repositioning. This could lead to a postoperative dehiscence and healing by secondary intention with likely scarring. Similarly, the coronal aspects of the releasing incisions should be placed a safe distance of roughly six to eight millimeters mesial and distal to the extraction site, thus ensuring that postoperatively, the incisions will lie over intact bone. See Figures 2.17A and 2.17B. If this is not accomplished, the flap

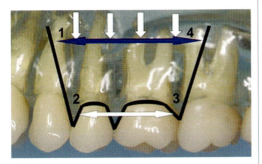

Figure 2-16. This picture shows a trapezoidal or four-cornered flap. The base of the flap (double-ended blue arrow) should be wider than the coronal aspect of the flap (double-ended white arrow) to allow adequate blood supply (single-ended white arrows).

might collapse into the bony defect, resulting in likely dehiscence and delayed healing. Additionally, the flap must be designed to avoid underlying vital structures such as the mental or lingual neurovascular bundles in the mandible or the superior alveolar bundles in the maxilla.

In soft tissues around the lower third molars, incisions should be well away from the lingual aspect of the ridge to avoid accidental severance of the lingual nerve, which may lie supraperiosteally in this tissue. Likewise, apical to the mandibular premolars lies the mental nerve. Incisions should be well anterior and/or posterior to this structure to

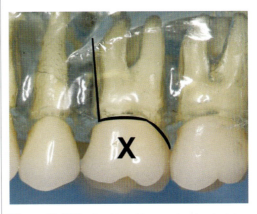

Figure 2-17A. Avoid making a releasing incision too close to or directly over the area of the extraction. An incision near a bony defect can result in a dehiscence and delayed healing. In this example, the release is too close to the tooth being extracted.

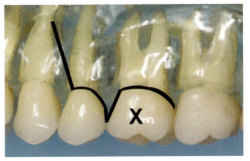

Figure 2-17B. The correct design. Releasing incisions should be 6–8mm anterior and/or posterior to the extraction site.

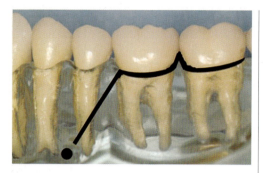

Figure 2-18. Avoid releasing incisions in the area of the mental nerve, as depicted here.

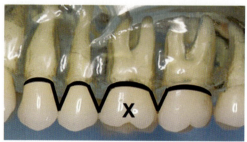

Figure 2-19. Envelope flap. Ideally, this type of flap should be extended one tooth posterior and two teeth anterior to the one being extracted in order to provide adequate reflection with minimal tension on the flap.

avoid accidental iatrogenic damage. See Figure 2.18. Also, an incision placed too high in the maxillary posterior mucobuccal fold could allow penetration into the area of the buccal fat pad. This becomes more of a surgical annoyance than a true complication. If this should occur, the pad can be repositioned easily, and the mucosa can be closed postoperatively; however, it will create a visual obstruction to the surgical field during the procedure.

When a palatal incision is necessary, attention must be paid to the greater palatine and incisive neurovascular bundles. The greater palatine artery provides the major blood supply to the palatal tissue, and therefore, releasing incisions should be avoided in this area. Anteriorly, if tissue must be reflected in the area of the incisors, transection of the incisive artery usually will not lead to significant bleeding, and the nerve tends to regenerate quickly. In addition, the altered sensation subsequent to this nerve's severance usually does not lead to significant morbidity for the patient. A good understanding of this underlying regional anatomy is mandatory to avoid inadvertent damage or exposure of vital structures. See Table 2.5.

With the preceding information kept in mind, the next decision is the design of the mucoperiosteal flap to be used. Intraorally, there are a number of flap designs to choose from, including the simple crestal envelope (see Figure 2.19); crestal envelope with one releasing incision (three-corner flap) (see Figure 2.17B); crestal envelope with two releasing incisions (four-corner flap) (see Figure 2.16); or semilunar design (see Figure 2.20.)

For surgical extractions, the most common flap is the sulcular envelope (with or without a releasing incision). For this flap, a full-thickness incision is created intrasulcularly around the buccal and lingual aspects of the teeth. The papillae are kept within

Table 2-5. Flap Design Considerations

Avoid	Result if not avoided
Incision over bony prominences	Tension, dehiscence, and delayed healing
Incising through papillae	Dehiscence, periodontal defect
Incision over facial aspect midcrown	Dehiscence, periodontal defect
Incision not placed over sound bone	Collapse and delayed healing
Vertical incision in area of mental foramen	Injury to the mental nerve
Lingual releasing incision in the posterior mandible	Injury to lingual nerve
Vertical releasing incision in the posterior palate	Bleeding, injury to the greater palatine artery or vein

SURGICAL EXTRACTIONS   29

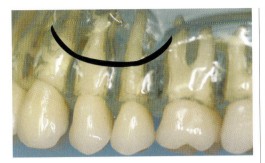

Figure 2-20. Semilunar flap.

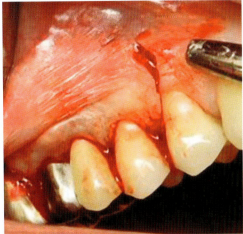

Figure 2-21A. Three-corner flap with the release anterior to the papillae (including the papilla in the flap). The releasing incision can also be placed posterior to the papilla (papilla not included in the flap).

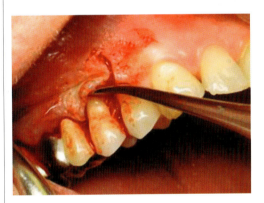

Figure 2-21B. A periosteal elevator is used to reflect the flap. Reflection is started with the sharp end.

the body of the flap, which is reflected apically in a full-thickness fashion. This flap provides great access to the coronal part of the tooth, allowing better visualization, instrumentation, bone removal, and tooth sectioning when needed. In addition, it can be easily converted into a three-corner flap if additional access is needed to the apical area.

Generally speaking, most surgical extractions can be performed without a releasing incision; however, occasionally additional reflection is necessary for tension-free visualization. The release can be created at either the mesial or distal end of an envelope, but in most cases, it is placed anteriorly and reflected posteriorly. See Figures 2.21A–E. Recall that this incision must run obliquely as it extends toward the vestibule to allow the coronal end of the incision (apex of the flap) to be narrower than the base (vestibular end of the flap). The releasing incision should be located at a line angle of a tooth and should not directly transect a papilla (see Figure 2.22) or cross over a bony prominence like the canine eminence in the maxilla. Papillary transection can lead to necrosis and loss of papillae postoperatively, thereby causing cosmetic and periodontal problems. Again, incising over a bony prominence should be avoided. When a procedure begins with a short envelope flap, the use of a release provides greater access, especially to the apical area. This is occasionally necessary in the posterior regions of the mouth, particularly in the maxilla, where visualization is often difficult.

When a release is necessary, it is very rare that a four-corner flap (two releases) will be needed. However, occasionally, with fractured roots in the posterior maxilla near the sinus, this flap design is beneficial—especially if there is the potential for an oral-antral communication requiring the advancement of tissue for primary tension-free closure. Semilunar incisions are of limited

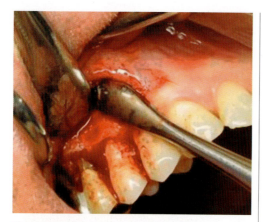

Figure 2-21C. Once started, reflection can be continued with the wider end.

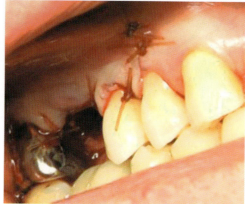

Figure 2-21E. To reposition the flap against the bone, the releasing incision portion is approximated first, then the papillae.

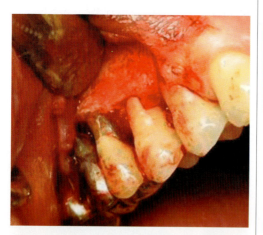

Figure 2-21D. The flap is held out of the way with a Seldin retractor.

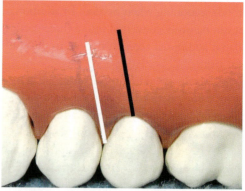

Figure 2-22. Releasing incisions should not transect the papilla (white line). Also, releasing incisions should not be placed in the midbuccal surface of the tooth (black line).

benefit in surgical extractions, as they provide limited access to the apical region of teeth. They are used more often for periapical surgery. Since this flap design is rarely used with extractions, it will not be discussed further in this chapter.

After all of the preceding information is considered, the technique for developing a surgical flap is relatively straightforward. Since the most common flap used for surgical extractions is the sulcular envelope with or without a release, this is the technique that will be described. Most incisions are created using standard #15 and/or #12 blades.

The incision is created intrasulcularly down to the alveolar bone. It begins at the distobuccal line angle, one tooth posterior to the tooth being extracted. The incision runs anteriorly in a single stroke. If an envelope flap is planned, the incision should be extended two teeth anterior to the tooth to be extracted. When a three-corner flap is planned, the incision is carried one tooth anterior, and a releasing incision is made to include or exclude the papilla in the design of the flap.

If a release is used, it is begun at the sulcus and extends in an anteroapical direction toward the vestibule. A standard Seldin or other broad retractor is used to tense the alveolar mucosa to allow a clean, smooth incision without tearing the tissue. When the incision is completed, reflection usually is conducted with the sharp end of a periosteal elevator. Reflection is begun at the anterior sulcular extent of the incision. The elevator is positioned underneath the full-thickness flap and run posteriorly along the sulcus, reflecting all of the papillae and buccal tissue down to the alveolar bone. The papillae are reflected by simply inserting the elevator against the alveolus and rotating the instrument—and concurrently the papillae—outward.

The crestal gingiva is always reflected first along the entire extent of the incision prior to reflecting the mucosa more apically. If any area of the crestal incision is difficult to reflect or it appears that the incision is not completely down to the alveolus, the blade is re-inserted to ensure a smooth full-thickness incision in the sulcus. Next, the sharp end of the periosteal elevator is run along the release incision against bone, and the tissue is elevated in a posteroapical direction—always in a full-thickness style. To ensure fullthickness, the periosteal elevator must always remain against the alveolar bone as the flap is reflected. When the anterior portion of the flap is raised, it is often helpful to place the broad end of a retractor under the flap and against the alveolus to assist in visualization while the remainder of the tissue is swept posteroapically. At this point, the broad end of the periosteal elevator is normally used to complete the reflection of the flap into the depth of the vestibule.

Following the surgical removal of the tooth, the final step is closure of the flap in a tension-free manner. If the flap has been designed and executed well, this portion of the procedure should be straightforward and done by repositioning the tissue using sutures to hold the tissue in place.

Creating an Adequate Path of Removal

Establishing a proper path of removal is one of the main principles in removing erupted or impacted teeth. Failure to achieve an unimpeded path of removal results in a failure to remove the teeth. This is commonly achieved either by sectioning the tooth or removing bone with a surgical handpiece next to the root to allow for delivery. The preferred sequence is to initially section the tooth, which will convert a multirooted tooth into single-root components. Elevation of each root separately will allow for removal of the tooth in the majority of the cases. If needed, bone can be removed to achieve a path of withdrawal. This sequence will preserve the most alveolar bone around the extraction socket. This preservation is important, especially when dental implants are planned.

Occasionally, reversing this sequence is needed (bone removal and then sectioning)—especially when the location of the furcation cannot be visualized. In these instances, bone should be removed on the buccal aspect to expose the furcation and allow sectioning of the tooth.

Use of Controlled Force

A key aspect of extracting teeth is the use of controlled force during elevation and forceps extractions. The dental surgeon needs to keep in mind that slow, steady movement should be used during extractions. Excessive force during extractions can result in the fracture of the tooth and possibly the alveolar bone. When the tooth cannot be extracted with reasonable force, the tooth should be surgically extracted. This is commonly accomplished by sectioning multirooted teeth and/or removing buccal bone, or a combination of both, to allow controlled removal of the tooth.

Technique for Surgical Extraction of a Single-rooted Tooth

The surgical extraction of a single-rooted tooth is relatively straightforward. After an adequate flap has been reflected and is held in proper position, the need for bone removal is assessed. Often, the improved visualization and access afforded by the flap makes bone removal unnecessary. This is because after a flap has been reflected, elevators can be used more effectively, and forceps can be seated more apically, creating a better mechanical advantage. The tooth then can be extracted without bone removal.

If bone removal is indicated, the tooth and, if necessary, a small portion of buccal bone may be grasped with the forcep. The tooth then is removed along with that small portion of buccal bone. See Figure 2.23. Other options when bone removal is necessary include removal of buccal bone using a bur or a chisel. The width of the bone removed should be approximately the same as the mesiodistal dimension of the root, and the most common vertical length of the bone removed is usually approximately one-third to one-half the length of the root. The tooth then can be extracted using a straight elevator and/or a forcep. See Figure 2.24. It is important to keep in mind that the amount of bone removed should be just enough to allow the extraction of the tooth. Excessive removal of bone should be avoided. This is especially critical in a patient who is treatment planned for implants.

If extraction of the tooth is still difficult after bone removal, a purchase point can be made. The purchase point should be made as apically as possible on the root, to create a better mechanical advantage. The purchase point should be large enough that an instrument such as a Crane pick or Cogswell B can be inserted and used to extract the tooth. See Figure 2.25. Adjacent bone is the fulcrum for the elevator.

After the extraction of a tooth, the surgical site should be inspected. All bony spicules should be removed, and all sharp bony edges should be smoothed. Sharp bony edges are assessed by replacing the flap and palpating it with a finger. A rongeur or a bone file may be used to smooth any sharp bony edges.

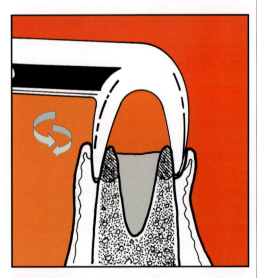

Figure 2-23. A forcep is shown being used to remove the root with a small portion of the alveolus.

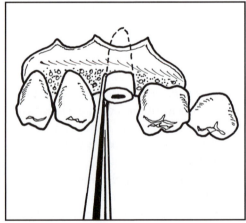

Figure 2-24. When adequate bone has been removed with a bur or chisel, the root is luxated and removed with an elevator, or a forcep can be seated onto sound root structure for its removal.

SURGICAL EXTRACTIONS

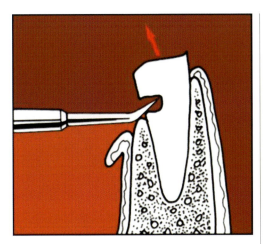

Figure 2-25. The placement of purchase point has three essential requirements: 1) The purchase point should be placed close to the level of the bone. 2) The purchase point should be deep enough to allow for placement of a Crane pick. 3) Enough tooth structure (3 mm) should be left coronal to the purchase point to prevent tooth fracture during elevation.

The surgical site then should be thoroughly irrigated with copious amounts of saline to remove all the debris. Special attention should be paid to the area at the base of the flap, as debris tends to collect in this area. Debris that is not removed can cause delayed healing or infection of the surgical site. The flap then is repositioned and sutured in position.

TECHNIQUE FOR SURGICAL EXTRACTION OF A MULTIROOTED TOOTH

The technique for the surgical extraction of a multirooted tooth is essentially the same as that for a single-rooted tooth. The main difference is that a multirooted tooth can be divided with a bur to convert it into multiple single-rooted teeth to facilitate its removal.

After an adequate flap has been reflected and held in proper position, the need for sectioning of the tooth and bone removal are assessed. As in the case for a single-rooted tooth, the improved visualization and access afforded by the flap might make bone removal and tooth sectioning unnecessary. In such cases, the more apical (to the bone level) application of elevators and forceps allows for a more effective extraction. The tooth then can often be extracted without sectioning or bone removal.

If further measures are deemed necessary in order to remove the tooth, it is preferable to initially section the tooth without removing any bone. Using this approach will either eliminate the need for bone removal or decrease the amount of bone removal. As in the case for a single-rooted tooth, it is important that the amount of bone removed be just enough to allow the extraction of the tooth or root. Excessive removal of bone should be avoided, especially in a patient who desires implants.

Bone removal prior to sectioning of the tooth is usually not necessary when the furcation of the tooth can be visualized after reflection of the flap. Sectioning of the tooth is accomplished with a bur. The roots are then separated. The roots are elevated and extracted with root forceps.

After the extraction of a tooth, the surgical site should be inspected. All bony spicules should be removed, and any sharp bony edges should be smoothened. Sharp areas of bone are assessed by replacing the flap and palpating it with a finger. A rongeur or a bone file may be used to smooth these areas.

The surgical site then should be thoroughly irrigated profusely with saline to remove bone or tooth chips—especially in the fold at the base of the flap. As mentioned, with single-rooted teeth, such debris can cause delayed healing or infection. The flap then is repositioned and sutured in position.

Case 1: Surgical Extraction of a Mandibular Molar

A flap is reflected. A bur then is used to section the tooth into mesial and distal segments. Adequate space should be created in the furcation area (by bone removal) to allow for an adequate path of removal. The mesial segment is first elevated with a straight elevator and removed with a forcep. If the root fractures or if there is inadequate mobility of the mesial segment, bone can be removed on the buccal aspect to facilitate the extraction. After the mesial segment has been extracted, the distal segment is elevated with a straight elevator and extracted with a forcep. Alternatively, the distal segment can be extracted using a Cryer elevator. The Cryer elevator takes advantage of the space created by the extraction of the mesial segment. All sharp bony edges are then smoothed, the area is irrigated, and the flap is repositioned and sutured. See Figures 2.26A–M.

Case 2: Surgical Extraction of a Maxillary Molar

A flap is reflected. A bur is used to cut off the crown of the tooth horizontally. The roots are then sectioned between the palatal root and the two buccal roots. The two buccal roots are then sectioned into a mesiobuccal root and a distobuccal root. If the maxillary sinus extends into the furcation area of the tooth, care must be taken when sectioning the tooth. The bur should extend just short of the furcation area and not into the furcation and the sinus. The straight elevator is used to complete the separation between the buccal and palatal roots. The straight elevator is then placed in between the mesiobuccal and distobuccal roots to complete the separation between the buccal roots. The straight elevator then can be used

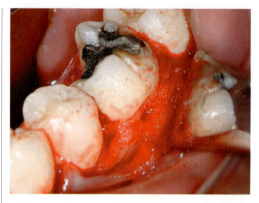

Figure 2-26B. The flap is retracted and held in position with the help of a Seldin retractor.

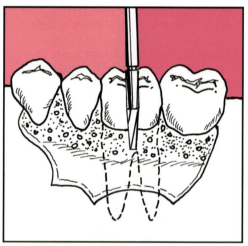

Figure 2-26C. This drawing shows a bur ready to remove a small amount of bone on the buccal surface of the tooth down to the furcation. Exposing the furcation allows visibility and access to use the bur for a section cut between the roots.

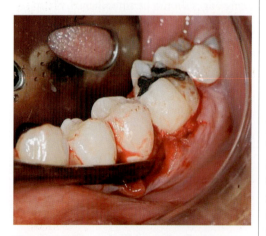

Figure 2-26A. Surgical extraction of a lower molar. Commonly an envelope flap is reflected with a periosteal elevator. Soft tissue is being detached and reflected on the buccal and the lingual.

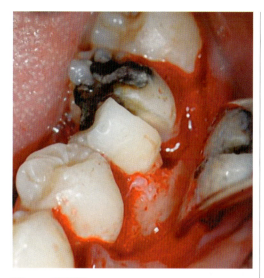

Figure 2-26D. This is a photograph showing how a small amount of bone can be removed on the buccal to the furcation, thus facilitating the section cut that has been made into the tooth.

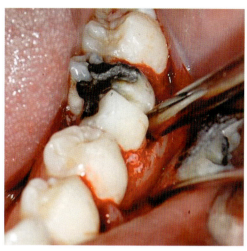

Figure 2-26F. A straight elevator is used to separate the mesial from the distal root. The elevator should be placed as apically as possible and rotated toward the part to be fractured.

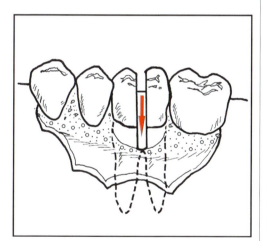

Figure 2-26E. The tooth is sectioned with a fissure bur on a surgical drill. The sectioning should extend into the furcation area and about three quarters of the way through the tooth in a bucco-lingual dimension—avoiding the lingual plate. Note the cut extending into the furcation area (red arrow). Also, in the drawing, some buccal bone has been removed.

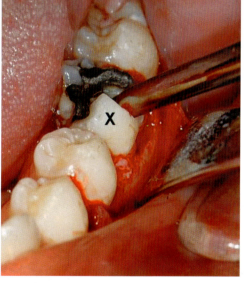

Figure 2-26G. If the elevator is placed too far coronally before being rotated this will commonly result in fracture of the crown only and, therefore, should be avoided. The X on the mesial part of the crown indicates enamel that might break off from the elevator being positioned too high.

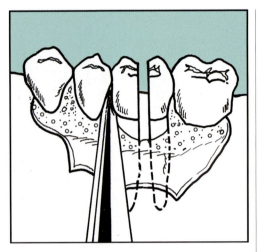

Figure 2-26H. After separating the mesial and distal roots, each root is elevated separately.

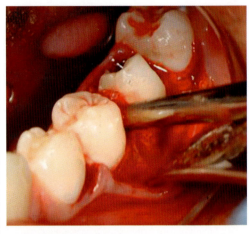

Figure 2-26J. This figure shows a clinical view of a lower first molar mesial root being luxated by a straight elevator.

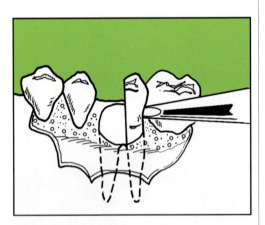

Figure 2-26I. After removal of one of the roots, the remaining root can be removed by luxation/elevation with a straight elevator.

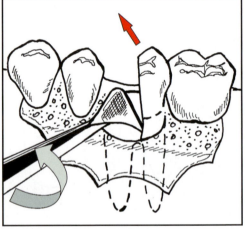

Figure 2-26K. Alternatively, an east/west elevator could be used.

to luxate the buccal roots. Following this, the buccal roots are extracted using a bayonet forcep or a fine-tip rongeur. Finally, the palatal root is removed in a similar manner. See Figures 2.27A–N.

Considerations for the Removal of Root Tips

No matter how experienced and careful the practitioner, roots fracture during extractions. If root fracture occurs during an extraction, the practitioner should make a determination as to whether the root tip can be left in place or whether it should be removed. If removal of the root tip is indicated, the operator must be comfortable with removing it. Otherwise, appropriate referral should be made.

If a small root tip fractures during extraction, if attempts at retrieval of the root tip are unsuccessful, and if further attempts at retrieval of the root tip are excessively traumatic, then consider leaving the root tip in

SURGICAL EXTRACTIONS   37

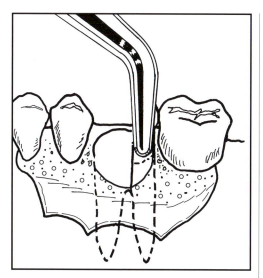

Figure 2-26L. An extraction forcep also could be used.

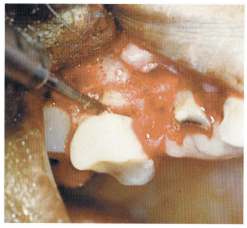

Figure 2-27A. Surgical extraction of an upper molar. After failed attempts with a forcep, a flap was reflected, and a fissure bur was used to section through the crown.

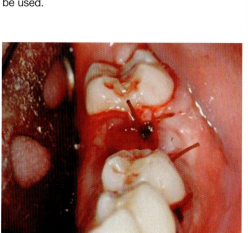

Figure 2-26M. The area is irrigated, especially under the flap, and then sutured.

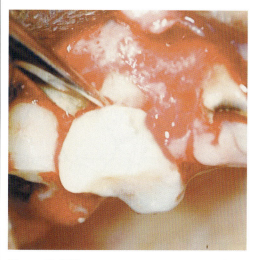

Figure 2-27B. The sectioning was completed by using a straight elevator. Note that when sectioning the crown, the dentist should leave enough coronal tooth structure for extraction of the roots.

place. The risks of continued, more aggressive attempts at retrieval of the root tip might outweigh the benefits.

Certain conditions must exist for a root tip to be left in place. The root tip must be small—less than 4 to 5 mm in length. In addition, it must be deeply embedded in bone and not near the crest of bone, so that subsequent bone resorption will not expose the root tip and interfere with the prosthesis that will be constructed to replace the extracted tooth. The root tip should also not be infected, which could cause subsequent flair-ups. If these conditions exist, then consider leaving the root tip in place. See Table 2.6.

In leaving a root tip, the risks of retrieval of the root tip must be greater than the benefits. One condition in which the risks out-

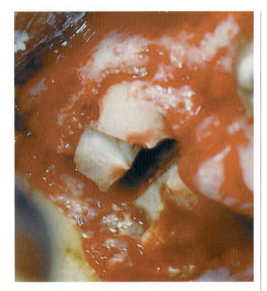

Figure 2-27C. Removing the crown better facilitates sectioning of the roots as shown here.

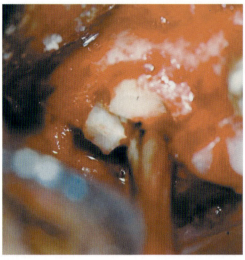

Figure 2-27E. A straight elevator can be placed between the buccal roots and the palatal root to complete the break.

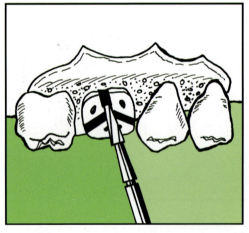

Figure 2-27D. The tooth is sectioned into two buccal roots and a palatal root (inverted T or Y).

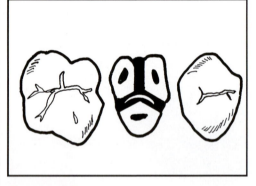

Figure 2-27F. Drawing of a straight elevator inserted between the buccal roots and the palatal root.

weigh the benefits in retrieving a root tip might be the need for a large amount of bone removal in order to retrieve a root tip. Another might be if retrieval of the root tip endangers anatomic structures such as the inferior alveolar neurovascular bundle or the maxillary sinus.

If a root tip is to be left in place, the patient must be informed that the risks of retrieval of the root tip outweigh the benefits. The reason for this is that there is the possibility of a future complication with the retained root segment. The fact that the patient was informed that a decision has been made to leave the root tip must be recorded in the patient's record.

Radiographic documentation of the root tip should be obtained and recorded in the patient's chart. The patient should also be instructed to contact the practitioner immediately should any problems develop in the area. It is also prudent to schedule a follow-

SURGICAL EXTRACTIONS 39

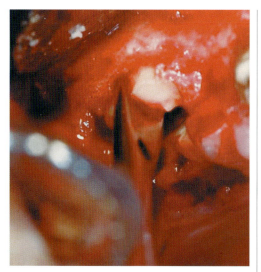

Figure 2-27G. Similarly, the straight elevator can also be placed and turned while between the buccal roots to facilitate complete separation of those two roots.

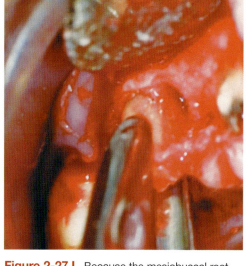

Figure 2-27J. Because the mesiobuccal root was adequately luxated, a forcep can be used to remove the root.

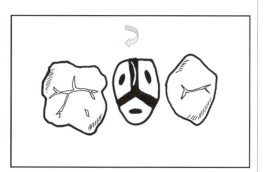

Figure 2-27H. Drawing showing positioning of the straight elevator between the buccal roots.

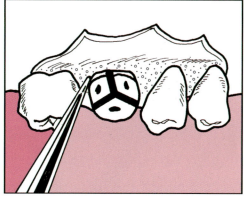

Figure 2-27K. An elevator could also have been used on the distobuccal root as shown in the drawing.

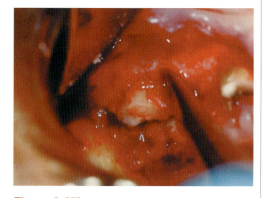

Figure 2-27I. The straight elevator is placed mesially to pry out the mesiobuccal root, using adjacent bone as a fulcrum.

up evaluation of the root tip six months or so in the future.

Surgical Technique for the Removal of Root Tips

Good lighting, access, and suction are critical for the successful removal of root tips. Most complications, such as displacement into adjacent anatomical structures like the maxil-

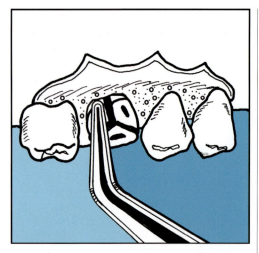

Figure 2-27L. A forcep could have been used on the distobuccal root as well.

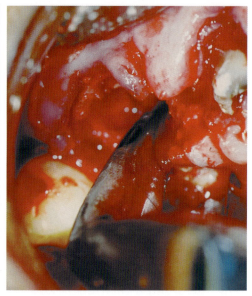

Figure 2-27N. The palatal root is then elevated and extracted with a root forcep.

Table 2-6. Indications for Leaving a Root Tip

1—Small root tip less than 4 mm in size
2—No evidence of periapical pathology or infection associated with root tip
3—Inability to visualize root tip
4—Removal of root tip will cause destruction to adjacent structures
5—Proximity to the inferior alveolar nerve
6—Proximity to the maxillary sinus
7—Ill-feeling patient
8—Uncontrolled hemorrhage

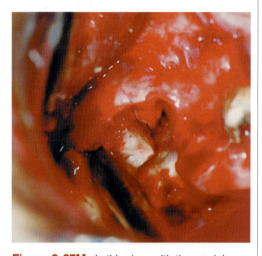

Figure 2-27M. In this view, with the mesiobuccal root removed, the operator can concentrate on the distobuccal root. This root is elevated into the space that was created by removing the mesiobuccal root. Careful evaluation should be made regarding the location of the maxillary sinus in the furcation area.

lary sinus, arise from attempts at removal of root tips under poor conditions.

A systematic approach is key in the removal of root tips. The practitioner should evaluate the part of the tooth that has been removed and determine the location and size of the fractured segment. This is especially critical for a multirooted tooth. If the location and size of the root tip cannot be determined clinically, a radiograph (preferably a periapical radiograph) should be obtained.

For small root tips (less than 4 to 5 mm in length), the irrigation-suction technique may be used for retrieval. This technique is useful only if the tooth was well-luxated and mobile before the root was fractured. The socket is irrigated vigorously and suctioned with a fine suction tip. In this way, the root tip may occasionally be irrigated from the socket and retrieved with the suction.

If the irrigation-suction technique is unsuccessful, a root tip pick may be used to retrieve the root tip. The root tip pick is inserted into the periodontal ligament space and the root tip gently teased out of the socket. Care must be taken not to exert excessive apical or lateral force when using the root tip pick. Excessive apical force could result in the displacement of the root tip into other anatomic locations such as the maxillary sinus or the mandibular canal. Excessive lateral force could result in bending or fracture of the root tip pick.

An endodontic file might also be used in the retrieval of root tips. The file can be inserted into the canal to engage the root tip. The root tip is subsequently removed by grasping the endodontic file with a hemostat. This technique is useful only if the root tip has a visible canal and if it does not have a severe dilaceration that prevents access to the canal.

If attempts at removal of the root tip using the preceding techniques are unsuccessful or if visualization or access is impaired, and if a flap has not been reflected, one should be reflected at this time to facilitate retrieval.

Following the reflection of a flap, bone may be removed from the buccal aspect of the root tip until it is exposed. It then can be retrieved with a root tip pick or a straight elevator.

Alternatively, the bone overlying the buccal aspect of the apex (on the outer buccal plate) of the root tip may be removed. In order to locate the exact location of the apex of the root tip, a periodontal probe is used to measure the distance from the crest of the bone to the root tip. This measurement is transferred to the bone. The size of the root tip is also measured on a periapical radiograph. A window or fenestration then is created in the bone at the apex of the root tip. The tip can be retrieved by inserting a root tip pick through this window. This technique is especially useful when bone on the buccal aspect is thin and must be preserved, such as when implants or orthodontic movement of a tooth into the area are planned. See Figures 2.28A–D.

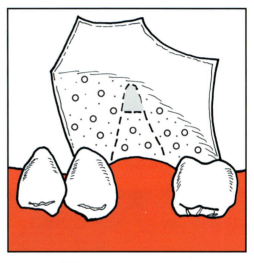

Figure 2-28A. To remove a small, inaccessible, buccal root tip in the maxillary arch, a flap should be reflected with adequate exposure to the tooth's apical portion.

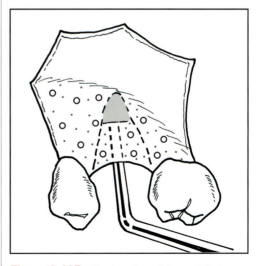

Figure 2-28B. The location of the root tip is measured.

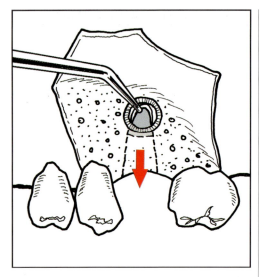

Figure 2-28C. This measurement is transferred to the buccal bone, and a window is created through which a root tip pick or similar instrument can push the root tip coronally.

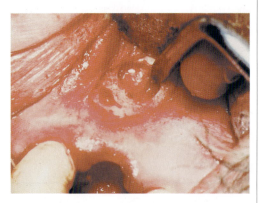

Figure 2-28D. Clinical example of the procedure only using a semilunar flap.

Technique for Extractions of Multiple Teeth

It is common for a patient to require extractions of multiple adjacent teeth or of all remaining teeth. If this is the case, certain principles should be followed so that the transition from a dentulous state to an edentulous state is as smooth as possible. The goal is to allow proper functional and esthetic rehabilitation with removable or fixed prostheses after the extractions.

The order in which the teeth should be extracted is important. In general, maxillary teeth should be extracted before mandibular teeth for several reasons. Local anesthetics tend to have a more rapid onset and a shorter duration of action in the maxillary arch. This means that surgery in the maxillary arch can begin sooner after the administration of local anesthetics, but also it means that the surgery should not be delayed. In addition, extractions of maxillary teeth first prevent debris, such as portions of teeth or restorations, from falling into mandibular extraction sockets if extractions of the mandibular teeth were performed first. Adequate hemostasis should be achieved in the maxillary arch before starting extractions in the mandibular arch. This improves visualization during extractions of mandibular teeth. Extractions should also progress from a posterior to an anterior direction. This allows for the more effective use of straight elevators in luxating and mobilizing the teeth before using forceps to extract them. However, since the canine tends to be the most difficult tooth to extract due to its long root, it should be extracted last. Extractions of the teeth on either side of the canine weaken its bony housing, potentially making the canine easier to extract.

In cases of extractions of multiple adjacent teeth or of all remaining teeth, the reflection of a flap improves access and visibility during the extractions. This allows for the more effective use of straight elevators and forceps, making the extractions easier. Reflection of a flap also allows for bone removal and sectioning of teeth if needed.

Selective alveoloplasty is usually required following extractions of multiple adjacent teeth or of all remaining teeth. This is especially true in the area of the canine prominence. The goal of the alveoloplasty is to remove all sharp bony edges. Areas of large undercuts should also be removed in patients who are to receive removable prostheses. Unjudicious removal of bone should be

SURGICAL EXTRACTIONS   **43**

avoided. Adequate height and width of the alveolar ridge should be maintained as much as possible to allow for proper rehabilitation. The alveoloplasty may be performed with a rongeur or bur, with the final smoothing performed with a bone file.

The surgical sites then should be thoroughly irrigated with saline. As mentioned previously, attention should be paid to the area at the base of the flap, as debris tends to collect there. The flap then can be replaced and sutured in position. An attempt should not be made to obtain primary closure of the surgical sites by advancing the flap toward the extraction sockets. This will only decrease the vestibular depth, which is to be maintained—especially if the patient is to receive a denture. If the flap has excess tissue at the time of closure, this excess tissue should be trimmed off. See Table 2.7.

Principles of Flap Closure

When the surgical procedure is completed and the surgical site has been irrigated, the flap can be sutured. Suturing the flap holds it in position and reapproximates the wound margins.

Various types of suture needles and suture material are available. Some common suture types used intraorally include silk, chromic or plain gut, or vicryl. With respect to size, recall that the larger the number, the thinner the suture. For instance, a 2-0 silk is thicker than a 5-0 silk. The most common type of suture used for the closure of a surgical extraction envelope flap is either a 3-0 or 4-0 chromic gut. This type of suture is resorbable and normally will take anywhere from one to two weeks for resorption.

A number of techniques can be used to successfully close a flap including a simple or interrupted technique, a running stitch with or without locking, and mattress style either vertically or horizontally. Each of these techniques has a place in appropriately closing an incision; however, the majority of envelope

Table 2-7. Multiple Extractions Sequence

1—Maxillary teeth

2—Mandibular teeth

3—Posterior to anterior

4—Achieve hemostasis prior to moving from one quadrant to the next

5—Reflection of a minimal buccal flap will facilitate extractions and allow for alveloplasty.

6—Alveoloplasty

7—Irrigation

8—Suturing

9—Postoperative instructions

flaps are closed with a standard interrupted suture technique.

Certain principles must be followed when suturing the surgical site. It is important that the suture needle is perpendicular to the surface of the mucosa as it penetrates the mucosa. This creates the smallest possible hole in the soft tissue and decreases the risk of tearing the soft tissue as the knot is tied. An adequate bite or width of soft tissue must also be taken to prevent the suture from pulling through and tearing the soft tissue. When tying the knot, it must be kept in mind that the purpose of the suture is to reapproximate the tissue. The knot, therefore, should not be tied too tightly. A knot that is too tight can cause ischemia of the soft tissue, resulting in soft tissue necrosis and wound dehiscence. In addition, the knot should not be positioned directly on the wound margin, as this causes additional pressure on the knot. Rather, it should be positioned to the side of the margin. The knot should have three throws so that it does not become undone. The suture material can then be cut. Nonresorbable sutures are generally left in place for approximately 5–7 days.

ENVELOPE FLAP CLOSURE

For the surgical extraction of a single tooth with reflection of an envelope flap, reposition the envelope flap into its correct location and suture the papillae. This is done by first passing the suture through the buccal gingival just apical to the base of the papilla and continuing the suture under the interproximal contact and out through the lingual gingiva. In many cases, it is not possible to obtain a good bite in the lingual tissue, and if this is the case, the suture needle is then grasped and a second pass is made from the lingual and extended back beneath the contact point and out the buccal. This suture is then tied using a standard knot. The entire process is repeated on the other papillae. The papillae adjacent to an extraction socket may be approximated using the simple interrupted sutures. See Figure 2.29.

A figure-eight suture or a horizontal mattress suture should be used if the extraction socket is packed with material to aid in hemostasis. For the figure-eight suture, the suture is passed through the buccal portion of the first papilla. It is then brought diagonally across the socket and passed through the lingual or palatal papilla on the opposite side of the socket. The suture is then passed diagonally again through the lingual papilla toward the buccal. The knot is tied on the buccal aspect of the ridge. See Figure 2.30A-E.

For the horizontal mattress suture, the suture is passed through the buccal portion of the first papilla. The suture is then passed through the lingual or palatal papilla. Then

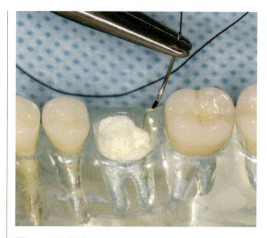

Figure 2-30A. Figure-eight suture. This is commonly used when the socket is packed with Gelfoam™ or Surgicel™. The needle is passed at the distobuccal papilla.

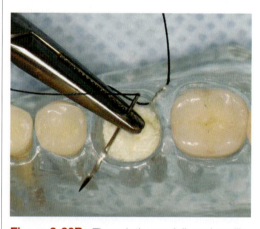

Figure 2-30B. Through the mesiolingual papilla.

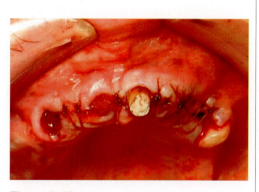

Figure 2-29. Interrupted sutures.

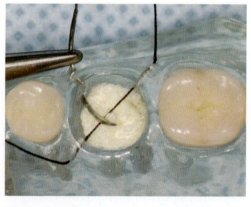

Figure 2-30C. Through the mesiobuccal papilla.

SURGICAL EXTRACTIONS   45

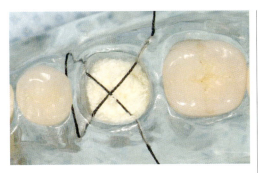

Figure 2-30D. Through the distolingual papilla.

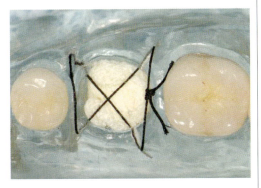

Figure 2-30E. Then the suture is tied.

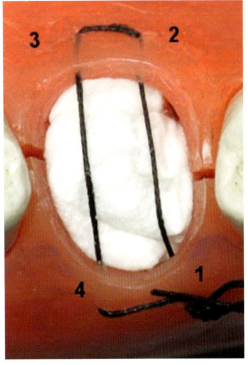

Figure 2-31. Sequence of placement of the horizontal mattress suture.

from the lingual side of the arch, the suture is passed through the lingual or palatal portion of the papilla on the other side of the socket. The needle is directed buccally through the last remaining papilla—from its inside to the outside (buccal). The knot can then be tied. See Figure 2.31.

CLOSURE OF A THREE-CORNER FLAP

The papilla at the site of the releasing incision should be sutured first. In order to facilitate the suturing at the site of the releasing incision, the soft tissue at the nonflap (fixed) side of the releasing incision may be lifted up slightly. The papillae on the remainder of the envelope portion of the flap should then be reapproximated. The anterior release is inspected. Many times it is necessary to place an additional stitch or two to ensure that the flap has enough support to prevent normal masticatory forces from displacing it postoperatively. See Figure 2.32. Usually, however, only two sutures are required to reapproximate the releasing incision.

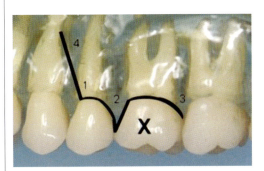

Figure 2-32. Closure of a three-corner flap. The releasing incision is closed first to reorient the tissue.

Continuous Suture

The simple continuous suture can be either locking (see Figure 2.33A–E) or non-locking (see Figure 2.34). For the simple continuous suture, the first papilla is reapproximated, and the knot tied in the usual fashion. The short end of the suture is then cut while leaving the long end of the suture intact. The adjacent papilla is then sutured, without tying a knot, but merely reapproximating the tissue as the suture is being placed. Succeeding papillae are then sutured in the same fashion until the final papilla is sutured and the knot tied. The final appearance is of the suture going across each extraction socket. The advantages of the simple continuous suture is that it takes less time to perform, and there are fewer knots—usually making it more comfortable for the patient. The disadvantage of the simple continuous suture is that if one suture pulls through, the entire suture line becomes loose.

Technique for Extractions of Teeth Using Periotomes

A periotome is a fine, straight elevator with a sharp, narrow blade that is designed to slice the periodontal ligament and displace the

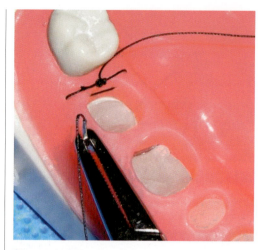

Figure 2-33B. Then the needle is passed through the adjacent buccal and lingual papillae.

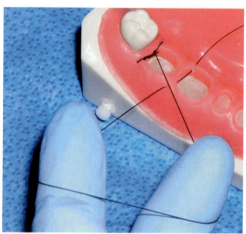

Figure 2-33C. A loop is created. That loop is twisted, and a needle is passed through it, after which the loop is pulled tight.

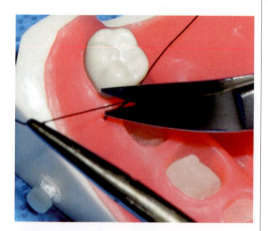

Figure 2-33A. Continuous locking suture. Initially a simple interrupted suture is tied. Only the short end of the suture is cut.

tooth as the instrument is manipulated apically. It is not a true dental elevator since it is not inserted and rotated to expand the bone and subluxate a tooth. It is, however, used when the postextraction site is to be reconstructed with a dental implant. The goal in these cases is to remove a tooth with minimal alveolar expansion or alteration in the bony housing. This is especially true if immediate implant placement is planned and

SURGICAL EXTRACTIONS 47

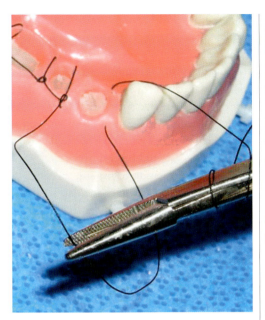

Figure 2-33D. The procedure is repeated until the last pass, where a final loop is made—which is used to place the final knot. This last loop functions as the short end of a simple interrupted suture.

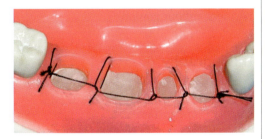

Figure 2-33E. Final continuous locking suture.

trauma to the surrounding alveolar bone must be avoided. The periotome is used by inserting the blade into the periodontal ligament space and gently rocking the instrument buccopalatally while applying gentle apical pressure. In this way, the periodontal ligament is cut, allowing the tooth to be gently lifted out of the socket without trauma or damage to the alveolar bone. Straight periotomes are indicated for use on single-rooted teeth, and angled periotomes are indicated for use on multirooted or posterior teeth.

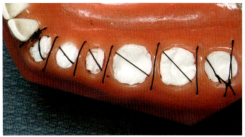

Figure 2-34. Continuous suture.

Common Mistakes during Surgical Extractions

The principles of surgical extraction as discussed previously should be followed to decrease the incidence of complications. Common mistakes that are made during extractions of teeth include attempting a forcep extraction when the preoperative evaluation had indicated that a surgical extraction was required, poor flap design, inadequate reflection of a flap, use of uncontrolled force, inadequate seating and adaptation of the forceps, attempting the removal of root tips without adequate access and visualization, inadequate irrigation of the surgical site prior to reapproximation of the flap, and poor reapproximation of the flap.

If the preoperative evaluation indicates that a surgical extraction, rather than a forcep extraction, is required, the practitioner should proceed with the surgical extraction. Attempts at extracting the tooth with a forcep in this situation might result in loss of valuable coronal tooth structure that would have facilitated the surgical extraction of the tooth. Using forcep extraction when a surgical extraction is indicated could also lead to excessive trauma of the soft tissue, fracture of the tooth, fracture of the adjacent bone, and patient fatigue from the extended length of the procedure.

When designing a flap, principles should be followed as discussed previously. Poorly designed flaps lead to complications such as wound necrosis, wound dehiscence, periodontal defects, damage to the papillae, and prolonged healing time.

The flap must be adequately reflected to permit adequate access and visibility during the extraction. Inadequate flap reflection could lead to excessive tension on the flap or a tear that is difficult to reapproximate. Inadequate flap reflection also prevents instruments from being seated properly.

The use of uncontrolled force in the extraction of a tooth should be avoided. Slow, deliberate movements, instead of rapid, jerky movements, should be used to expand the bone. Excessive force should not be used as it leads to fracture of the tooth or adjacent bone. If heavy force seems necessary to extract a tooth, bone should be removed or the tooth sectioned (in cases of multi-rooted teeth) to allow for a more controlled extraction.

The forcep should be adequately seated and adapted for a successful extraction. It should be placed as apically as possible and reseated periodically during the extraction. The beaks of the forcep should be shaped to adapt to the root of the tooth. If it doesn't, a different forcep should be used. The beaks of the forcep should be held parallel to the long axis of the tooth so that the forces generated are delivered along the tooth's long axis. This provides maximal effectiveness in expanding the bone. If a cowhorn forcep is used, the beaks should be properly seated in the area of the furcation, so that the tooth that is being extracted is squeezed out of the socket. Buccolingual movement should be avoided until the beaks of the cowhorn forcep are properly seated.

Attempting the removal of root tips without adequate access or visualization should be avoided. This is especially important in the maxillary arch as complications such as root displacement into the maxillary sinus can occur if excessive apical pressure is used. If access to and visualization of the root tip is inadequate, further reflection of the flap or bone removal should be performed.

Adequate irrigation of the surgical site prior to reapproximation of the flap is critical. As discussed previously, debris tends to collect at the base of the flap. This area should be thoroughly irrigated prior to repositioning of the flap. Inadequate irrigation of the surgical site can lead to an infection, which will require the surgical site to be reopened for irrigation and debridement.

Proper reapproximation of the flap is important to prevent wound necrosis, wound dehiscence, periodontal defects, damage to the papillae, and an extended healing time. Adhering to proper suturing techniques is important. The flap should always be held in position without tension.

Bibliography

1. J. R. Hooley, and D. B. Golden. *Surgical Extractions.* Dental Clinics of North America 38 (2): 217–236. 1994.
2. H. Dym and O. E. Ogle. *Atlas of Minor Oral Surgery.* Philadelphia, PA: W.B. Saunders. 2001.
3. L. J. Peterson. *Principles of Complicated Exodontia.* In *Contemporary Oral and Maxillofacial Surgery,* edited by Larry J Peterson, 3rd edition. St Louis: Mosby, pp. 178–214, 1998.

Chapter 3

Surgical Management of Impacted Third Molar Teeth

Dr. Pushkar Mehra and Dr. Shant Baran

Introduction

Removal of impacted third molars or "wisdom teeth" is one of the most common surgical procedures performed in a dental office. **Impaction** refers to the lack of eruption of a tooth into the dental arch within the expected time. The tooth becomes impacted because eruption is prevented by a physical barrier such as an adjacent tooth, dense overlying bone, or excessive soft tissue. The National Institutes of Health (NIH) Consensus Development Conference, held in 1979, established a series of guidelines that provides information for clinicians who treat patients with impacted third molars. Teeth most often become impacted because of inadequate arch length (total alveolar arch length is less than the total dental arch length). The most common impacted teeth are maxillary and mandibular third molars, followed by maxillary canines and mandibular premolars.

As a general rule, **all** impacted teeth should be **evaluated for treatment**, which could mean either observation, removal or surgically assisted eruption. Dentists must use knowledge acquired from their education, training, and experience and combine it with clinical and radiographic examinations before deciding whether to retain or remove the impacted teeth. For the most part, removal of impacted teeth is indicated unless a specific contraindication exists. This philosophy is based on the fact that removing impacted teeth becomes more difficult and complicated with advancing age. A fundamental precept of the philosophy of dentistry is "prevention of problems." Preventive dentistry indicates that impacted teeth be removed before complications arise.[1–5]

Certain standards of care and expectations have been established for all dental and surgical procedures, and third molar surgery is no exception. Whether a general dentist or a specialist performs the surgery, these standards remain the same. The patients benefit from an accurate diagnosis, good presurgical planning, sound execution of surgery, and well-managed postoperative care. This chapter discusses the basic principles for management of impacted third molars. It is designed to provide a basic framework for the dental surgeon interested in performing third molar surgery and provides information that will help in assessing surgical difficulty and managing impacted third molar patients in their practices.

Indications for Third Molar Removal

Many indications for removal of impacted third molars exist.[1-9] However, elective removal of third molar teeth should not be performed if potential risks outweigh the benefits of surgery. The following paragraphs list certain conditions that are routinely considered as indications for removal of third molars.

PERICORONITIS

Pericoronitis is an infection of the soft tissue that usually occurs around the crown of a partially impacted tooth (see Figure 3.1). This infection is caused by the normal flora of the oral cavity as the presence of bacteria in excessive pericoronal soft tissue presents a challenge to the delicate balance between host defense and bacterial growth. Transient decreases in host defenses can precipitate a bacterial surge and subsequently cause infection that results in moderate to severe pain and/or trismus. If left untreated, the infection may spread to adjacent head and neck fascial spaces. Recurrent trauma from traumatic of an opposing maxillary molar often causes the area around the mandibular third molar to swell, which leads to a vicious cycle of further traumatic occlusion and continued infection. Another common cause of pericoronitis is entrapment of food under the operculum. This provides a haven for streptococci and the anaerobic oral microbes to grow.

Initial treatment should include mechanical debridement to cleanse the area, prescribing oral rinses such as chlorhexidine to reduce bacterial load, and the use of antibiotics

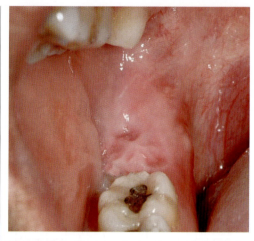

Figure 3-1. Photograph showing pericoronitis around an impacted third molar tooth. Note the erythema of the gingival surrounding the third molar.

with oral flora coverage. Patients should be instructed in the use of strict oral hygiene measures. Early intervention is advantageous because of the potential for rapid spread from this area to fascial spaces, which would require hospitalization and, possibly, major invasive surgery.

PERIODONTAL DISEASE

Periodontal disease of the adjacent second molar is often a concern when an impacted third molar is present (see Figure 3.2). Retention of an impacted third molar can compromise the bone housing the second molar and might predispose it to periodontal defects. This situation can progress to clinical recession and pocketing—leading ultimately to possible root caries and/or mobility.

CARIES

Due to its posterior position, a third molar presents a hygiene challenge to the most meticulous of patients. A third molar that is not in its correct position relative to the arch creates a more cumbersome situation with regard to hygiene. The susceptibility of such

SURGICAL MANAGEMENT OF IMPACTED THIRD MOLAR TEETH

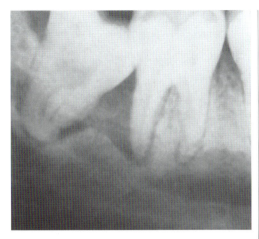

Figure 3-2. Radiograph showing severe bone loss around the second molar secondary to periodontal disease caused by an impacted third molar.

a third molar to carious involvement is, therefore, high, and it is not uncommon to see this in clinical practice (see Figure 3.3). Even when an obvious communication of the tooth may not exist with the oral cavity, the potential still exists for subsequent bacterial invasion. Dental caries and pulpal necrosis contribute to an increasing number of third molar extractions with increasing age.[9]

ROOT RESORPTION

As with periodontal disease, the mere presence of an impacted third molar in close proximity to a second molar predisposes the second molar to a myriad of problems. One problematic situation is that of resorption of the roots of the second molar. Root resorption associated with an impacted third molar is common in the 21- to 30-year age group, and the most common site for root resorption is the middle third of the distal surface of the adjacent second molar.[10] This presentation may, unfortunately, result in extraction of the second molar, which is news not often pleasing to the patient.

REMOVABLE PROSTHESES

When planning treatment for dentulous patients with removable prostheses, close attention should be paid to the presence of impacted third molars. Retention of these teeth under such prostheses may lead to their "eruption." Continued pressure over these areas caused by the prosthesis can initiate remodeling of the bone overlying the tooth, eventually leading to ulceration of the soft tissue and exposure of the previously unerupted tooth. The patient is then at risk for a problem that could present at at any time.

Figure 3.4 shows a radiograph of a 70-year-old patient with third molars exposed to the oral cavity due to prolonged denture wear. This patient had recurrent episodes of

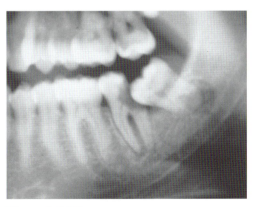
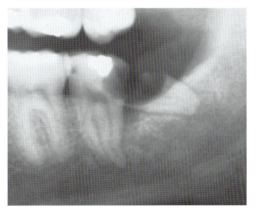

Figure 3-3A,B. Radiographs showing caries on the distal aspect of the second molar secondary to an impacted third molar.

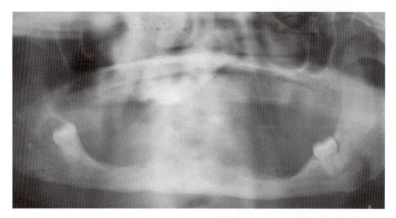

Figure 3-4. Radiograph of a 70-year-old patient with third molars exposed to the oral cavity due to prolonged denture wear. This patient had recurrent episodes of pericoronitis and was treated by removal of the offending teeth. Performing third molar extractions in this kind of patient is complex due to the presence of an atrophic mandible. There is increased risk of jaw fracture and inferior alveolar nerve injury during surgery.

pericoronitis and was treated by removal of the offending teeth. Performing third molar extractions in this type of patient is more complicated due to the presence of an atrophic mandible. There is increased risk of jaw fracture and inferior alveolar nerve injury during surgery at this age.

Pathology

Certain types of tumors and cysts have been associated with the follicles of impacted teeth. Although the overall incidence of odontogenic cysts and tumors is not particularly high, the correlation between pathology and impacted teeth cannot be ignored. It is recommended that if impacted teeth have pathology associated with them, they should be removed, and the pathologic cyst or tumor sent for histopathological examination.

Figure 3.5A shows a panoramic radiograph of an impacted third molar in a 17-year-old female with a pericoronal radiolucency, causing root resorption of the second molar. Upon histopathological examination, this radiolucency was found to be an ameloblastoma.

Figure 3.5B shows a panoramic radiograph of a 46-year-old male with an impacted maxillary molar, which has been displaced superiorly and posteriorly toward the infratemporal fossa by expansion of an associated dentigerous cyst. The patient required a Le Fort 1 osteotomy procedure for removal of the impacted tooth and cyst.

Management of Dental Crowding/ Adjunct to Orthodontic Treatment

Patients who undergo orthodontic treatment spend a great deal of time and money in pursuit of attractive looking teeth. The presence of impacted wisdom teeth may interfere with orthodontic movement and is suspected to provide a long-term mesially directed force that may contribute to relapse. The removal of impacted third molars may also create some additional space in the posterior jaws for orthodontic distalization of teeth. Consideration should be given to removal of any impacted wisdom teeth prior to initiating orthodontic treatment or, in some cases, upon completion. The orthodontic treatment plan, age of the patient, and stage of development of the teeth are some factors

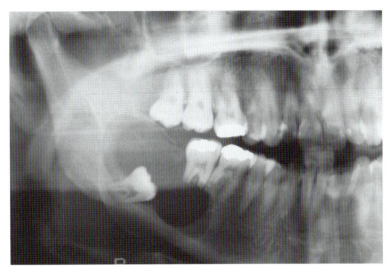

Figure 3-5A. Panoramic radiograph of an impacted third molar in a 17-year-old female with a pericoronal radiolucency causing root resorption of the second molar. Upon histopathological examination, this radiolucency was found to be an ameloblastoma.

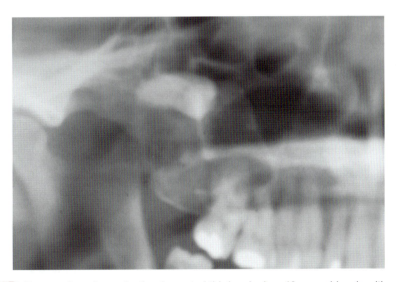

Figure 3-5B. Panoramic radiograph of an impacted third molar in a 46-year-old male with a large pericoronal radiolucency in the maxillary sinus area. The impacted third molar has been displaced into the sinus and towards the infratemporal fossa. Upon histopathological examination, this radiolucency was found to be a dentigerous cyst.

that might dictate the timing. The NIH consensus conference concluded that although significant orthodontic reasons exist for the early removal of third molars, the practice of early surgical enucleation of third molar buds between the ages of 7 to 9 years is not recommended.[11]

Preparation for Orthognathic Surgery

When a patient is being evaluated for orthognathic surgery, the presence of impacted teeth should be noted. In patients where a mandibular sagittal split osteotomy is recommended, the presence of such teeth may complicate the surgery. It is recommended to remove such teeth at least 6–9 months prior to undertaking such a surgery to permit adequate healing of the bone. The newly formed bone will allow for a more predictable bone separation during surgery as well as providing more osseous bulk for rigid fixation and stability.

In the authors' experience, impacted maxillary third molars can be removed safely concomitantly during a maxillary Le Fort I osteotomy procedure. Access for removal of the third molar is unrivaled, and usually the extractions are a relatively straightforward procedure. Some surgeons, however, prefer that the third molars be removed prior to surgery if the surgeon is osteotomizing the maxilla in multiple segments. Removal of the third molars approximately three to six months prior to this orthognathic surgery is often sufficient to avoid subsequent surgical complications.

Management of Facial Pain

Patients may present complaining of radiating pain stemming from the area of an impacted third molar. Due to the proximity of the temporomandibular joint (TMJ) and associated musculature, the third molars may be a possible source of pain. However, it should be emphasized that the third molars may not be the source of the pain. If the patient has no absolute contraindications as outlined later in this chapter, removal of the impacted teeth may be considered. The patient should be informed of the risks of undertaking such a procedure with no clear resolution in sight. Patients should understand the possibility of not experiencing relief despite removal of the impacted teeth.

Prevention of Pathologic Mandible Fracture

Although the purpose of the alveolus is to house the teeth, the presence of teeth invariably lessens the osseous bulk. When a tooth is embedded within the mandible, it occupies space that would otherwise be bone contributing to its strength. If the position of the impaction is such that it permits minimal continuity of bone, it might represent a point of weakness. This situation could predispose an individual to fracture of the mandible in the area of the impaction (Figure 3.6). Moreover, the presence of such a tooth complicates the treatment of a mandibular fracture. Therefore, it has been suggested that these impactions be removed prior to such incidents. Although iatrogenic fractures may occur during removal, the incidence is low, and a controlled setting with a systematic approach minimizes this as a complication.

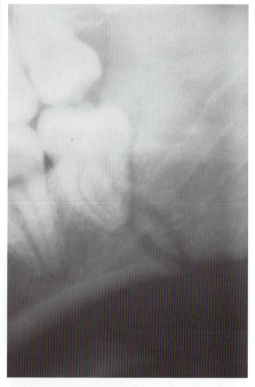

Figure 3-6. Panoramic radiograph demonstrating a left mandibular angle fracture which runs through the impacted third molar area.

Contraindications to Removal of Impacted Third Molars

The removal of teeth comes with a number of risks and potential complications. One reason to consider not removing impacted wisdom teeth is that the potential for subjecting a patient to these complications outweighs the potential gain achieved by their removal.

Damage to Adjacent Structures

A number of vital structures surround third molars, and with varying degrees of impactions come varying degrees of risk to these areas. Careful clinical and radiographic analysis is required to assess the proximity of the teeth to these structures of concern as well as an understanding of the extent of surgery required to remove these teeth. This analysis plays a significant role in determining the extent of morbidity associated with any procedure. If, after careful evaluation, it is determined that extensive damage may occur from the removal of such teeth, then a decision to remove them may not be justifiable.

Figure 3.7 shows a radiograph of a 48-year-old male with clinically asymptomatic third molars. The impacted teeth were discovered on routine panoramic radiographic examination. No surgical treatment was recommended. Clinicians must understand that surgical removal of the impacted lower tooth in this patient would risk serious complications including, but not limited to, nerve injury and jaw fracture.

In contrast to the preceding scenario, Figure 3.8 shows a panoramic radiograph of a 39-year-old male with symptomatic impacted second and third molars ("kissing molars"). Like the case in Figure 3.7, these extractions are very difficult, and in an asymptomatic patient, a very strong case can be made for close observation without surgery. However, this patient had recurrent bouts of infection, and consequently, despite the risks of surgery, the teeth were removed. Due to the extent of surgery, the procedure was performed in a hospital setting, and the

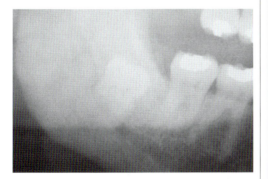

Figure 3-7. Deeply impacted mandibular third molar in very close proximity to the inferior alveolar nerve in a 48-year-old male. Note the dense bone overlying the impacted tooth. In view of the difficulty of the surgery, age of the patient, and asymptomatic nature of the impaction, elective extraction was not recommended.

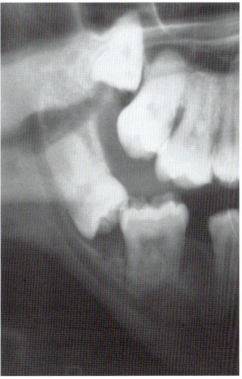

Figure 3-8A. Panoramic radiograph of a 39-year-old male with symptomatic impacted second and third molars ("kissing molars").

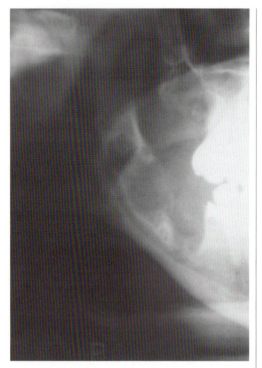

Figure 3-8B. The patient had recurrent infections so despite the risks of surgery, the impacted teeth were removed. The procedure was performed in a hospital setting. A bone graft was harvested from the hip and placed into the large surgical defect to augment the weakened mandible. Maxillomandibular fixation (wiring of jaws) was applied for four weeks postoperatively to prevent jaw fracture.

patient was bone grafted and placed into maxillomandibular fixation for four weeks postoperatively to prevent jaw fracture.

AGE OF PATIENT

Age might become a significant factor in deciding whether or not to remove an impacted wisdom tooth. There exists some controversy as to the most optimal time for removal. A general consensus, however, does exist in one area: "Removal of third molar teeth should be deferred until one can determine whether or not they may remain impacted."

The surgeon must understand that although third molars can be removed at any age, surgery itself is easier and associated with less morbidity when performed in patients who are in their late teens or early 20's.[1, 3, 11, 13, 14] With regard to advanced age, older patients tend to respond less favorably to the removal of teeth, particularly impacted third molars. Bone becomes increasingly calcified with age, leading to rigidity, and becomes less forgiving of the forces required to remove these teeth. This yields a situation in which more bone must be sacrificed, and the procedure becomes more traumatic. In the case of asymptomatic impactions, an approach is favored that requires the watchful eye of the general dentist and frequent radiographic checks to rule out pathology.

MEDICAL COMPROMISE

Oftentimes, practitioners may find themselves so focused on the patient's dental condition that they neglect the patient's medical condition. A thorough review of the patient's medical history must be performed and the patient informed of any issues that may preclude the removal of a tooth or the need for further preoperative preparation. Removal of asymptomatic impacted teeth must be viewed as "elective." If a patient has uncontrolled cardiovascular or respiratory conditions, immune compromise, or a significant coagulopathy, serious consideration must be given to deferring surgery in these cases. In nonelective cases, further preoperative preparation, involvement of the patient's physician, and possible hospitalization may be required.

Surgical Instrumentation

When a dentist attempts any procedure, having the correct instruments can make the difference between success and complication. This is particularly true with surgical procedures. The following armamentarium is sug-

SURGICAL MANAGEMENT OF IMPACTED THIRD MOLAR TEETH

gested as a "basic template" for the surgical removal of third molars:

- #15 Bard-Parker blade
- Periosteal elevator (example: #9 Molt)
- Retractors
  - Flap (example: Seldin, Minnesota, Herman)
  - Cheek (example: Minnesota, Bishop, Herman)
- Dental elevators
  - Straight (preferably one each of a small, medium, and large size)
  - East-West
  - Crane pick
  - Pott's or Miller's (if required)
- Bone file
- Extraction forceps
  - Upper universal
  - Lower universal
- Rongeurs
  - End cutting
  - Side cutting (if needed)
- Needle holder
- Suture scissors
- Suture (resorbable or nonresorbable)
- Rotary instrument for cutting bone and tooth
  - Drill
  - Burs (round, straight, or cross-cut fissure)

The exact choice of equipment may vary among practitioners. Various blades, suture material, retractors, and elevators are available, and it is recommended that operators use those with which they are most comfortable. The rotary instruments chosen should be of the type that do not exhaust air into the surgical field, which will minimize complications such as intraoperative or postoperative air emphysema and/or foreign body entrapment.

Presurgical Considerations

After it is decided to perform the surgery, several factors need to be addressed prior to commencing the procedure. Attention to these areas will allow the surgery to proceed more smoothly and safely.

INFORMED CONSENT

When planning for the surgical removal of third molars, one must always inform the patient of the risks that are involved and the potential complications that may arise. These should be explained to the patient in terms that the patient can comprehend, highlighting aspects that may be of particular concern in each respective case.

It should be discussed that during any procedure, a time of discomfort or pain is to be expected, and appropriate medication will be provided. Infection can arise postoperatively with any surgical procedure, as can "dry socket." Damage to adjacent structures can occur, but to prevent this, the utmost care should be exercised. When maxillary third molars are to be extracted, sinus exposure is often possible. When extracting mandibular teeth, issues involving the inferior alveolar, mental, and lingual nerves should be discussed. The neural aspect should be stressed because of its associated morbidity—despite its rare occurrence. There are times where noninfected root tips might be retained given that retrieval can cause further harm with little benefit. The patient should be made aware of this.

Informed consent is a vital aspect of one's practice. When a patient is caught off-guard by an unexpected mishap, it can lead to unnecessary stress for the patient and practitioner. Patients have the right to be informed, and it is the professional's responsibility to use their knowledge to guide the patient through decisions about which they know very little.

RADIOGRAPHIC EXAMINATION

Thorough radiographic analysis is imperative in assessing difficulty and planning the surgical approach. Panoramic radiographs are the "workhorse" in impacted third molar surgery, and in the authors' opinion they should be obtained for all surgical cases. They conveniently demonstrate a large area of the face in one view. The relation of third molars to the inferior alveolar nerve and approximate proximity of maxillary teeth to the sinus can be evaluated, as can potential pathology that would otherwise be missed in more focused fields. This is not to discount the use of other dental radiographs. Greater detail can be visualized in periapical films, and the bucco-lingual dimension can be appreciated only with occlusal films. In extremely complex cases, computerized tomography (CT) scans or magnetic resonance imaging (MRI) scans might be indicated, as they may provide more detailed information about hard and soft tissue structures, respectively. Oftentimes, the clinician may need to use a combination of radiographs and other modalities to arrive at a diagnosis or plan.

Mandibular Third Molar Impactions

Mandibular impactions are classified based on three criteria: angulation, position relative to the anterior ramus, and position relative to the occlusal plane.

Assessing Difficulty

These classification systems are not mutually exclusive, and when used together, can aid the surgeon in assessing difficulty and extent of surgery, and also to plan a surgical approach for patients with impacted mandibular third molars.

Angulation refers to the angle of the long axis of the third molar relative to the long axis of the second molar. A mesioangular direction is the most common impaction and is one in which the crown of the molar is tilted mesially. The second most frequent is the vertical impaction in which the long axis re-

mains parallel to that of the second molar, but the tooth has not erupted. A severe mesial inclination may occur, leading to a perpendicular relationship of the second and third molars; this is referred to as a horizontal impaction. Finally, if the crown of the third molar faces away from the second molar, it is known as a distoangular impaction.

The Pell and Gregory system of classifying impacted third molar teeth (see Figure 3.9) uses the position of the tooth relative to the anterior ramus and occlusal plane. When classifying teeth relative to the anterior ramus, if the mesio-distal dimension of the third molar is completely anterior to the anterior aspect of the ramus, the molar is referred to as Class 1. Class 2 is a situation in which approximately half of the crown remains covered by the bone of the anterior ramus. Class 3 presents with the entire crown posterior to the anterior ramus. It is fair to say that Class 3 will likely present a greater challenge than a Class 1 impaction.

The other aspect of the Pell and Gregory classification is the position of the tooth relative to the occlusal plane (see Figure 3.9). Class A depicts a situation in which the occlusal surface of the third molar is flush with the second molar. Class B describes a tooth that has its occlusal surface located between the occlusal plane and the cervical line of the second molar. In the Class C impaction, the third molar presents with its occlusal surface below the cervical line of the second molar. Again, a class C impacted tooth will be deepest in bone and can be expected to be surgically more difficult than Class A and B impacted teeth.

Facial Form

Facial form has been implicated as an additional factor in assessing difficulty (see Figure 3.10). This stems from anatomy and can highlight specific concerns potentially influencing surgical access. Patients exhibiting a square or compact facial form tend to have

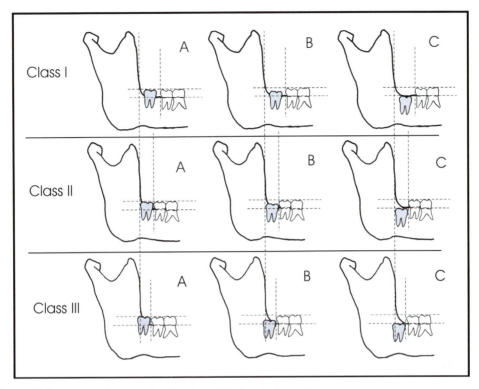

Figure 3-9. Pell and Gregory classification of third molar impactions.

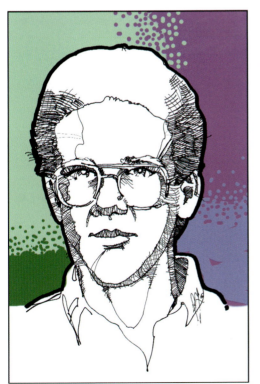
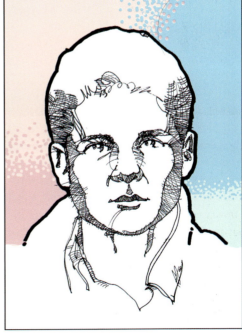

Figure 3-10. Different types of facial form can affect difficulty of surgery. **A.** Tapering facial form. **B.** Compact facial form.

zygomatic arches that are relatively low and maxillary tuberosities that are in close proximity to the coronoid process when in an open-mouth position. These factors make surgical access to maxillary third molars more difficult than in a patient with a tapering facial form whose zygomatic arches are high and whose coronoid processes do not encroach upon the tuberosities. With regard to the mandible, patients with a tapering facial form tend to have an anterior ramus that is more lateral when compared to the square form. These observations may seem trivial but can make a difference in technique, instrumentation, and modification of approach.

Root Morphology

Root morphology plays a major role in determining the degree of difficulty in the removal of impacted teeth. The first factor is the length of roots. In general, the most optimal time for removal of impacted teeth is when the roots are one-third to two-thirds formed (Figure 3.11A). At this stage the roots are generally blunt and rarely fracture during removal. They are also not embedded as deep as teeth with fully formed roots and, thus, are most likely more distance away from vital structures when compared to teeth with long, fully formed roots. If the roots are not developed at all, the extraction is usually more difficult since the tooth tends to rotate within its own crypt during elevation (Figure 3.11B).

The next factor to take into consideration is whether the roots are fused into a conical shape or whether the roots are separate and distinct. Teeth with fused conical roots are easier to remove than teeth with separate, divergent roots (see Figure 3.11C). Root cur-

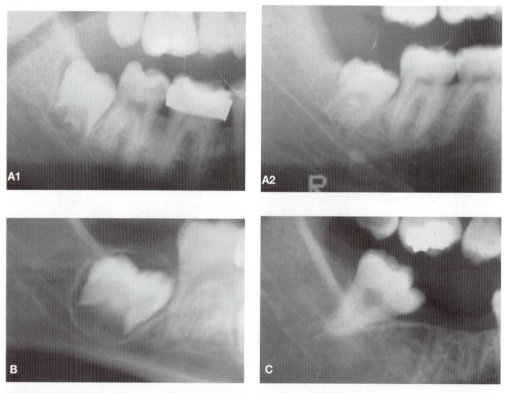

Figure 3-11. Root morphology affecting complexity of surgery. **A1, A2.** Roots are approximately 1/3 to 2/3 developed, therefore, these are easier extractions. **B.** Roots have not developed—may be a difficult extraction. **C.** Conical roots morphology—easier extractions.

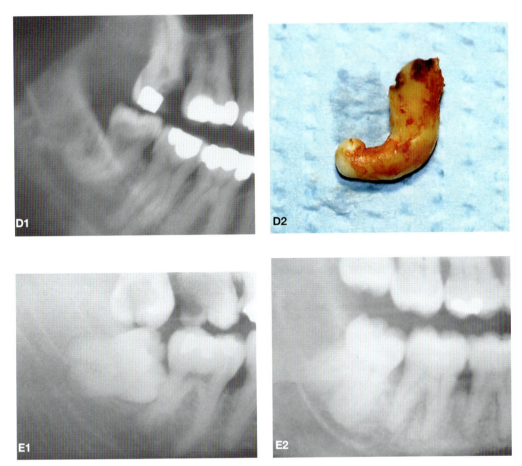

Figure 3-11. (*continued*) **D1,D2.** Dilacerated roots—more difficult extractions. **E1,E2.** Bulbous roots—more difficult extractions.

vatures must be assessed. Dilacerated roots can complicate a relatively simple extraction procedure, as the curved root will often fracture in the apical dilacerated portion (see Figure 3.11D). The direction of curvature also is important and must be assessed in relation to the direction of delivery of the tooth. Teeth with bulbous roots often require extensive bone removal for successful removal (see Figure 3.11E).

MISCELLANEOUS CONSIDERATIONS

Certain other factors like density of the overlying bone, size of follicular sac, proximity to the second molar, and relationship to vital structures (inferior alveolar nerve, maxillary sinus, and so on) must also be taken into consideration, as they can help in determining the difficulty of the extraction. Figure 3.12 shows an extracted third molar in which the mandibular canal traversed through the roots.

SURGICAL TECHNIQUE

Although the surgery itself, in large part, dictates the postoperative course, certain accommodations can potentially improve it. Patients undergoing third molar surgery may benefit from gross debridement of the periodontal tissues. A healthy environment can create more optimal conditions for healing. Preoperative rinsing with chlorhexidine glu-

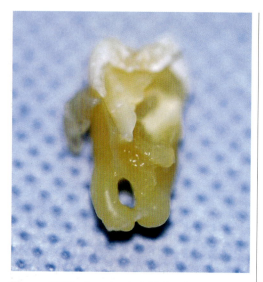

Figure 3-12. An extracted third molar demonstrating the course of the mandibular canal through the tooth roots.

conate, an antimicrobial rinse, has been shown to improve the postoperative course, specifically lowering the incidence of alveolar osteitis, or dry socket. Anecdotal "evidence" suggests that patients with a history of pericoronitis have benefited from preoperative antibiotic prophylaxis with a continued postoperative course. Ultimately, the removal of impacted third molars consists of local anesthetic administration, flap design, bone removal, luxation, sectioning of teeth, tooth delivery, and closure.

Anesthesia

When preparing for any extraction, adequate and profound anesthesia is paramount. The preferred technique for maxillary third molar extractions is buccal infiltration and a palatal nerve block in the area of the greater palatine nerve. Inferior alveolar nerve blocks combined with long buccal infiltration are the preferred anesthesia for mandibular third molar extractions.

The anesthetic standard upon which dental recommendations are based is 2 percent Lidocaine with a 1:100,000 concentration of epinephrine in a 1.8-ml cartridge. However, other types of anesthetic may be used as per the surgeon's preference. Each preparation and type of anesthetic has its own time of onset, duration of action, and specific toxicity levels, and attention should always be paid to such characteristics. Occasionally, circumstances may dictate the use of a local anesthetic preparation without epinephrine. In these cases, one can expect somewhat more bleeding intraoperatively due to lack of vasoconstrictive properties of epinephrine. Since patient comfort is the ultimate goal, many surgeons inject a long-acting local anesthetic either preoperatively or postoperatively. Bupivicaine, at a 0.5 percent concentration, is routinely administered for this purpose.

Flap Design

The type of flap used in third molar surgery is classified as **full thickness**, which describes an incision that is made from the epithelial surface to the underlying bone. A periosteal elevator is then placed with the concave surface against the bone to raise the mucoperiosteum from the bone.

The surgeon may find numerous classifications of flap design and varying nomenclature in articles and textbooks. However, in the setting of impacted third molar surgery, three main types of flap designs exist, and basically, all are modifications of one of the following flap designs (see Figure 3.13):

1. Flaps without a releasing incision (envelope flaps)
2. Flaps with an anterior releasing incision (three-cornered or triangular flaps)

It should be noted that these designs are not meant to limit the operator but are meant to provide a basic foundation from which to work. Based on experience and preference, surgeons might use a myriad of modifications of these fundamental flaps.

SURGICAL MANAGEMENT OF IMPACTED THIRD MOLAR TEETH

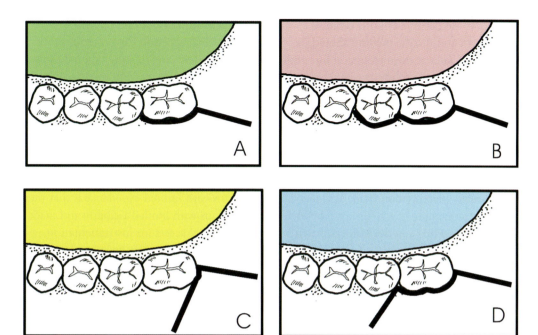

Figure 3-13. Common flap designs for mandibular third molar surgery. **A.** Short envelope flap. **B.** Long envelope flap. **C.** Short triangular flap. **D.** Long triangular flap.

Practitioners are encouraged to use a technique that they are comfortable with, provided the following fundamentals are not violated (see Figure 3.14):

- The base of the flap should be larger than the apex. Essentially, the releasing incision(s) should be divergent in relation to the site of exposure so as to not undermine the blood supply of the raised flap.
- The flap should be raised and released in such a manner as to prevent tearing of the flap. Tearing might lead to a compromised blood supply and necrosis.
- The ratio between the height of releasing incision(s) and length of base should not exceed 2:1.

Envelope flap: This flap can further be divided into a short envelope (see Figure 3.13A) or a long envelope flap (see Figure 3.13B).

When exposing a mandibular impacted tooth, the envelope flap begins with a distal

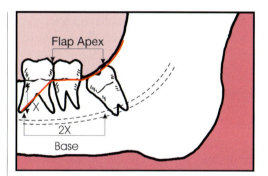

Figure 3-14. Basic principles of flap design: The base of the flap should be wider than the apex of the flap. The releasing incision(s) should be divergent in relation to the site of exposure so as to not undermine the blood supply of the raised flap. The ratio between the height of releasing incision(s) and length of base should not exceed 2:1.

incision. This incision should be placed buccally, because most impacted teeth are found buccally positioned in the jaws, and there is a decreased chance of complications like iatrogenic injury to the lingual nerve, bleeding, and so on. The distal incision commences at the external oblique ridge area posteriorly, and the the incision should be placed anteriorly at the distobuccal line angle of the second molar tooth or even just lingual to this area. More lingually placed incisions may increase the possibility of lingual nerve injury. Kiesselbach et al[15] found that in approximately 17 percent of the population, the lingual nerve lies at or above the alveolar crest. Thus, if the tissue lingual to the correctly placed incision line is violated, it could cause lingual nerve injury. The incision is then carried anteriorly intrasulcularly around the second molar (short envelope flap) or further anteriorly as desired (long envelope flap).

Three-cornered (triangular) flap: Very often, a fully submerged impaction will require more exposure than an envelope can provide. In such cases, a three-corner flap may be necessary. A three-corner flap is an envelope flap with the addition of a vertically oriented releasing incision. For a lower impacted third molar, the incision is started similarly to the envelope flap. A retractor is used to palpate the external oblique ridge and then tense the tissue. A #15 blade is placed at the point where retractor meets tissue, and an incision made to the distobuccal corner of the second molar. From this point, two variations exist (see Figures 3.13C and 3.13D): The releasing incision can be made posterior to the second molar (short triangular flap) or anterior to the second molar (long triangular flap). In both cases, the releasing incisions **must** be made at an obtuse angle to maintain a wide base for adequate perfusion of the triangular flaps.

As with any surgical procedure, access is of paramount importance. Although not all impactions require the elevation of a full-thickness mucoperiosteal flap, the limited visibility in the posterior oral cavity compounded by the nature of an impaction often mandates its use. A fresh, sterile blade should always be used. The envelope flap is the most common but often may not provide sufficient access in the posterior of the oral cavity. Releasing incisions should, however, be used judiciously. Although sometimes unavoidable, extending a releasing incision into unattached mucosa is not optimal and may complicate repositioning of the flap.

The authors have consistently found that one of the most common mistakes made by clinicians with limited experience is that they design flaps with limited visibility and inadequate surgical access for instrumentation. One must remember that in general, envelope flaps give lesser exposure and access when compared to flaps with releasing incisions. It is sometimes prudent to start with flaps with large access and visibility (for example: a long envelope flap versus a short envelope flap). However, the greater the amount of elevated tissue, the greater will be the degree of postoperative discomfort. Thus, the caveat is to exercise prudent surgery: to have enough visibility for adequate access without compromising the procedure and to discourage unnecessary reflection of tissue. As the surgeon gains more experience, it is only natural that he or she will modify flap length and design for each individual case based on clinical and radiographic examination, personal preference, and the operator's level of expertise.

Bone Removal

After careful reflection of soft tissue with a periosteal elevator, a bur should be used to expose the crown of the tooth, from the buccal. Careful attention should be paid to protecting the soft tissues of the flap, the lip, and the cheek. If the surgeon is intently focused on the tooth, damage to these structures can occur very easily. The goal of bone removal is to create a path for the delivery of the tooth, but not entirely at the expense of the alveolus.

The **first step** of bone removal provides

SURGICAL MANAGEMENT OF IMPACTED THIRD MOLAR TEETH 65

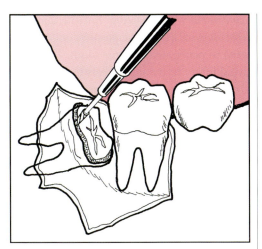

Figure 3-15A. Bone removal for a mesioangular impacted mandibular third molar surgery. Bone removal from the occlusal aspect.

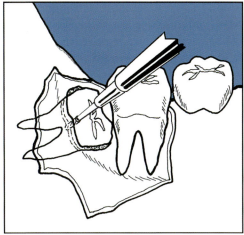

Figure 3-15C. Troughing of bone on the buccal aspect with a straight handpiece.

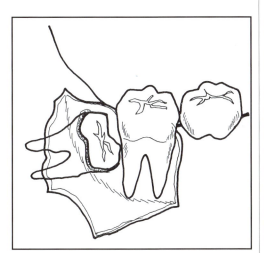

Figure 3-15B. Bone removal from the buccal aspect.

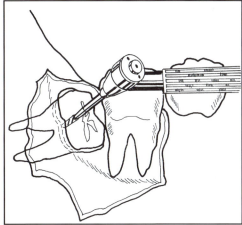

Figure 3-15D. Troughing of bone on the buccal aspect with a surgical high-speed handpiece.

exposure and visualization of the tooth surface. This includes bone removal from the occlusal aspect (see Figure 3.15A) and then from the buccal aspect to expose the tooth (see Figure 3.15B). Distal bone also can also be removed if needed. Bone is not removed from the lingual except when using the "lingual split-bone" technique of third molar removal. This technique is not commonly used in the United States and is not recommended because of the high incidence of surgical trauma and lingual nerve injury as compared to the standard buccal approach.

After the tooth has been exposed, the **next step** in bone removal is **troughing** (see Figures 3.15C and 3.15D). Troughing refers to bone removal into bone adjacent to the tooth, which provides a ledge of bone for use as a fulcrum for tooth elevation purposes. The trough should be made wide enough to accommodate a straight elevator but not so wide as to permit spinning of the instrument. This can be accomplished by cutting the buccal bone at its interface with the tooth. Directing the bur in a manner parallel to the long axis of the tooth will create a groove while removing minimal buccal bone. This will begin to free the tooth from its osseous housing without relinquishing mechanical advantage. The depth of the groove should be extended to approximate the "furcation" of the tooth. This generally corresponds to the length of the cutting surface of a fissure bur. The practitioner should not take too much comfort in being on the buccal, with its great leeway for cutting, because the inferior alveolar canal may be positioned buccally.

Troughing is generally confined to the buccal and, occasionally, the distal. The distal should be approached with great care. Owing to the potential crestal position of the lingual nerve, one should exercise caution along the distal and not venture past mid-distal. Also, given that the lingual nerve is entirely soft-tissue borne, an instrument should be placed along the distal bone, ensuring no contact of the bur with soft tissue. Cutting bone on the mesial side of the third molar should be avoided, as it can violate the second molar or create a periodontal defect if the interdental bone is sacrificed.

Luxation

When the crown of the tooth has been exposed and an appropriate amount of bone has been removed, an attempt to elevate the tooth from the socket may be made, keeping in mind the anatomy of the area and the vector of the directed force. In some instances, this may allow removal. If not, consideration should be given to sectioning the tooth.

Tooth Sectioning and Delivery

Tooth sectioning refers to splitting of the tooth from its buccal aspect, using a rotary instrument with irrigation. Initially, a groove is made with a bur. The groove does not need to penetrate the entire tooth. This is to avoid injury to the lingual soft tissues and the lingual nerve. In many cases, the lingual surface of the tooth is in very close proximity to a very thin lingual cortical plate. It is not uncommon that there may be accidental perforation of the rotary bur through the plate, thereby injuring the soft tissues including the lingual nerve. Thus, most surgeons will invariably stop their bur cut slightly short of the lingual surface of the tooth, and instead, use a straight dental elevator to fracture (split) the last remaining lingual aspect of the tooth into the desired portions. A narrow straight elevator is usually placed within the cut, and the blade rotated toward the aspect to be removed.

Mesioangular impactions are the most common type of mandibular third molar impaction. In many instances of a mesioangular impaction, the mesial aspect of the third molar may lie beneath the distal contour of the second molar. This poses a mechanical obstacle to delivery of the crown. A bur may be used to section the tooth in a number of ways that might permit removal of the crown followed by a path for removal of the roots (see Figure 3.16). One simple method is to longitudinally split the tooth into mesial and distal halves (see Figure 3.16A). Occasionally, the mesial aspect of the crown may still be trapped under the second molar and might require an additional cut (see Figure 3.16B). Many surgeons prefer to make a transverse cut parallel to the cementoenamel junction (CEJ) of the third molar, thereby separating the crown from the root trunk (see Figure 3.16C). The crown can be grasped with a forceps or ronguer. Another attempt should be made to elevate the remainder of the tooth. If unsuccessful, further troughing of the bone surrounding the roots may be considered. If a furcation exists, a second cut may be placed to split the roots from one another, facilitat-

SURGICAL MANAGEMENT OF IMPACTED THIRD MOLAR TEETH 67

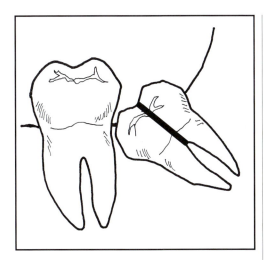

Figure 3-16A. Sectioning options for mandibular mesioangular third molar impactions. This view shows a cut longitudinally through the furcation.

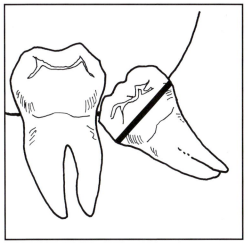

Figure 3-16C. Crown and root separation. The crown is removed and then the root is delivered into the original crown space.

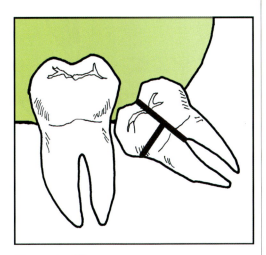

Figure 3-16B. Same as 16A, but with an additional cutting of the mesial crown, which is wedged under the second molar.

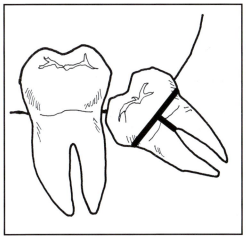

Figure 3-16D. Crown removal as in option 16C, but then the roots are divided longitudinally through the furcation and moved into the crown space for removal.

ing removal by creating two single roots (see Figure 3.16D).

One important principle to remember while making cuts within teeth is to keep the width of the cut as close as possible to the width of the dental elevator. This will provide for a clean separation of the crown from the root trunk. After the elevator is placed into the surgically made groove, the surgeon should give it a controlled twist. He/she will feel the tooth separate into the two segments as planned. An often overlooked option for tooth delivery is the use of the drill to place a purchase point in the buccal surface of the tooth structure. It should be deep enough to engage with a Crane pick or Cogswell B elevator without further fracturing the tooth. With correct placement and appropriately directed force, these instruments can exert a substantial rotational force (given a small lever-arm) that can elevate the most stubborn of teeth.

Horizontal impactions are treated much the same way as mesioangular impactions. A few adjustments are made based on the inclination. For instance, one usually elects to remove the crown prior to the root(s). This requires a cut wider superiorly than inferiorly to free the crown for withdrawal. On occasion, distal bone of the ascending ramus may need excision. This should be attempted cautiously. Protecting the lingual soft tissues is of paramount importance. Fortunately, the lingual nerve is entirely in soft tissue. With careful use of the drill and shielding of the lingual soft tissue by placing a retractor on bone, one may safely relieve small amounts of distal bone. The drill should approach, but never touch, the distolingual corner of the third molar. These modifications will aid in extracting horizontal impactions but may also be used for other types of impactions as well. Figure 3.17 shows common sectioning techniques for removal of horizontally impacted third molars.

Another common presentation is the **vertical impaction** of a lower third molar. A vertical impaction requiring removal often encroaches on the roots of the second molar and should be approached carefully. If the crown is clear of any undercuts, delivery can

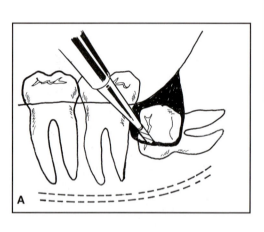
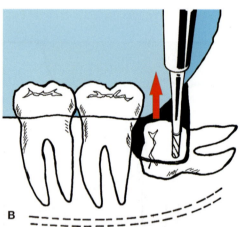
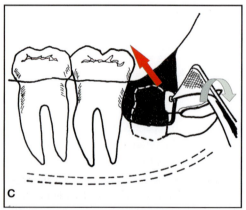
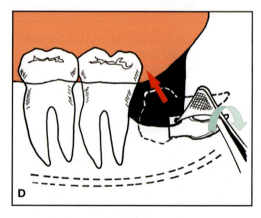

Figure 3-17. Common surgical technique for the removal of horizontally impacted mandibular third molars. **A.** Bone is removed from the superior surface of the tooth and from the buccal—and also perhaps from the occlusal aspect of the crown if there is sufficient bone thickness distal to the second molar. **B.** Crown is sectioned from root, and then removed. **C.** Roots are delivered together. Occasionally, a purchase point can be made to facilitate delivery. **D.** Roots have been split and delivered separately.

be accomplished by either elevating the tooth and/or placing a purchase point to allow for delivery with a crane pick. Oftentimes the crown is either limited by the distal of the second molar anteriorly or by the ascending ramus posteriorly. The operator might elect to section the roots vertically if a furcation exists. This allows for removal of the unencumbered portion, thereby creating a space into which the trapped segment may be directed. Occasionally, relieving bone along the distal of the crown is necessary to allow delivery. This should be performed with the utmost care owing to the likely presence of the lingual nerve near the lingual crest. As earlier described, careful use of the drill and shielding of the lingual soft tissue by placing a retractor on bone will enable one to relieve small amounts of distal bone. An alternative is to remove the distal portion of the crown in an oblique fashion, leaving the mesial for leverage. One may elect to remove the entire crown horizontally from the buccal if a substantial amount of distal bone would otherwise be required for removal. This would allow delivery of the crown followed by the root trunk because of clearance created. Figure 3.18 shows common sectioning techniques for removal of vertically impacted third molars.

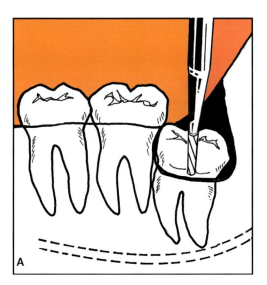

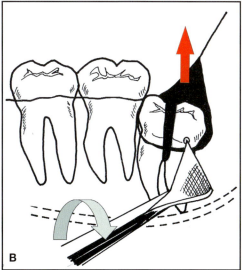

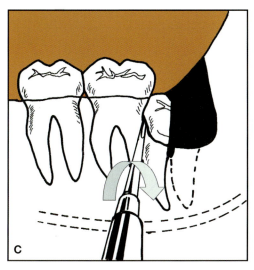

Figure 3-18. Common surgical technique for removal of vertically impacted mandibular third molars. **A.** Bone is removed on the occlusal, buccal, and distal aspects. **B.** After sectioning lengthwise through the tooth the posterior aspect is delivered first with purchase point and an elevator. **C.** The mesial part of the tooth is delivered with a straight elevator using rotary and a lever-type of motion.

Distoangular impactions can, at times, present a challenge for even the most experienced surgeon. When facing such a tooth, one must thoughtfully weigh the risks and benefits—knowing full well that this is often the most difficult type. Due to the inclination, both access and delivery are compromised. The same principles apply—soft tissue reflection, hard tissue removal, and sectioning of tooth structure. What differs is the approach to sectioning. One always tries to remove portions that present a mechanical obstacle, creating a pathway for removal. This is the "divide and conquer" approach. The sequence of sectioning may differ. In the distally inclined tooth, the ramus will be the obstacle to withdrawal. Because one cannot remove the ramus, adopt a strategy that employs removing crown and bone or sectioning of roots in a manner that permits delivery. Figure 3.19 shows a common sectioning technique for removal of distoangularly impacted teeth. Many times, removal of the distal portion of the crown is sufficient to clear any undercuts, but such a tooth will still require a substantial amount of force for delivery. Frequently, placing a purchase point as apically as possible and attempts at luxation from within that purchase point will provide enough leverage to deliver the tooth.

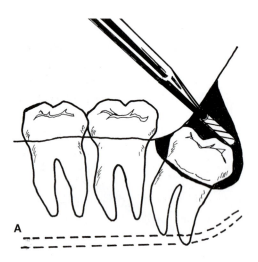

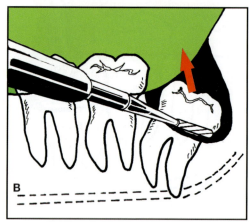

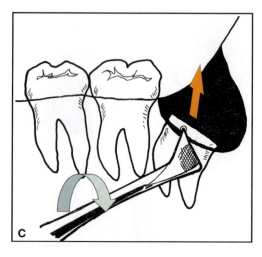

Figure 3-19. Common surgical technique for the removal of distoangularly impacted mandibular third molars. **A.** Bone is removed on the occlusal, buccal, and distal aspects. More distal bone removal is usually required in these cases. **B.** The crown of the tooth is sectioned from the root and delivered with straight elevators. **C.** A purchase point is made and an elevator is used to deliver both roots. Sometimes, roots may need to be split into separate halves and delivered separately.

CLOSURE

Upon removal of all tooth fragments, careful examination of the socket is warranted to ensure the complete removal of the tooth and fragments, as well as to inspect for any associated pathology. Prior to re-approximating the soft tissues, thorough irrigation of the socket and also irrigation beneath the raised flap should be done to flush any fragments or debris that may pre-dispose the patient to infection—especially subperiosteal abscess formation.

Prior to suturing, certain "housekeeping" operations might need attention. One must ensure the safe and complete removal of any follicle if it is visualized. Enucleation or thor-ough curettage followed by removal with a hemostat should be accomplished. Unerupted teeth will usually present with a follicle, and often the mesial and lingual as-pects require attention. Retained follicles have the potential to develop into pathologi-cal cysts and tumors. Removal should be done with care due to the proximity of the adjacent structures including nerves. Infected or granulomatous tissue should also be treated in this fashion. Bone contour should also be evaluated, and any sharp edges, tooth fragments, or loose bone fragments should be eliminated with a ronguer and/or bone file. This will permit better soft tissue ap-proximation and an improved postoperative course. Irrigation should be performed once again before closure.

When suturing a flap, one must first align known landmarks such as corners of the re-lease and/or papillae, if involved. This will provide the best closure due to the internal anatomy having changed postextraction and will be less likely to cause an advancement of the flap while suturing. The choice of suture material is at the discretion of the practi-tioner, although 3-0 chromic gut suture on a reverse cutting, half-circle needle is com-monly used owing to its rapid breakdown and ease of manipulation in the oral cavity.

Maxillary Third Molar Impactions

In comparing the removal of maxillary to mandibular impactions, there are similarities but also some salient differences. Both the similarities and the differences need to be well-understood by the operator.

CLASSIFICATION

When discussing maxillary third molars, the classification system is modified to exclude the position relative to the ramus since this anatomic marker is irrelevant. The only sig-nificance of the relative position of the tooth to the ramus is in assessing access.

Generally speaking, with regard to diffi-culty, the same angle of impaction yields the opposite degree of difficulty in the maxilla when compared to the mandible. Mesio-angular impactions pose a greater challenge compared with distoangular impactions in the maxilla, whereas in the mandible, the sit-uation is reversed. Also, the bucco-lingual di-mension of the alveolus limits the position-ing of the mandibular third molar lingually, but maxillary impacted third molars can, in some cases, be quite palatally positioned.

When compared with mandibular im-pacted third molars, maxillary procedures tend to be more straightforward. The aspect that complicates matters the most in maxil-lary impactions is that visibility can be a greater limiting factor. With that in mind, a prudent practitioner should approach the ac-cess preparation somewhat more aggressively.

FLAP DESIGN

Envelope and triangular flaps are also used for maxillary surgery (see Figures 3.20A–D). As with mandibular surgery, either the short or long versions of the flaps can be used. A new, sterile #15 blade should be used for the incision. The posterior extension of the inci-sion will be determined by the relative posi-tion of the tooth to the tuberosity. The inci-

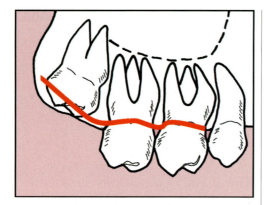

Figure 3-20A. Envelope flap showing the extent of the nearly linear incision.

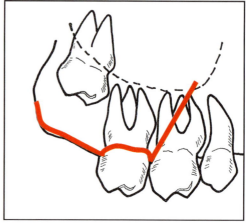

Figure 3-20C. This drawing shows the outline of a typical triangular flap.

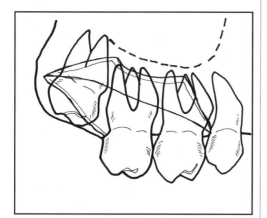

Figure 3-20B. When the envelope flap is reflected, this is the access that is achieved.

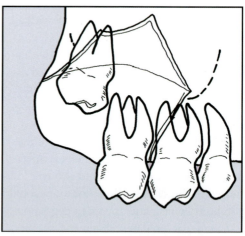

Figure 3-20D. When the triangular flap is reflected, this is the access that is achieved. It allows greater visibility than the envelope flap.

sion is begun on the anterior aspect of the tuberosity distal to the second molar. This slightly buccally positioned crestal incision is extended anteriorly to include the gingiva surrounding the first and second molar (envelope flap) or just the second molar (triangular flap).

As previously indicated, visibility is greatly reduced in the maxilla, and the use of a releasing incision is encouraged—especially for the surgeon with limited experience and for full bony impactions. By maintaining a wider base with the release, one can hope to overcome the obstacle of limited visibility. Frequently, another complicating factor in this surgery is the coronoid process of the mandible. As the mouth is opened, it translates anteriorly and often comes to lie buccally opposite to the impacted maxillary third molar. If this anatomic structure limits visibility or access, the mouth opening should be reduced, and then the surgeon should have the assistant manually shift and stabilize the lower jaw toward the surgical side.

Utilizing a periosteal elevator and the appropriate leverage, a full-thickness mucoperiosteal flap is reflected, elevating in an anterior to posterior direction. The same soft tissue precautions as in mandibular surgery should be used. Attention must be paid to protecting the soft tissues with adequate retraction. It is wise to reflect some of the palatal soft tissue, especially the crestal portion, as this will aid in smooth delivery of the tooth.

BONE REMOVAL

The buccal bone in the maxilla is less dense than in the mandible; therefore, removal of bone is often more conservative. In general, unlike mandibular third molar surgery, impacted maxillary teeth require bone removal only on the buccal and occlusal aspects. It is rare to ever remove significant distal bone. Bone can sometimes be removed either with hand instruments like a sharp periosteal elevator or, alternatively, with rotary instruments. The aim of bone removal is to visualize most of the crown of the tooth and establish access for extraction instruments. A straight dental elevator may be applied to assess mobility and access.

TOOTH SECTIONING, LUXATION, AND DELIVERY

The practitioner should be cognizant of the presence of the maxillary sinus and tuberosity and be careful with the forces directed superiorly or posteriorly. An attempt should be made to place the elevator from the mesiobuccal and engage the tooth from a point that will permit movement of the tooth in a distobuccal and buccal direction. Consideration should be given to the use of a curved elevator that is meant to engage the interproximal contour of the tooth and impart a force from the palatal. See Figure 3.21A and B.

Due to the location of the maxillary third molar, a vertical vector of force for luxation is necessary, and a slightly misdirected force can have drastic consequences. The potential

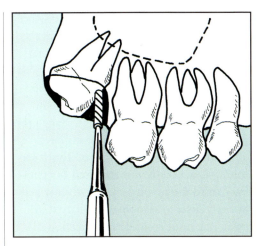

Figure 3-21A. Surgical technique for extraction of maxillary impacted third molars. If the tooth is not visualized once soft tissue has been reflected, bone is removed from the buccal and occlusal aspects. This can be accomplished with hand instruments (such as a periosteal elevator) or with rotary instruments.

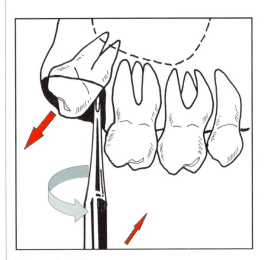

Figure 3-21B. The tooth is delivered with straight elevators applied on the mesiobuccal with rotational and lever types of motions. The tooth is always delivered in a distobuccal and occlusal direction.

to dislodge the maxillary third molar superiorly is a very likely one. Therefore, the careful placement of a Seldin retractor posterior to the tuberosity is advised. This provides a tactile sense of how posterior and superior one's force is being directed, a mechanical barrier to aid in preventing displacement, as well as the potential for a wedge effect that forces the tooth toward the oral cavity.

It should be stressed that maxillary third molars are known to have the most anomalous root morphology. Although many present with conical formations, others have rather strange root arrangements. **Tooth sectioning is generally not required for maxillary third molar surgery.** However, when the need arises to section a maxillary third molar, one must consider the direction the tooth is to be delivered. The presence of a second molar prohibits an anterior path and the dense palatine bone is quite unforgiving, and forces directed in this direction are marred by complications. If a trifurcation exists, then the procedure can be similar to that of any maxillary complicated exodontia in which a "T" formation will split the three roots and facilitate removal. If such a furcation does not exist, as is often the case, removal of the distal portion of the crown in an oblique fashion will provide enough clearance to allow the molar to escape in a distobuccal direction.

In the case of a distoangular impacted maxillary wisdom tooth, a few modifications might be required. The steps outlined throughout this discussion are sufficient to address this situation, but a few anatomic concerns need be covered. With a distoangular maxillary impacted third molar, the crown often undermines the tuberosity and poses a significant risk of fracture and the loss of tuberosity bone. This could become a concern for the patient later in life, if dentures are necessary, and it can also predispose the patient to a maxillary sinus exposure. Understanding these implications necessitate a slightly modified approach. One hopes to deliver the tooth in the direction in which it faces; that is, posteriorly. If tuberosity must be relieved to allow this, it is preferable to do this conservative excision (with minimal bone removal) rather than risk fracture of

the entire segment. Consideration should also be made to sectioning the crown from the root trunk, as done in many other instances. This may allow for root removal with posterior elevation. If relief of buccal bone is indicated, it should be done judiciously so as to not eliminate all leverage access.

When fracture of a bone segment such as buccal cortex or tuberosity is expected, one should attempt to reflect the least amount of soft tissue so as to preserve blood supply. If the operator anticipates such a fracture, avoiding reflection of the overlying periosteum will preserve the blood supply to the detached segment and will provide the best chance of survival postoperatively. If the overlying tissue has been reflected and a fracture is subsequently noted, removal of the fractured segment is advocated due to the high incidence of postoperative infection stemming from the retained fragment.

CLOSURE

As described earlier, upon completion, thorough examination of the socket followed by irrigation of the area beneath the flap is advised so as to flush any and all debris. Closure of the flap then is accomplished with the same principles described in the removal of mandibular teeth, beginning with approximating known markers.

POSTOPERATIVE MANAGEMENT

It is important for patients to understand what to expect during the postoperative course. Unexpected events can hamper one's recovery. If adequate preoperative consultation appointments and informed consent are an integral part of the treatment planning, then the patient knows approximately what they will experience during the postoperative course.

Patients should expect moderate discomfort following surgical removal of impacted third molars and should be informed of such. In the authors' experience, recovery after removal of impacted mandibular third molars is far more complex than recovery from maxillary third molar surgery. Adequate analgesic medication should be prescribed, and if indicated, the proper use of antibiotics should be employed. Patients should also be informed of specific activities and foods that they should avoid. The postoperative period can be marred by many complications, the most notable of which are pain, infection, dry socket, slow healing, and the formation of bony splinters. Smoking should be discouraged completely, and preferably avoided, for as long as the socket remains open. Forceful spitting may dislodge the blood clot and disrupt healing, as can the use of straws. Patients should be instructed to avoid these practices. Ice application for the first 24–48 hours is highly encouraged as it minimizes swelling and pain. After three days, warm moist heat compresses can be used to aid in the resolution of soft tissue swelling, decreasing joint stiffness, and increasing jaw mobility. A diet comprised of cold and soft foods is preferable as long as the socket areas remain tender. Hot and spicy foods tend to irritate the surgical sites. Caution should be used to not consume foods that are extremely brittle or flaky as they may remain in the sockets—precipitating pain and slow healing. Careful rinsing with saline should be encouraged beginning the following day to ensure cleansing of the areas without aggressive mechanical irritation. A follow-up appointment should always be given for all impacted third molar surgery patients.

Management of Postoperative Complications

Many postoperative complications are avoided by performing careful surgery. Still, some occur, even with the most meticulous operators.

DAMAGE TO SOFT TISSUE

Soft tissue damage can take the form of a tear or puncture in the flap or an abrasion or laceration of the lip or mucosa during the course of the procedure. The reason for such injuries is usually excessive retraction of the flap. If one sees that the tissue is tensing and providing resistance, consideration should be given either to extending the flap or to making a releasing incision. Inadvertent tearing of a flap markedly increases postoperative pain and delays healing. Furthermore, parts of a torn flap are prone to necrosis.

Puncturing of flaps often results from inappropriately controlled forces caused by the slippage of an instrument. This can also predispose a patient to the issues noted previously. The careful use of instruments and the knowledge that these untoward events can happen will help in their prevention.

Placing one's fingers along the shank of an elevator, using finger rests when indicated, and having adequate jaw and facial support (with the operator's other hand or an assistant) all can aid in preventing such occurrences.

The lips and mucosa can be iatrogenically harmed during the course of a surgical procedure. Retraction for a long period of time can cause splitting of the commisure of the lips. Heating of rotary instruments (the drill) can cause burns on the lips. Care must be taken to use a burguard and appropriately shield the soft tissue from the handpiece. These burns and/or abrasions must be treated palliatively with moisturizing ointments. Lacerations, if encountered, should be evaluated for the need of sutures. The typical healing period for such injuries is 5 to 10 days. In rare cases, such problems might require plastic surgical repair and should be referred to a specialist for evaluation and definitive treatment.

Pain and Swelling

Postoperative swelling is often expected with the surgical removal of third molars, particularly when the procedure requires soft tissue manipulation, bone removal, and a significant amount of time. Swelling is generally noted to worsen through the second day after the procedure and typically begins to subside soon after. Persistent or increasing swelling beyond three days warrants a re-evaluation.

Patients often encounter some degree of pain or discomfort after these procedures. Generally, they will require approximately two to three days of narcotic analgesic medication followed by a brief course of over-the-counter analgesics. It may be a good idea to prescribe nonsteroidal anti-inflammatory medications like ibuprofen since they decrease inflammation and provide analgesia—thereby decreasing narcotic use and potential abuse. Severe pain persisting beyond the first few days that begins to worsen after initial improvement needs reexamination by the practitioner.

Infection

Dentoalveolar procedures are usually not marred by postoperative infections, but whenever soft tissue flaps are elevated or bone is removed, the susceptibility to infection increases. The prudent practitioner will try to incorporate practices that will help minimize such risks. These steps include care not to tear a flap, thorough irrigation when removing bone with a drill, and copious irrigation prior to closure of the soft tissue.

Infections are rare within the first two days but might present after the third or fourth day. Persistent or worsening edema, erythema, increasing tenderness, and onset of trismus are signs that warrant investigation. These signs may also present as part of the normal healing process so differentiating between the two is essential to prevent a poor outcome. Fever, chills, and worsening trismus with dysphagia/odynophagia often signify potentially serious infection and require immediate evaluation.

The use of prophylactic antibiotic treatment or preoperative antibiotic mouth rinses is a highly debated topic. Opinions vary, and results of studies echo these varying opinions.

The offending microorganisms in dentoalveolar infections are usually a mixed oral flora with streptococci predominating. Unless a contraindication exists, empirical treatment of oral infections with an oral antibiotic (Pen VK or amoxicillin—clindamycin if allergic to penicillins) should be initiated and continued for one full week. If the swelling presents with a fluctuant character, incision and drainage with placement of drains should be considered with concomitant administration of antibiotics. These patients should be observed closely and frequently to ensure resolution. Referral to a specialist is indicated if the infection worsens or does not respond to usual treatment.

Alveolar Osteitis (Dry Socket)

The phenomenon of alveolar osteitis, otherwise known as dry socket, has been attributed to multiple factors including smoking, difficulty of extraction, bacterial contamination, birth control pills, and aberrant host healing. These predisposing factors may or may not be present. In any given case, it is difficult to determine the cause. Simple extractions can also suffer from alveolar osteitis.

The exact pathophysiology of dry socket is not known, but numerous theories have been given. Patients often present after the third or fourth postoperative day has passed and complain of sudden, progressively worsening of pain in the affected area. A characteristic mal-odor may be accompanied by a foul taste. There is an absence of fever, edema, erythema, or lymphadenopathy.

Examination of the socket yields an open socket with no clot present, with the area being extremely tender.

The treatment of alveolar osteitis is aimed at establishing the comfort of the patient. The process is self-limiting and must run its course. Pain relief often requires careful irrigation of the socket with saline an obtundant dressing inside the socket, and the short-term use of a narcotic analgesic. A number of commercially available obtundant preparations exist for these situations. These preparations usually contain a combination of anesthetic, eugenol, and balsam of pine or balsam peru. Other commercial variants exist, and their ingredients should be checked and used accordingly. A small strip of gauze conservatively covered with one of these preparations should be placed inside the affected socket. The act of placement can be painful, but relief sets in within minutes.

Patients treated for these symptoms should be seen 24 to 48 hours later for removal of the packing. Replacing the dressing is often the prudent choice for most patients. Many patients require two to three packings before experiencing complete relief.

BLEEDING

Some postoperative bleeding may be expected for up to 72 hours after a surgical procedure. This takes the form of "oozing" rather than pulsatile bleeding. Pulsatile bleeding warrants an evaluation in an emergency setting. Oozing beyond 72 hours may not be a benign finding, rather, it may be a sign of an underlying coagulopathy. If local measures are not successful, a medical and hematological work-up may be indicated.

Local measures to control bleeding postoperatively are similar to those used intraoperatively. Intraoperative options include the use of direct pressure, sutures, local hemostatic agents like Gelfoam (absorbable gelatin sponge), Surgicel (regenerated oxidized cellulose), topical thrombin, and collagen. A figure-eight suture is usually placed for retention.

Direct pressure is the mainstay of controlling bleeding, regardless of location. Firm, direct, digital pressure or biting on moist gauze over the site will provide adequate hemostasis in the majority of cases. Bleeding that appears after a few days have transpired will still often respond to direct pressure with gauze or with a tea bag. The tannic acid in tea has been anecdotally noted to have success in providing hemostasis. The previously mentioned measures (Gelfoam etc.) are also at one's disposal, but care must be taken because to treat a socket with more than direct pressure will often require the administration of local anesthesia to ascertain the source.

If bleeding continues, the placement of sutures may be indicated. If the soft tissue is not firmly bound to the bone, this may be the cause of bleeding and will often respond well when reapproximated.

Patients with good general health will generally respond to such measures. If such minimal treatment does not reveal the source, referral for further medical or surgical treatment is indicated to avoid ongoing problems. Patients who have systemic medical issues that predispose bleeding or are taking medication that prevents adequate hemostasis may require surgical intervention.

DAMAGE TO TEETH AND/OR ADJACENT STRUCTURES

Third molar surgery presents the challenge of having the most limited accessibility of all extractions, hence raising the associated risk of damage to adjacent structures. Adjacent teeth are always at risk due to the nature of the luxating forces applied during instrumentation, and therefore, the careful use of applied force is mandatory. Examination of the adjacent teeth and opposing teeth should be done, noting those teeth with extensive caries, extensive restorations, and those with root canal therapy. Although all teeth are subject to these forces and may succumb, these characteristics increase their susceptibility. The patient should be made aware of this. Patients should be notified if a problem arises (that is, fractured adjacent tooth, crown coming loose, and so on), and steps should be taken to rectify it.

NERVE DYSFUNCTION

Although rare, inferior alveolar or lingual nerve dysfunction is one of the most devastating complications that can arise from the removal of a mandibular tooth. Most nerve injuries are usually preventable. Careful diagnosis, treatment planning, and sound surgical principles can be of paramount importance in preventing these injuries. The authors recommend that all patients undergoing surgical removal of impacted third molars should receive a follow-up appointment one week postoperatively. During this evaluation, nerve function should always be evaluated. If a sensory deficit exists, the area of deficit should be noted. Sensory deficits associated with the removal of teeth warrant evaluation by a specialist. Treatment and thorough evaluation of nerve injuries is beyond the scope of this text.

DISPLACEMENT OF TEETH OR ROOTS

Nothing is quite as unnerving to a practitioner as realizing that the tooth or fragment that is being extracted is no longer visible. In the mandible, third molar roots can displace into the submandibular space or into the inferior alveolar canal. Maxillary teeth or their roots can be displaced into the maxillary sinus, the infratemporal space, or the buccal space.

Mandibular teeth or their roots can be displaced through the lingual cortical plate into the submandibular space if there is a thin cortex and significant force. If such a situation is suspected, one should place an index finger along the lingual aspect of bone and attempt to locate the fragment. Oftentimes, compression from an apical position can propel the fragment back up and facilitate retrieval; otherwise a lingual dissection may be necessary. This procedure risks injury to the lingual nerve and has the potential for excessive bleeding from the floor of the mouth. In the authors' experience, this should only be attempted if the practitioner has significant surgical experience. Usually, a referral should be considered.

Displacement of a tooth, root, or fragment into the maxillary sinus is managed differently. Upon discovery of displacement, one should review the previous condition of the tooth. If the tooth was not infected and the fragment is relatively small, leaving the root in place can be considered if minimal attempts at recovery prove fruitless. Larger fragments or those with preexisting apical pathosis require removal. Radiographs should be attained to ascertain position. Thorough irrigation and suction will improve visibility. Irrigation and suction of the socket may flush the fragment out. The suction tip and trap should be checked to ensure this. The oroantral communication within the extraction socket should **never** be enlarged. If minimal exploration proves unsuccessful, access via a Caldwell-Luc procedure may be necessary. This procedure to access the maxillary sinus should be performed by a specialist.

If referral is necessary, the patient should be informed and be placed on **sinus precautions**: avoid smoking and using straws for drinking. Sneezing or nose blowing should be with the mouth open. An antibiotic like amoxicillin, clindamycin, or a comparable cephalosporin should be prescribed for approximately 10 days. Decongestants should also be prescribed along with nasal saline sprays to help maintain a patent sinus ostium.

Displacement into the infratemporal space is a situation that requires surgical retrieval and should be performed only by a specialist in a hospital setting. Specialized radiography and equipment is needed for this procedure.

Occasionally, a tooth or fragment might be lost down the posterior oropharynx. If noted, the patient should be placed mouthdown and encouraged to cough. Suction should be placed to facilitate recovery of the fragment. If unsuccessful at retrieval, either aspiration or swallowing of the fragment has occurred. If violent coughing or difficulty breathing is encountered, this likely indicates aspiration. EMS must be activated, and basic life support principles should be followed. If these signs do not develop, it is likely that the fragment was swallowed and will pass within two to four days. The standard of care is to refer the patient to an emergency room, where chest and abdominal radiographs can be performed.

Oroantral Communication

An oroantral communication describes a situation in which the integrity of the membrane lining of the maxillary sinus has been disrupted. This can be noticed during a procedure which requires immediate closure, or it can develop up to a few weeks postoperatively. Patients will complain of congestion, diffuse face pain on the affected side, and the sensation of liquid entering the nose while drinking.

If an oroantral communication is suspected upon removal of a maxillary molar, the practitioner should occlude the patient's nose and ask the patient to **gently** express air through the nose with his or her mouth open. With direct vision and a mouth mirror, one should look for air bubbles and/or condensation of the reflective surface of the mirror and also attempt to hear any passage of air. If a perforation is suspected, patients should be placed on sinus precautions and an antibiotic with sinus flora coverage (see the "Tooth Displacement" section). The

communication within the extraction socket should **never** be enlarged iatrogenically by instrumentation. Small perforations (<5 mm) generally heal by themselves in cooperative patients. Large perforations require surgical repair and are best referred to a specialist. Description of the surgical procedures for repair of oroantral communications are beyond the scope of this text.

Jaw Fracture

Jaw fractures, although uncommon, can complicate impacted third molar surgery. The clinician must be cognizant of the factors listed here, as these could predispose this unfortunate complication: difficult (deeply impacted teeth) extractions, older-age patients, atrophic jaws, systemic disease affecting bones (for example, osteoporosis), associated jaw pathology causing weakening of bone (for example, bone defect due to a cyst), and use of inappropriate surgical technique (excessive extraction force or extensive bone removal). With careful treatment planning and the execution of sound surgical techniques, the majority of jaw fractures can be prevented.

Dentists should be aware of the fact that after surgical bone removal, the defect remodels for a few weeks before final bone deposition starts to takes place. This initial remodeling includes osteoclastic cell activity—which further weakens bone for approximately four weeks after surgery. Thus, it is more common to see a jaw fracture in a postoperative patient at 2–4 weeks after surgery rather than immediately postsurgery. Patients at high risk for postoperative jaw fracture (for example, those patients requiring extensive bone removal) must be closely followed and should be instructed to stay on a full-liquid diet or, preferably, put in maxillomandibular fixation (wiring of jaws) to decrease the chance of a jaw fracture.

If a jaw fracture occurs during surgery, it must be recognized clinically and a baseline postoperative radiograph (panorex) taken. The patient should be informed of the occurrence and instructed to stay on a liquid diet with minimal jaw function. All patients with jaw fractures should be referred immediately to an oral and maxillofacial surgeon for definitive treatment. Antibiotics (penicillin or clindamycin) and chlorhexidine oral rinses should be prescribed.

Maxillary fractures are generally confined to alveolar process fractures and can usually be treated with splinting of segments with composite-wire splints, with or without maxillo-mandibular fixation. However, mandibular fractures most often extend into basal bone and may need more complex treatment.

Bibliography

1. A.F. Fielding, A.F. Douglas, and R.D. Whitley. Reasons for early removal of impacted third molars. *Clin Prev Dent* 3:19. 1981.
2. E.C. Hinds, and K.F. Frey. Hazards of retained third molars in older persons: report of 15 cases. *J Am Dent Assoc* 101:246. 1980.
3. R.A. Bruce, G.C. Frederickson, and G.S. Small. Age of patients and morbidity associated with mandibular third molar surgery. *J Am Dent Assoc* 101:240. 1980.
4. G.W. Pederson. *Oral Surgery*. Philadelphia, PA: W.B. Saunders Company. 1988.
5. L.J. Peterson. Principles of management if impacted teeth. In *Contemporary Oral and Maxillofacial Surgery*. L.J. Peterson (ed), 3rd edition, pp. 215-48. St. Louis: Mosby Year Book. 1998.
6. Amercian Association of Oral and Maxillofacial Surgeons. Position paper on impacted teeth. Chicago: AAOMS. 1983 and 1989.
7. K.R. Koerner. The removal of impacted third molars: principles and procedures. In *Basic Procedures in Oral Surgery. Dent Clin North Am*, pp. 255. Philadelphia, PA: W.B. Saunders Company. 1994.
8. H. Dymm. Management of impacted third molar teeth. In Atlas of minor oral surgery, pp. 80–92. Philadelphia, PA: W.B. Saunders Company.
9. A. Khanooja, and M.P. Powers. Surgical management of impacted teeth. In Oral and Maxillofacial Surgery (vol 1). R.J. Fonseca (ed), pp. 245–80. Philadelphia, PA: W.B. Saunders Company. 2000.
10. D. Nitzan, J.T. Keren, and Y. Marmary. Does an impacted tooth cause resorption of an adjacent one? *Oral Surg Oral Med Oral Pathol* 51: 221. 1981.
11. NIH Consensus Development Conference for removal of third molars. *J Oral Surg* 38: 235. 1980.
12. M.H. Amler. The age factor in human extraction wound healing. 35: 193. 1977.
13. K.R. Koerner. Clinical procedures for third molar surgery. St Louis, MO: PennWell Books. 1986.
14. T.P. Osborn, G. Frederickson, I.A. Small, et al. A prospective study of complications related to mandibular third molar surgery. *J Oral Maxillofac Surg* 43: 767. 1985.
15. J.E. Kiesselbach, and J.G. Chamberlain. Clinical and anatomic observations on the relationship of the lingual nerve to the mandibular third molar region. *J Oral Maxillofac Surg* 41:565. 1984.

Chapter 4

Pre-prosthetic Oral Surgery

Dr. Ruben Figueroa and Dr. Abhishek Mogre

Introduction

Patients who are partially or completely edentulous will have esthetic and biomechanical concerns that need to be addressed before prostheses can be fabricated. The rehabilitative goal of an edentulous patient is to restore oral function and facial form. Approximately 10 percent of the American population, including 35 percent of those above age 65, are edentulous, and millions are partially edentulous.

After the natural dentition is lost, the patient can have an alveolar ridge with irregularities, undercuts, scarring, and insertion of perioral muscles that interfere with the stability of the prosthesis. Changes in the soft tissues are related to the degree of underlying jaw atrophy. Subsequent to extractions, nature steps in to begin the process of alveolar ridge resorption. This process is rapid following extractions and then slows down to achieve a balance between osteoblastic and osteoclastic activity. Over a period of years, patients often end up with an edentulous bony ridge that lacks adequate prosthetic support. Immediate and late consequences of edentulism require a careful evaluation of the intraoral supporting structures in order to

provide proper rehabilitation and to minimize the ongoing process of bone loss.

Irregular alveolar ridges, undercuts, tori, large maxillary tuberosities, and shallow vestibules are some of the problems that can interfere with dental prosthetic rehabilitation. This chapter covers surgical techniques to solve some of these problems.

Patient Evaluation

The patient evaluation is the most important aspect of treatment. Before any surgical or prosthetic procedures are performed, it is important to evaluate the patient's overall situation.

The evaluation begins by obtaining a detailed understanding of the patient's medical and dental history (including any previous success or failure associated with dental treatment) and a thorough physical examination of the patient. During this initial evaluation, it is important to obtain a clear picture of the patient's chief complaint and his or her expectations in order to determine whether you can meet those expectations. The medical history should provide information on the presence of any risk factors for surgery including medical conditions that might affect bone or soft tissue healing.

The extraoral examination should include an assessment of any facial deformities, such as previous trauma or surgeries, that might affect treatment. The intraoral examination includes an assessment of remaining teeth, bone, and soft tissue covering denture-bearing areas, muscle attachments, jaw relations, and the presence of soft tissue or bony pathology.

INTRAORAL EXAMINATION

An intraoral examination of osseous structures includes visual inspection, palpation, and radiographic examination, as well as looking at stone models of the mouth. During the visual inspection, an assessment of ridge contours, height, undercuts, and muscle attachments as well as soft tissue health is determined. Palpation of the denture-bearing areas might reveal sharp bony areas that need surgical correction. A radiographic examination is necessary in the diagnosis of any underlying bony pathology. Retained roots along with radiolucent and/or radiopaque lesions have to be identified and differentially diagnosed in order to plan appropriate treatment. Retained roots that are embedded in the bone, but asymptomatic, are usually left untouched. Attempts to remove them are usually only partially successful, and the bony defect left behind can be more problematic for denture retention and comfort than simply leaving them alone. However, patients should be informed of the presence of roots and the rationale of not removing them surgically.

Maxilla

The maxillary denture-bearing area is evaluated for undercuts or bony protuberances on the buccal and palatal sides. Of particular interest are palatal tori and tuberosity hypertrophy. Any areas that interfere with the insertion of the maxillary denture should be corrected surgically. It is important to evaluate posterior tuberosity notching for its importance in denture stability and posterior seal.

Mandible

The mandibular ridge is evaluated for ridge form and contour, irregularities, buccal exostoses, and tori (see Figures 4.1 and 4.2). Be careful when examining severe mandibular bone resorption since in these cases the ridge cannot be assessed by visual inspection alone. Muscle attachments as well as a lack of vestibule may obscure the actual underlying bone anatomy. Using palpation, one

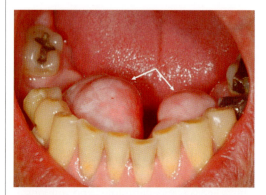

Figure 4-1. The arrows are showing massive mandibular tori. Tori are found bilaterally on the lingual side in the premolar canine area.

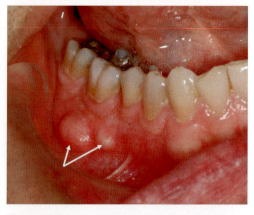

Figure 4-2. The arrows are pointing towards bony exostoses. Exostoses are usually found buccally, in contrast to tori, which are located lingually.

should palpate and identify the mental foramen and the mental neurovascular bundle, especially if it is located on the superior aspect of the mandibular ridge, since this situation is prone to neurosensory disturbances.

Maxilla/Mandible Relationship

The relationship between the arches is extremely important. During examination, anteroposterior and vertical relationships along with the possibility of any skeletal asymmetry should be evaluated. This evaluation must be done with the patient in a normal resting position. Overclosure of the mandible might give the impression of a pseudo Class III malocclusion. Lateral cephalometric radiographs with the patient closing down in a normal position are helpful to determine anteroposterior relationships of the jaws. Interarch distance, particularly in the posterior area, should be carefully evaluated. In addition, any amount of vertical excess in the tuberosity region, either bony or soft tissue, might impinge on the space necessary for the placement of dentures.

Soft Tissue Importance

Soft tissue covering the denture-bearing area needs to be carefully evaluated. The health and quality of soft tissue is one of the most important determinants of success with complete dentures. Ideally, there should be healthy keratinized tissue, which is firmly attached to the underlying bone. The presence of any hypermobile, fibrous tissue is inadequate for providing a stable denture-bearing area (see Figure 4.3).

The vestibular area should be free of inflammation secondary to an existing or previous ill-fitting denture. Tissues at the depth of the vestibule should lack any irregularities in order to provide maximal peripheral seal. The vestibular assessment should include an evaluation of muscle attachments. Muscle attachments that come onto the bony ridge might

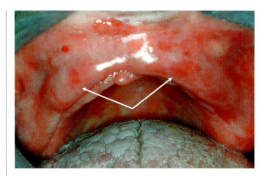

Figure 4-3. The arrows are showing hyperplastic tissue over the maxillary ridge. This tissue will make the denture base unstable.

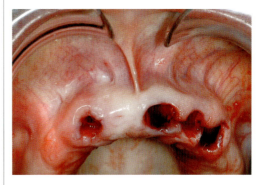

Figure 4-4. A labial frenum extending toward the alveolar crest, thus interfering with buccal flange extension.

interfere with denture retention due to the loss of peripheral seal during speech and mastication (see Figure 4.4). The linguovestibular area of the mandible should be inspected to determine the location of mylohyoid muscle and genioglossus muscle attachments in relation to the crest of the ridge. The myohyoid and genioglossus muscles will elevate during tongue movement, so if their attachments are high, they will cause movement and displacement of the lower denture.

Treatment Planning

After recording the medical/dental history and completing the physical examination, a treatment plan should be formulated. This will always precede any surgical intervention.

Benefits and possible complications of the surgery should be discussed with the patient. Alternative treatments, such as implant-supported dentures, should be presented when indicated. Surgical procedures involving bone contouring or augmentation should be addressed first, followed by soft tissue procedures.

The following surgical procedures will be presented in this chapter:

- Immediate dentures
- Alveoplasty
- Maxillary tuberosity reduction
- Maxillary torus
- Mandibular tori
- Epulus fissuratum
- Papillary hyperplasia
- Vestibuloplasty
- Labial frenectomy
- Lingual frenectomy
- Palatal graft
- Ridge augmentation

Armamentarium

The following is a list of basic surgical instruments needed to perform pre-prosthetic surgery.

- #15 and #11 surgical blades
- Bard Parker scalpel handle
- Molt periosteal elevator
- Seldin retractor
- Tissue forceps (pickups)
- Chisel and mallet
- Blumenthal bone rongeurs
- Straight fissure bur
- Large round or oval nongouging bur
- Dean scissors
- Needle holder
- Bone file
- Allis forcep

Immediate Dentures

Many patients can be treated with an immediate denture on the day of their extractions.

However, this procedure requires careful planning before performing extractions and insertion of the dentures. Inflamed and bleeding gingival tissue with heavy deposits of plaque and calculus are a definite predisposition for postoperative bleeding and infection. Patients with severe periodontal disease and inflammation of the gums should be treated by scaling and root planing before extractions.

In rare cases and with adequate planning, all remaining teeth can be extracted in one patient appointment, with the denture being inserted the same day. More commonly, it is recommended that complicated extractions (that is, posterior teeth) should be done and the ridges be allowed to heal before taking final impressions. Considerable alveolar ridge changes occur after such extractions that would affect retention and adaptability of the denture.

The sequence of extractions is an important aspect of overall treatment. Usually, mandibular and maxillary molars are removed first, leaving premolars for the assessment and maintenance of vertical dimension. About two months later, when fabrication of the immediate denture is complete, extraction of the remaining teeth is performed and the denture is inserted.

At the time of the extractions, contouring of the ridge can be done as planned on the patient's model. A clear surgical stent can be positioned to determine any pressure points that need further bone reduction. Care must be taken not to pull sutures too tightly.

Following surgery, pain medication should be prescribed. Antibiotics are usually unnecessary unless there is evidence of infection or if the patient has other medical indications. The patient is instructed not to remove the denture(s) until follow-up the next day. During this next-day appointment, the dentist will remove and clean the dentures and perform any needed denture adjustments. Sutures should be removed in five to seven days.

PRE-PROSTHETIC ORAL SURGERY   85

Table 4-1. Immediate Dentures Treatment Sequence

Steps	Notes
1. Prophylaxis prior to extractions	Minimize bleeding and infection probabilities
2. Complicated extractions	Bony changes may affect final impressions and denture fit
3. Extractions of maxillary and mandibular molars	After extractions allow six weeks for healing before making final impressions
4. Final impressions	
5. Model surgery	Remove teeth that are visible above the gingiva, contour gingival tissue, and remove undercuts
6. Construction of clear surgical stent	Will guide the surgeon during the procedure for alveolar contouring
7. Extraction of remaining teeth	Minimal alveolar contouring should be necessary
8. Denture insertion	Denture adjustments

ALVEOPLASTY

Alveoplasty is contouring of the alveolar ridge to remove any irregularities and undercuts. Most alveoplasties are performed on the maxilla and anterior mandible. The goals are to provide a stable base for the prosthesis and preserve as much alveolar bone as possible. Always be conservative when removing bone. Remember that if the patient desires to have implants in the future, every little bit of preserved bone counts.

Surgical Technique for an Alveoplasty in an Edentulous Patient

After adequate local anesthesia is obtained, a crestal incision is made over the area. A vertical release incision should be made when there is a risk of tearing the soft tissue flap. Be careful with anatomical structures such as the mental nerve and always maintain a wide-base flap. A thin ridge in the anterior mandible presents a challenge because it is possible to end up in the floor of the mouth.

Use a periosteal elevator to raise a full-thickness flap. Keep the pointed edge of the elevator against bone at all times to mini-mize tissue perforation. If a vertical release incision was made, start the reflection where it joins the crestal incision. Reflect the flap enough to identify the areas needing to be smoothed. When the full-thickness flap is reflected, use a Seldin or Minnesota retractor to retract and protect the flap.

Contouring of the bone is accomplished with a bone file, rongeurs, and/or round bur mounted on a slow-speed handpiece. Undercuts and sharp edges are eliminated, but the contouring does not have to be perfectly smooth. Frequently reposition the flap and try to feel the bone (with a gloved finger through soft tissue) for irregularities. Never perform digital palpation of the bone directly because some irregularities are minimal and will not be noticeable or significant enough to remove with the flap in position. Use the bone file for final contouring and smoothing of the bone. Before suturing, irrigate the area—especially at the bottom of the flap, where bone debris frequently accumulates. When the alveoplasty is finished, the flap is repositioned to its original position and sutured with interrupted or continuous sutures. Analgesics should be prescribed, but antibiotics are usually not necessary (see Figures 4.5A–B).

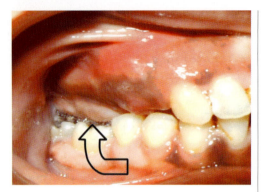

Figure 4-5A. The arrow in the picture shows a severe loss of inter-ridge distance. There is no space to restore the edentulous span.

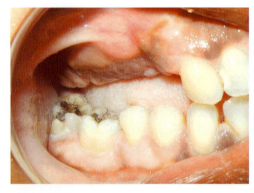

Figure 4-5B. Increased inter-ridge distance after alveoloplasty.

Maxillary Tuberosity Reduction

A maxillary tuberosity can increase in the vertical dimension, decreasing the vertical space between the maxilla and the mandible. The resultant problem is not having enough space for the denture base. To determine adequacy of the space, a dental mirror should be placed between the tuberosity and the ascending ramus of the mandible. If it fits and the patient is not uncomfortable with the pressure of the mirror in place, then there is enough space. A maxillary tuberosity could also have significant undercuts that would interfere with the path of denture insertion.

INDICATIONS

- Decreased intermaxillary space
- Decreased freeway space
- Severe undercut that interferes with denture fabrication steps (including impression techniques) and denture insertion
- Mobile soft tissue that interferes with denture stability

Presurgical radiographs should be taken. The ideal radiograph for this purpose is a panoramic film. This kind of film will show the proximity of the maxillary sinus and will help determine whether the enlargement is fibrous or bony in nature. Usually a communication with the maxillary sinus during surgery is of no consequence because primary soft tissue closure is easy to obtain.

FIBROUS TUBEROSITY

The objective of the correction of a fibrous enlargement is to surgically reduce the enlarged tuberosity and create enough vertical space for the denture. Wedge resection is the technique of choice. After the area is properly anesthetized, an elliptical incision is made down to the bone with a #15 scalpel blade. Wedge incisions should start on the crest of the ridge at the junction of the normal ridge with the fibrous tissue. The incisions extend posteriorly toward the hamular notch, removing one third of the bulbous mass. The wedge of tissue is grasped with an Allis forceps and freed from the cortical bone with sharp and blunt dissection. When the wedge is removed, the operator proceeds with the submucous lateral resections with a #15 blade. Submucous cuts are made parallel to the bony surface on either side, being careful not to perforate the flaps. The buccal and palatal flaps are repositioned and trimmed until they meet without overlapping and with no tension. When removing tissue, always preserve the vestibule and attached gingiva. Close with continuous 3.0

PRE-PROSTHETIC ORAL SURGERY

sutures. Prescribe analgesics as needed, but antibiotics are usually not necessary.

BONY TUBEROSITY

With a #15 blade, a single crestal incision is made starting at the hamular notch and coming forward to 10 mm beyond the intended area of reduction. At the anterior end of the crestal incision a vertical release incision is made. The angle of the release incision should be approximately 135° to the crest to provide a wide-based flap. This full-thickness flap is reflected with a periosteal elevator—remembering to keep the pointed edge against bone. In areas of an undercut, care should be taken not to perforate the flap. Reflect enough to expose the bone area to be removed. Use a Seldin or similar retractor to reflect and protect the flap. Contouring of the bone can be performed with a side-cutting roungeur or a large oval bur (such as a bone bur, available through companies like Brasseler). After the cortical bone is removed, be careful with the underlying medullary bone since it is softer. Lack of caution could lead to a postoperative defect. Reposition the flap to visualize the result and evaluate the area. Finish contouring with a bone file and irrigate with normal saline. Any excess tissue can be trimmed away with scissors. Be careful to preserve the vestibule and hamular notch, which are important for denture retention.

If you have a communication with the maxillary sinus, irrigate the area well and then suture without tension. The patient should be informed of the communication and instructed not to blow his or her nose, sneeze, or cough unless the mouth is open. Antibiotics (Amoxicillin 500 mg tid for seven days) and a nasal decongestant should be prescribed.

Maxillary Torus

A maxillary torus consists of a sessile mass of cortical bone in the middle of the palate.

Most often, maxillary tori do not need surgical removal. Satisfactory dentures can be constructed over most of them. However, there are some situations where their removal is indicated:

- Constant trauma
- When they prevent a good postdam seal or have large undercuts that interfere with impression techniques
- Speech impediment
- Psychological phobia

A radiographic evaluation should be performed in order to determine the proximity of the nasal cavity and the maxillary sinus. Lateral radiographs will generally supply this information. One of the possible complications of this procedure is the exposure of the nasal cavity, creating an oronasal communication.

TECHNIQUE

A maxillary impression is made, and a cast is poured. The torus is removed from the cast and a clear stent is made. The stent will protect the area, prevent hematoma formation, and provide postoperative comfort to the patient. The authors recommend using the stent, even though some surgeons do not consider it essential.

Local anesthesia with a vasoconstrictor is administered for the greater palatine and the nasopalatine nerves. Infiltration is suggested around and into the torus to facilitate elevation of the thin mucoperiosteum. Allow enough time for the anesthesia and vasoconstrictor to work.

A #15 blade is used to make an incision in the form of a Y in order to expose the bone of the torus. Reflection of the flap is performed with a periosteal elevator—being careful not to tear the extremely thin mucosa. The flap is then held open with 3-0 silk sutures.

After the entire torus is exposed, it is

scored (depth cuts) with a fissure bur in a crisscross pattern, using copious irrigation. The depth of the cuts should be approximately 1.0 to 2.0 mm down from the level of the horizontal palatal shelf (toward the oral cavity). After the cutting pattern has been established, a chisel and a mallet are used to remove the individual segments. (If the operator is uncomfortable using the chisel/mallet method, a bur can be used.) Stay superficial in order to avoid perforation into the nasal cavity. The final smoothing of the bone is accomplished with a large oval bur and copious irrigation. There is no need to remove the entire torus. The area is irrigated and sutured with 3.0 silk or chromic gut using interrupted sutures. The stent is tested intraorally, and if unstable, it can be relined with soft tissue relining material. The stent can be made from thermoplastic material with a vacu-form device, or alternatively, an acrylic stent may be fabricated by a lab.

The stent is retained for 48 hours, after which it is removed by the surgeon in order to clean and inspect the surgical area. It can be worn during the healing period of approximately two weeks, but after the first 48 hours, the stent should be removed after each meal for cleansing.

It is not unusual for the palatal flap to slough off. This is not a problem, and granulation tissue will eventually cover the defect with secondary epithelialization (see Figures 4.6A–J).

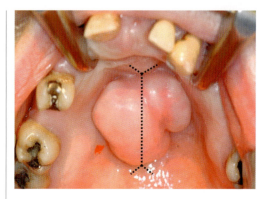

Figure 4-6B. This picture shows an outline of a surgical incision for torus removal. The incision is placed over the torus and extended beyond its anterior/posterior borders. The typical incision appears like two Ys joined in the midline.

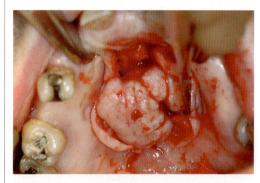

Figure 4-6C. Flaps are reflected and the torus is exposed.

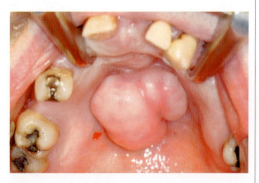

Figure 4-6A. A palatal torus that interferes with fabrication of a maxillary denture.

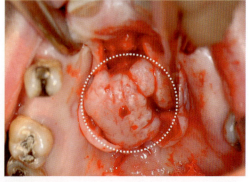

Figure 4-6D. The bony torus is outlined in the above picture.

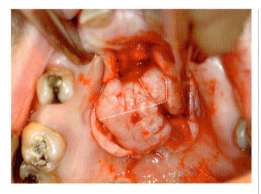

Figure 4-6E. Tori are surgically removed in small segments. An attempt to remove a palatal torus in one piece could lead to a perforation into the nasal cavity. The outline shows the surgeon's choice of sectioning the torus before its removal.

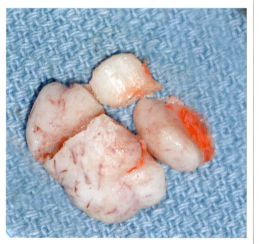

Figure 4-6F. The excised bony torus is shown.

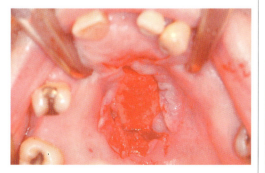

Figure 4-6G. Tori can be removed using hand instruments, rotary instruments, or both. The picture shows the appearance of the site after surgery. It is not necessary to completely remove the bony growth. The extent of removal can be assessed by frequent closing of the flaps and feeling the area for sharp edges of bone.

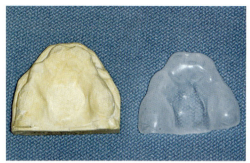

Figure 4-6H. Surgical templates can be used to create pressure for hemostasis and provide a method of delivering soft tissue liners as a surgical dressing. In this case, since the patient was also scheduled for full arch extractions, a complete upper clear surgical template was fabricated. An immediate denture could also have been used.

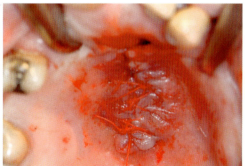

Figure 4-6I. Flaps are then closed with sutures.

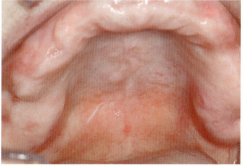

Figure 4-6J. This eight weeks postoperative picture shows healthy mucosa and excellent healing.

Mandibular Tori

Mandibular tori are usually bilateral and located on the lingual aspect of the mandible. They are normally found in the premolar and molar area. Before construction of a mandibular removable denture, they frequently need to be removed. The mucosa covering them is thin and prone to irritation and ulceration.

TECHNIQUE

Local anesthesia consists of inferior alveolar nerve blocks and infiltration subperiosteally over the torus (which helps with dissection). An incision is made along the crest of the ridge, extending the equivalent of two teeth beyond the torus on each end. In dentate patients, the incision is placed in the lingual gingival sulcus. Release incisions are usually not necessary.

With extreme care, a full-thickness envelope flap is raised. Because the mucosa is thin, perforation of the flap can easily occur, with the consequence of delayed and painful postoperative healing. The flap is extended below the torus enough to place a Seldin retractor, which will protect the area while the torus is being removed. With a fissure bur, create a groove on the superior margin of the torus where the torus meets the mandible. The depth of the groove is approximately halfway through the vertical dimension of the torus. If the torus is large, create some additional vertical cuts to help facilitate removal. A monobevel chisel is then placed into the groove that was created with the angle facing the mandible. While the chin is being supported manually, the chisel is tapped with the mallet. Alternatively, the initial bur cut can be extended all the way through the vertical dimension of the torus, following which it can be removed with a needle holder. After the torus is removed, its surface is smoothed with a bone file or a large, round nongouging bur. At all times protect the flap with the retractor.

The surgical area is irrigated with normal saline. Close with either interrupted or continuous 3-0 silk or Vicryl sutures. Using moist gauze, the operator can place digital pressure on the flap for a few minutes to help initiate fibrin adhesion and prevent subsequent hematoma formation.

Even when careful, postoperative bleeding with hematoma formation is a possible complication. Bleeding in the floor of the mouth could pose a threat to the airway (see Figures 4.7A–D).

Ridge Augmentation with Hydroxyapatite (HA)

The basic concept behind using particulate hydroxyapatite (HA) for bone augmentation is that HA is a dense nonresorbable material that seems to show negligible foreign body reaction. It is placed subperiosteally by a special technique called subperiosteal tunneling. There is evidence that during the healing process, bone forms around particles of HA that are in contact with alveolar bone. Remaining, more internal HA particles are densely suspended in a connective tissue matrix that does have some vascularization. The amount of bone augmentation depends on how careful the operator is to minimally stretch and tunnel the periosteum. The disadvantage of this technique includes particle escape and movement and a lack of adequate density as compared to autogenous bone grafts.

Epulis Fissuratum

Epulis fissuratum is a hyperplastic growth of the mucosa secondary to denture irritation. This constant irritation eventually develops submucosal fibrosis. This condition interferes with denture stability and comfort. Patients usually see great benefit from surgical treatment. However, before surgery either the patient should discontinue wearing the denture for two weeks or the dentist should relieve the denture in the area(s) of irritation.

PRE-PROSTHETIC ORAL SURGERY 91

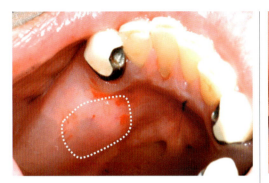

Figure 4-7A. Outline of a mandibular torus. Mandibular tori can create undercuts, thereby making denture fabricaton and insertion cumbersome. The mucosa covering the torus is thin and prone to pressure ulceration from dentures.

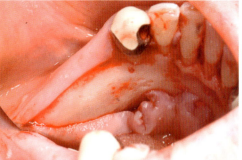

Figure 4-7C. The torus is removed and the surface smoothed. Smoothness can be checked by replacing the flaps and then feeling for rough bony areas.

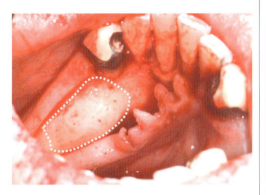

Figure 4-7B. Mandibular torus after surgical exposure. An incision was made over the crest of the ridge, extending the equivalent of two teeth beyond the torus on each end.

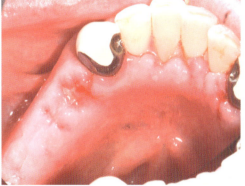

Figure 4-7D. This postsurgical result shows a great improvement in the shape of the mandibular ridge and absence of any undercuts.

As a result of this chronic irritation, there is often also a loss of underlying bone. If there is significant bone loss after removal of the epulis, the patient might not have an appropriate vestibular depth, and retention of the denture could be compromised. During the evaluation appointment, the patient should be informed of this possibility.

SURGICAL TECHNIQUE

Local anesthesia with vasoconstrictor should be used. If excessive infiltration is done, the anatomy of the epilis fissuratum will be distorted. Identify the epulis and use as many Allis forceps as necessary to grasp the tumor-like growths. The surgeon holds the forceps, and the assistant retracts the lip to ensure that the lip muscles are not excised. The superior border of the epulis is incised first with a #15 blade, electrosurgery, or laser. The epulis is raised by the surgeon, and then the inferior cut is made. Both incisions are made superficial to the periosteum. The entire mass is removed. It is important to retain as much healthy attached mucosa as possible. Bleeding points are controlled with electrocautery or laser. The removed tissue should be sent for histopathologic examination.

Primary closure is not necessary in all cases, and it should be avoided whenever possible. Primary closure tends to roll the lip inward, decreasing the amount of vermillion that shows. The denture should be trimmed as needed and lined with soft tissue reline material after surgery. This dressing should be removed in 48 hours and the denture cleaned. The denture can be relined again if necessary. It takes about six weeks for complete healing—after which the denture can be remade or relined. Pain medication should be prescribed, and antibiotics are usually not needed.

Papillary Hyperplasia

Papillary hyperplasia or denture stomatitis is generally secondary to ill-fitting dentures. Other factors that contribute to this condition are poor oral hygiene, fungal infections, and around-the-clock denture use.

This condition is not premalignant but inflammatory in nature, and total full-thickness removal of the mucosa is not needed. Before performing invasive surgical treatment, the maxillary denture should have a soft reline, and the patient should be instructed not to wear the denture at night. Suspected candidiasis should be treated with appropriate antifungal agents. If this conservative therapy is not successful, surgical therapy should be considered.

Surgical Technique

Local anesthesia with vasoconstrictor is used to block the greater palatine and nasopalatine nerves. A biopsy specimen should be taken, avoiding the area of the greater palatine vessels. Removal of the hyperplastic tissue can be accomplished with an antral curette. Scraping of the tissue is performed until the dense white tissue (corium) below the epithelium is exposed.

Electrocautery with a loop electrode can also be use for the removal of the hyperplas-

tic tissue. Care should be taken not to burn the perioral tissues. Always leave the periosteum intact. Mucoabrasion with a large, nongouging round bur mounted on a slow-speed handpiece could also be used. Irrigation should be performed when using the handpiece/bur technique.

Laser surgery is perhaps the most ideal technique to use for removing this hyperplastic tissue. As it removes redundant tissue, it coagulates the blood at the same time. Adjacent areas should be covered with moist sponges for protection.

Following excision, the denture should be relined with a soft material (for example, Coe-Comfort) for hemostasis and to prevent discomfort. Healing by secondary epithelization is usually completed within three to five weeks. Pain medication is recommended, but antibiotics are usually not needed.

Vestibuloplasty

The goal of a vestibuloplasty is to remove unwanted muscle insertions into the alveolar ridge. This is done by exposing bone at the place where these muscles formerly attached. The vestibuloplasty surgical technique requires an adequate amount (height) of alveolar bone. The basic problem here is usually not the lack of bone but rather that the shallow vestibule prevents the denture flange from extending to provide adequate stability and retention. If the patient does not have enough bone height, then a ridge augmentation procedure might need to be done before the vestibuloplasty.

During the presurgical evaluation it is important to evaluate the proximity of anatomical structures such as nerves and the location of muscle insertions. A panoramic radiograph will help to evaluate the bone height and identify structures such as the mental foramen.

Nerve blocks and infiltration should be used to obtain profound anesthesia and hemostasis. The incision is placed at the junction of attached and unattached mucosa with a #15 blade. A partial-thickness flap is raised with the blade or Dean scissors, preserving the periosteum. Any muscle fibers attached to the periosteum should be removed. Small perforations of the periosteum will not cause major problems but should be avoided. The mucosal edge is sutured to the bottom of the dissected area.

The resulting denuded periosteum may be handled in different ways. If the operator decides to let it heal by secondary intention, the relapse rate is about 50 percent. Another method is to graft the area with palatal mucosa, a collagen membrane, or cadaveric mucosal membrane. Grafts should be perforated with the tip of a #11 blade after suturing in order to prevent blood clots from forming between the graft and the periosteum. Light pressure on a graft is desirable in order to prevent blood clot formation, and also to immobilize the graft. This can be accomplished with the patient's denture after it has been relieved and a soft tissue relining material placed inside. One should be careful that the soft tissue relining material does not get lodged under the graft. Another alternative would be the use of a soft clear splint kept in place with two titanium screws. Screws are simple to place and to remove. The denture or splint should not be removed for a week.

When the splint is removed, the grafted tissue will look white and avascular. This is normal. It usually means that the superficial layer of the graft has been lost, but one should not worry because the rest of the graft will be vital. Angiogenesis into the graft occurs within 48 hours, and healing takes up to 5–6 weeks (see Figures 4.8A–F).

Labial Frenectomy

Frenal attachments consist of thin bands of fibrous tissue attached to the bone. If the frenum is close to the crest of the alveolar

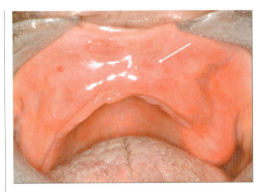

Figure 4-8A. The arrow is pointing towards unattached alveolar mucosa and a shallow labial vestibule. These conditions affect denture stability and retention.

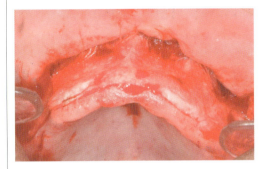

Figure 4-8B. The recipient site is prepared with a partial-thickness flap. The periosteum is preserved, but any muscle or fatty tissue is removed in order to have a nonmovable graft after healing.

ridge, it can interfere with the extension of the denture flange and, consequently, with retention and comfort.

Surgical Technique

Three surgical techniques are effective in removing labial frenal attachments. Simple excision and Z-plasty techniques are effective when the mucosal and fibrous band is relatively narrow. When the frenal attachment has a wide base, a localized vestibuloplasty with secondary epithelialization is preferred.

Local anesthesia with a vasoconstrictor is infiltrated. Avoid injecting excessive anesthetic solution because it might obscure the

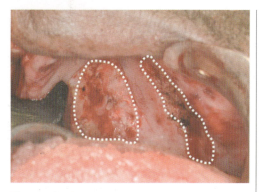

Figure 4-8C. Outlined areas represent a palatal graft donor site.

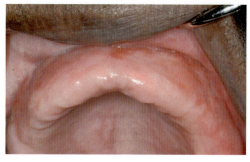

Figure 4-8F. Three months postsurgical picture showing excellent vestibular depth and healthy keratinized tissue.

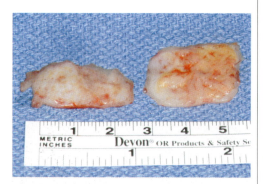

Figure 4-8D. Palatal grafts of the required size are obtained from the donor site. Yellowish areas in the graft represent fatty tissue, which should be removed before adapting the grafts to the recipient site.

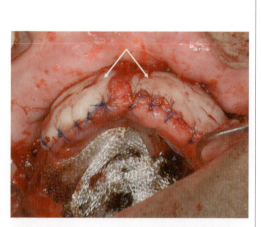

Figure 4-8E. The arrows are showing palatal grafts sutured in place. There is a corresponding increased depth of the labial vestibule.

anatomy. It is convenient to have an assistant to elevate and evert the lip.

For the simple excision technique, a narrow elliptical incision is done around the frenum down to the periosteum. The frenum is removed with sharp and blunt dissection from the underlying periosteum and soft tissue. The margins of the incision are undermined with Dean scissors. The first suture is placed at the maximum depth of the vestibule including both edges of the mucosa and the underlying periosteum. This suture, called an **anchor** suture, will maximize the depth of the vestibule. The remainder of the incision should be sutured with interrupted sutures. Sometimes, part of the wound cannot be closed primarily and is left to granulate secondarily (see Figures 4.9A and 4.9B).

For the Z-plasty technique, the lip is everted to expose the frenum, and with a #15 blade, an incision is made along the frenum. At each end of the incision, two small incisions are made in a Z fashion. The two flaps are undermined and rotated to close the original vertical incision in a horizontal manner. This technique minimizes the amount of vestibular ablation as seen after the previously described simple technique (see Figures 4.10A–C).

The final method is the vestibuloplasty with secondary epithelialization. In cases

PRE-PROSTHETIC ORAL SURGERY   95

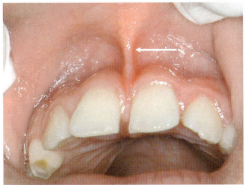

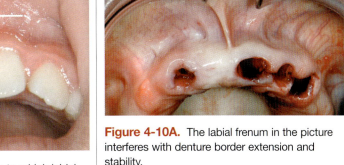

Figure 4-9A. The arrow points to a high labial frenum attachment in a child. Such freni can lead to development of a diastema between the central incisors.

Figure 4-10A. The labial frenum in the picture interferes with denture border extension and stability.

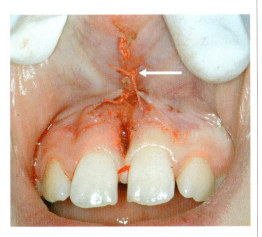

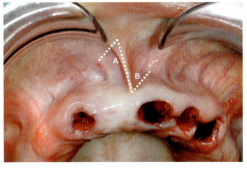

Figure 4-9B. The frenal attachment is corrected by simple excision technique. The arrow points to the part of the wound that was sutured. Below this area, sutures could not be placed because soft tissue could not be closed. It is left to heal by secondary intention. It is important to remove the fibrotic tissue between the centrals.

Figure 4-10B. The lines represent a Z-plasty technique. Areas marked as A and B indicate two flaps that will be surgically repositioned, thereby eliminating the frenum.

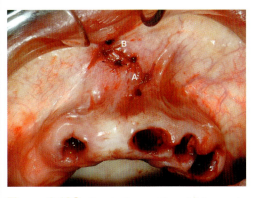

with a broad frenum attachment, a semi-lumar supraperiosteal incision is made at the junction of free and attached mucosa. The flap is undermined supaperiosteally and sutured to the periosteum, thus increasing the depth of the vestibule. Healing takes place by secondary epithelialization, and a denture with a soft liner is placed over it.

Figure 4-10C. Surgical correction of this prominent frenum attachment shows the dramatic improvement.

Lingual Frenectomy

Tongue-tie or ankyloglossia causes difficulty in denture construction due to the overextension of fibrous lingual attachments, which sometimes may be up to the crest of the ridge. They can also create difficulty in speaking.

SURGICAL TECHNIQUE

Local anesthetic with vasoconstrictor is used to infiltrate the area. A traction suture is placed through the tip of the tongue and then is used to stretch the tongue superiorly toward the palate. Bleeding can be minimized by clamping a hemostat at the base of the frenum for a few minutes before making a horizontal incision. Care should be taken to avoid injury to the submandibular gland ducts. As the incision is made, the tip of the tongue is simultaneously stretched to check the range of movement. The margins are undermined and are then sutured back with 3-0 chromic gut. The patient should be advised to not move the tongue very much during healing (see Figures 4.11A and 4.11B).

Palatal Graft

The hard palate is a useful donor site for grafting small defects in the oral cavity. It provides keratinized tissue around implant collars that lack attached gingival, for covering an area of vestibuloplasty (see previous), and to correct gingival recession.

SURGICAL TECHNIQUE

The area to be grafted should be prepared first. Measure the defect with a ruler or calipers to determine the size and shape of the graft or construct a template. A template can easily be made from the sterile cardboard in a suture envelope.

Local anesthesia is given at the donor site. Infiltration of local anesthetic with a vaso-

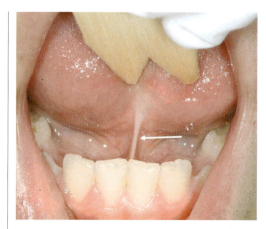

Figure 4-11A. An abnormal position of a lingual frenum close to the tip of the tongue can restrict its movement. The condition is called tongue-tie. The arrow is showing such a condition.

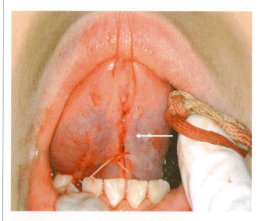

Figure 4-11B. The tongue is corrected surgically by a procedure called lingual frenectomy. The arrow shows an immediate postsurgical improvement in the range of tongue movement.

constrictor is preferred for hemostasis. It should be allowed to work at least 5–7 minutes before harvesting the graft. The ideal sites for the donor tissue are between the first premolar and the second molar. This area is free of anterior rugae and is thick enough to perform a partial-thickness flap procedure. The greater palatine artery runs closely attached to the periosteum above the second molar and should be avoided. To judge the depth of the incision, a #15 blade can be used and sunk to the depth of the bevel (1 mm). After outlining the incision, begin removing the graft from one of the anterior corners. If difficulty is encountered, one trick is to increase the depth of one of the anterior corners by 1 mm. Begin harvesting with a #15 blade, lifting the edge with Adson tissue pickup. Sharp dissection can be accomplished with a blade or Metzenbaum scissors. The graft is carefully dissected supraperiosteally away from underlying tissue and removed. The donor site is inspected for any bleeding, which can be controlled with electrocautery. Collagen may be placed to further control bleeding. If the patient wears a denture, soft tissue conditioner can be added to this area within the denture to increase pressure and provide hemostasis. If dissection has been performed without injury to the greater palatine artery, bleeding will be minimal.

Inspection of the graft is done, and any fatty and/or glandular tissue is removed with scissors. This is important for the nutrients to reach the graft from the host bed. The graft is adapted to the host site and sutured to snugly fit. Stability and adaptation of the graft are essential for success. The graft should have gentle pressure placed by pushing with a moist piece of gauze. This promotes graft adhesion to the recipient site and also helps prevent hematoma, which could lead to graft failure. After the graft is sutured, small stab incisions could be made with a #11 blade into the graft so as to allow drainage. Angiogenesis occurs within 48 hours, and complete healing takes up to five weeks (see Figures 4.8C–E).

Conclusion

Pre-prosthetics is an important part of oral and maxillofacial surgery. This chapter includes basic and simple pre-prosthetic surgeries that can be performed routinely—even by the general dentist. The purpose of the authors is to simplify the subject in a way that will provide greater confidence to the generalist wanting to perform these procedures.

Chapter 5

Conservative Surgical Crown Lengthening

Dr. George M. Bailey

Introduction

Crown lengthening procedures are an indispensable part of restorative dentistry, pocket maintenance, and enhanced oral esthetics. However, the surgical procedure itself is frequently avoided due to the perceived complex interplay between technique, tooth stability, and esthetics. Part of the problem is a slightly erroneous concept regarding the relationship between the tooth and soft tissue attachment. This chapter explores the clinical realities of that relationship, the indications for crown lengthening, the various surgical procedures that are available for crown lengthening, and specific surgical techniques.

Biologic Width

In order to develop conservative crown lengthening techniques, it is necessary to fully understand the relationship between the tooth and the soft tissue structures that support and protect it. The main rationale that answers the question "Why do crown lengthening?" lies in the term **biologic width**, a concept that is both clinical and histological.

The term biologic width was first introduced as "an epithelial attachment and the connective tissues which extend vertically from the bottom of the sulcus to the crest of the bone."[1] Additional findings indicated that there is a proportional relationship between the depth of the gingival sulcus, the epithelial attachment—now called the junctional epithelium (JE), the connective tissue fibers, and the crest of the alveolar bone around the tooth (see Figure 5.1).

This same study also measured this relationship, showing that in healthy gingiva, the sulcus is approximately 1 mm deep (obviously a **very** healthy environment), the JE is 1 mm, and the connective tissue overlying the alveolar bone is 1–2 mm in vertical thickness.[2] These studies have thus set the clinical basis for crown lengthening and suggest that there should be at minimum a 3-mm space between the restoration margin and the alveolar bone to accommodate the biologic width.

More recent findings by Vacek et al. basi-

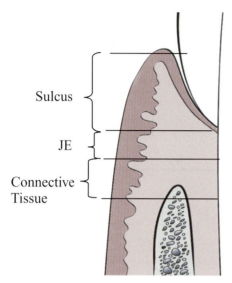

Figure 5-1. Normal relationship of the biologic width.

cally verified these original relationships but indicated a wider range of measurements and suggested to the clinician the importance of measuring these values for the individual patient rather than assuming that all measurements are the same.[3] The high variability of biologic structures from one patient to another must be kept uppermost in mind in treatment.

The author's clinical experience is that the connective tissue portion of the measurement overlying the bone is most often 2 mm or greater, with a sulcus depth in excess of 1 mm in a healthy site. Similar observations have led some to indicate that as much as 5.5 mm between the bony crest and the restorative margin/sound tooth structure must exist for proper restorative procedures (2 mm connective tissue, 1 mm junctional epithelium, 2 mm sulcus, and 0.5 mm for soft tissue rebound).[4]

It is this enhanced distance that is of concern for the clinical dentist since the issues of adequate tooth support and esthetics come into play. This distance ranging from a very conservative 3 mm to as much as 5.5 mm exposed root is a frequent deterrent to performing surgical crown lengthening. It is also important to remember that the term **biologic width** is as much a proportional relationship as it is just a vertical measurement. Additionally, biologic width appears to be a changing reality that is altered by the presence of inflammation, hormones, medications, tooth position, and age, just to name a few. It should be known that the original work was performed on human cadavers and not living patients.[5]

A clinical reality known to all in dentistry but seldom defined is that there is also a **horizontal** measurement to the biologic width. The chronic inflammation around an over-contoured crown with excessive labial-lingual dimensions, even though the vertical relationship of the biologic width is intact, is an all too common reminder of this principle. Figure 5.2 is a clinical example of a restoration that seemingly did not violate the vertical dimensions of the biologic width but is over-contoured on the labial, violating the horizontal dimensions and producing inflammation and spontaneous bleeding.[6]

A final note regarding biologic width concerns other terms that are commonly and interchangeably used to describe it. Although these are presented for the sake of linguistic accuracy, they do not have a tremendous negative clinical impact if used as synonyms (see Figure 5.3).

The foregoing was basically a discussion about average histological entities that are

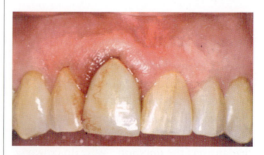

Figure 5-2. Inflammation when the **horizontal width** is violated.

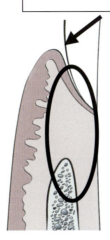

Figure 5-3. The dentogingival unit with junctional epithelium and gingival fibers.

determined by microscopic methods that are not readily available to clinical dentistry. It is important that the clinician use these measurements only as a guide and evaluate each clinical situation on its own realities.

A Treatment Plan for Surgical Crown Lengthening

Treatment planning for all procedures in dentistry follows similar steps leading up to the procedure itself. The process becomes nearly intuitive with the experienced practitioner. So much so that that person might need to pause and think if asked how the final decision was obtained, even though he or she probably used a step-by-step approach.

Table 5.1 indicates a typical process leading to a decision for surgical crown lengthening. It is meant as a directional guide only since each case has a myriad of modifying clinical factors. The individual elements with expanded information are presented in the following sections.

MEDICAL

Medical advances have sustained lives and in general improved the lives of our patients. However, determining the true medical status of the patient and the influence of medications on the body in general and the oral cavity in particular has become exceedingly complex. It is beyond the scope of this chapter to enter into the myriad possibilities of medications, medical conditions, and their influence on surgical crown lengthening procedures. Each practitioner should become knowledgeable in this area before any surgical procedure is undertaken. A localized surgical endeavor with a high degree of success can become disastrous if the body cannot heal properly.

ORAL CAVITY

As with all clinical determinations, the visual and tactile senses combine with experience to provide the most accurate diagnosis. Table 5.2 summarizes some of the common clini-

102   CHAPTER 5

Table 5-1. A Treatment Plan for Surgical Crown Lengthening

Data Collection

Medical—determination of influence of medical status/medications on crown lengthening. Potential of patient to successfully undergo surgery. Limitations imposed by medical conditions.

Oral—periodontal probings/sounding measurements, radiographic interpretations, notation of inflammation, amount of keratinized tissue, esthetic and structural concerns, and deviation from normal.

Diagnosis

A collation of all data into a statement of the problem (for example, subgingival decay 2 mm below the bony crest with insufficient space for the biologic width, which requires surgical crown lengthening before restorative procedures).

Presurgical Procedures

Consultation—presentation to the patient of the diagnosis; indicated corrective procedure(s); options, if any, and the pros and cons of each; explanation of the procedure; prognosis if performed; potential consequences if not; how procedure is performed; time requirements; postsurgical expectations; financial considerations; how the surgical procedure fits into the overall dental plan; and other items the patient needs to know and understand.

Debridement and Oral Hygiene—necessary cleaning procedures and oral hygiene techniques to reduce inflammation. Also includes proper use of antibiotics and other antimicrobials.

Informed Consent Form—serves as a legal document and as a review for the patient.

Surgical Procedures

Operatory Set Up—includes gathering necessary instruments, organizing clinical data, and creating a sterile surgical environment

Surgery—performing the actual surgical procedure, remembering always the goal of the technique.

Postsurgical

Immediate Postoperative—instructions to the patient on the care of the surgical site, dietary requirements, prescribing appropriate antibiotics and analgesics, and setting sequences for follow-up appointments.

Monitoring the Healing—when the patient is seen, what is done, and the time before restorative or other procedures can be accomplished is dependant on the type of surgery performed (for example, flap or gingivectomy, overall patient healing, and other factors).

Restorative Procedures

Determination of when restorative procedures can be effectively completed without negating the surgical result. Also applies to orthodontics.

---

cal methods for determining biologic width violations.

Periodontal Probings

Periodontal probings should be accomplished and recorded for not only the tooth/teeth in question but also the adjacent areas; particularly those that are healthy and can be used as comparative references. Notation from the probings should indicate pseudopockets, those with increased probings because of gingival enlargement versus a true pocket caused by inflammation. The preceding should also be differentiated from a true violation of the biologic width.

Table 5-2. Clinical Indications of Biologic Width Violations

Pain	Pain is frequently elicited upon gentle probing around a restoration margin.
Inflammation	Especially diagnostic when the surrounding areas are free of pathology.
Direct Measurement	Under local anesthetic, a periodontal probe is pushed vertically from the sulcus through the attachment tissues (JE and connective tissue) until the underlying bone is contacted. A measurement of 2 mm or less apical to the restoration margin/decay/fracture *may* indicate insufficient biologic width to maintain health, although there are many clinical variations. This process should be compared with similar measurements on adjacent healthy teeth.

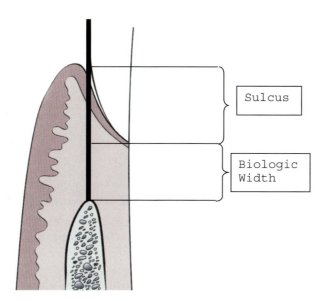

Figure 5-4. Sounding: the total sounding depth − suclus depth = biologic width.

Sounding

See Table 5.2 and Figure 5.4. Using a periodontal probe to determine the actual position of the bone remains **the** most accurate clinical method available. Once again, the total clinical probing depth (usually taken from the gingival margin to the alveolar bone) minus the pocket (sulcus) depth equals the vertical height of the biologic width. Local anesthetic is needed to provide adequate comfort for this procedure.

Although this technique actually perforates the sulcus and the underlying tissues, properly done there appears to be no sustained clinical damage. As with the general probings, adjacent healthy environments should be sounded and recorded as reference points.

An important addition to the preceding is a **horizontal** measurement of the associated gingival tissues. This measurement can be useful in determining whether excision of the tissue is indicated or an internal beveled flap with apical positioning is necessary. The periodontal probe is pushed horizontally through the gingival tissues until the tooth or the alveolar bone is encountered and then recorded. Similar horizontal measurements are made through surrounding healthy tissues. Since one of the objectives of crown lengthening is to produce tissues that are similar in horizontal thickness to those that are healthy, this is a particularly important measurement.

Radiographic Measurements

Radiographic evaluations are fairly accurate in determining interproximal bone levels and then, by extrapolation, adding in the vertical necessities for the biologic width. However, bone position on the labial and palatal aspects and possible biologic width violations in these areas are lost due to superimposition of oral structures (see figures 5.5 and 5.6).

Conventional periapicals/bite-wings should be taken via the paralleling technique to achieve the greatest accuracy. Use of a radiographic grid placed over a periapical x-ray before exposure can improve radiographic measurement accuracy[7] (see figure 5.7).

Digital radiographs have improved diagnostic interpretations since the image can be manipulated, magnified, and colorized to en-

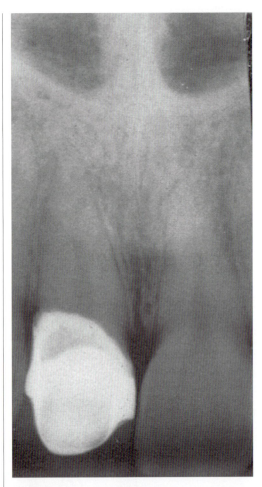

Figure 5-6. X-ray indicating violation of biologic width from extension of crown margin.

hance bone level identification; density determinations can be performed; reverse images can be created; subtraction radiographic images can be created; and so on. Digital radiography can greatly enhance the ability to determine bone/attachment relationships. As digital radiography technology advances, this may become a primary tool for bone location and its relationships with the overlying soft tissues (see Figure 5.8A–C).[8]

With both types of radiographs it is important to have x-rays of the surrounding areas with which to compare against the target area.

Radiographs can also be important in determining whether the lesion in a tooth is

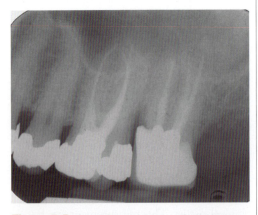

Figure 5-5. Paralleling technique. Periapical x-ray showing extension of decay into the biologic attachment area.

CONSERVATIVE SURGICAL CROWN LENGTHENING **105**

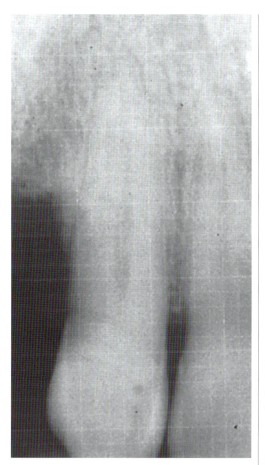

Figure 5-7. Use of measurement grid in a radiograph.

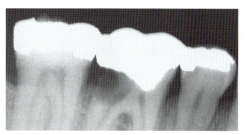

Figure 5-8A. Digital radiograph of a lower molar area.

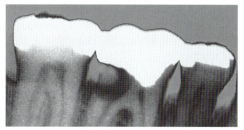

Figure 5-8B. Digital manipulation of the original radiograph, such as seen here with increased brightness and contrast, enables the operator to see another type of view. This can enhance clinical diagnostic capabilities

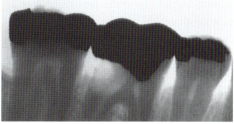

Figure 5-8C. Here is a digital radiograph with image reversal (positive view). This is especially good when looking at the alveolar crest of bone and furcations.

decay or resorption. The differentiation is important since stopping resorption is generally less predictable than stopping decay. This difference might lead to a treatment method other than trying to retain the tooth such as extraction and restorative tooth replacement (see Figures 5.9 and 5.10).

Subjective Considerations

An important part of data collection leading to a definitive diagnosis and treatment plan involves the motivations of the patient. Surgical procedures of all types produce wariness in our patients not commonly evident in routine dental procedures. An opinion should be formed **prior** to any surgery about the feelings of the patient relative to the surgical procedure itself.

Does the patient agree with the need for this procedure and/or want to have it performed? Can the patient emotionally undergo a surgical procedure? What is the perception of this patient's ability to tolerate pain? Are the patient's final outcome expectations realistic? What if these expectations

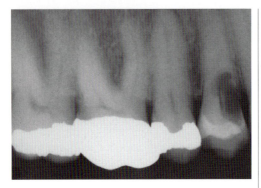

Figure 5-9. Radiographic evidence of resorption into the biologic width. X-ray shows relationship of resorption to the bony crest, shows endodontic involvement, and shows a low probability of restorability.

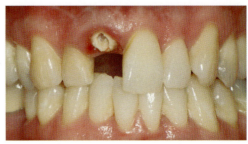

Figure 5-10A. Consider the consequences of crown lengthening in this case.

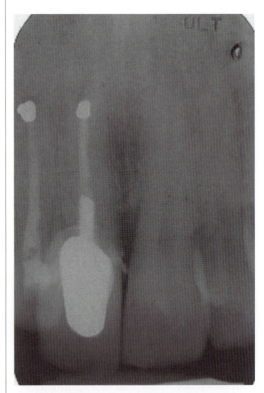

Figure 5-10B. Radiograph of tooth in 5-10A prior to fracture. There was decay around the post, a deep sliver of tooth (distal) came out with the crown, and the tooth is short from a previous apico. This tooth is not a good candidate for surgical crown lengthening.

are not met? Are there any phobias that might prohibit a successful surgical procedure such as needles, the sight of blood, and so on? Can the patient devote the requisite time for the procedure and the postoperative healing?

This is just a small sampling of questions that need to be answered before any surgery. It is important to have the patient with us not only medically but also emotionally. A positive attitude is a well-known necessity for all surgical procedures.

The Diagnosis

The importance of a definitive diagnosis can never be understated. The diagnosis embodies a mental organization of all the data collected and then put into a concise directed whole that includes the totality of one's education and experience. It should be considered **the** most important part of the treatment process since it is the director of technique and probable outcome. No amount of technical wizardly can compensate for an erroneous diagnosis.

The wife of one of my dental continuing education course participants once approached this author with some thoughts on the importance of the diagnostic process.

She (eminent and successful in her own field) was of the opinion that dentists were missing the point about the diagnostic procedure. She wondered why there was a tendency in dentistry to monetarily give away the diagnosis and charge so much for the technical procedure. In her field, the opinion (diagnosis) represented the totality and expertise that only she could give—thus, the diagnosis was more important than the actual procedure itself. Diagnosis sets the stage for everything else.

The definitive diagnosis leading to the need for surgical crown lengthening can encompass many factors but usually breaks down to just two statements: 1) a violation of the biologic width or 2) excessive gingival enlargement. Both of these two clinical situations will be explored in depth below.

PRESURGICAL PROCEDURES

Before the actual surgery procedure is performed, there are several factors that must be considered. They are all important in favorably influencing the outcome of a case.

Oral Hygiene

The two major indications for surgical crown lengthening, biologic width violations and gingival enlargement, both display characteristics of inflammatory periodontal disease. It is well established that meticulous oral hygiene is a necessary part in the control of this inflammation. It is also well known that surgical procedures in the oral cavity without control of the oral bacteria struggle at best.[9–11]

The patient should receive proper oral hygiene instructions and demonstrate an ability/willingness to keep the area free of bacteria prior to surgery. This is especially important when the surgical site is in an esthetic zone. Surgical healing in a highly inflamed area generally lacks predictability as to the final position of the soft tissue.[12–14]

Debridement

Ideally, a thorough debridement (the term used to include both hand instrumentation and mechanical cleaning methods) coupled with proper oral hygiene should precede the surgical procedure by three weeks. This period of time gives full soft tissue healing and can enhance predictability of the final position of the soft tissue after a surgery. This is also the time in which to evaluate the patient's ability and willingness to maintain the surgical area and keep it healthy.

Antimicrobials

Proper use of antimicrobials, which includes oral rinses, local release antimicrobials, and systemic antibiotics, may help to reduce inflammation presurgically. If indicated, these products can enhance the predictability of the final position of the soft tissue margin, an important issue when esthetics is involved. "The bang for the buck" occurs when antimicrobials are used concomitantly with proper oral hygiene and debridement, as indicated previously.

A Final Show and Tell

When the preceding has been accomplished and the surgical site is as healthy as it is likely to become, a final evaluation with the patient should be considered. Most patients have a limited understanding of oral anatomy (the why of the procedure) and might have forgotten or misunderstood the process and the intended final outcome.

This is the point in the process at which to visually show in the patient's own mouth what the procedure will accomplish and what it is likely to look like postsurgically. This can also be demonstrated via models, alterations of the patient's own models, photographs, and computer-generated designs. The intent and the need are to enhance the patient's understanding and truly have them with us in the process. Since many crown lengthening procedures are done largely for esthetic purposes, the show and tell becomes doubly important. Sometimes the patient's expectations are beyond reality.

This is also a time to answer questions, to allow the patient to express concerns, and to build confidence in the patient before the actual procedure. Most surgical crown lengthening is limited to small areas and is viewed by the dentist as a minor procedure. It is well to remember at this point the tongue-in-cheek definition of a minor surgery—any surgery that is performed on anyone other than oneself. Most patients view **minor** surgeries as something more major.

Informed Consent

The informed consent form is usually given immediately before beginning the surgical procedure. Informed consent forms are more than just a perceived legal requirement. As important as it is as a legal document, informed consent is an invaluable tool to make certain that the doctor and the patient are on the same page. A consent form given to the patient already in the dental chair with the surgical procedure looming over them can be quite intimidating to the patient.

Properly worded, the consent form can both serve the legal necessities and give the patient a final review. The patient should have the opportunity to ask final questions and receive clarifications. All too frequently the patient scribbles a hurried signature and dismisses the document as an irritation rather than an invitation for dialogue.

Form 5-1 is a typical consent form for a surgical crown lengthening procedure. Since there are many local, national, and international legal requirements, this sample should be viewed as a formation guide only. There are forms available from local dental societies, continuing education courses, or legal sources.

Gingival Hypertrophy and Crown Lengthening

As described previously there is a proportional relationship between the sulcus depth and the soft tissue attachment above the alveolar bone, which is necessary to maintain health around the tooth. An increased pocket depth due to increased gingival height (gingival hypertrophy or clinically noted as gingival enlargement), even though the soft tissue attachment is within normal limits, violates that relationship. This produces a pocket that may lead to periodontitis and/or create esthetic problems. Orthodontic appliances, medications, and genetics may play significant roles in producing gingival hypertrophy.

ORTHODONTICS AND GINGIVAL HYPERTROPHY

Young patients in orthodontic braces commonly produce gingival hypertrophy. This is more a result of poor oral hygiene and changing hormones than irritation from the brackets themselves. However, some studies have shown that orthodontic appliances and the food and plaque accumulation on them changes the microbiology in the sulcus, making gingivitis more common than in those not in braces (see Figures 5.11 and 5.12).[15, 16]

Clinical and radiographic measurements generally indicate a normal biologic width, but with greatly increased sulcus depth due to gingival hypertrophy. Initially the increase in gingival size can easily be reduced by debridement and enhanced oral hygiene. If not rapidly reduced by these nonsurgical methods, the gingival tissues become fibrotic and will need surgical crown lengthening procedures.

Some gingival enlargements during orthodontic treatment might be extensive enough to inhibit normal tooth eruption and/or prohibit normal orthodontic movement. A common problem encountered is gingival growth into diastemas, which prevents normal orthodontic closure. Gingival hypertrophy has become a major issue in dentistry with the increase in the numbers of young patients undergoing orthodontic treatment.

Patient Information / Consent for Crown Lengthening

1. I have been informed and I understand the purpose and the nature of the periodontal surgical procedure(s).

2. Dr. _____ has carefully examined my mouth. Alternatives (if any) have been explained.

3. I have been informed of possible risks and complications that may be involved with the surgery, which may include: pain, swelling, infections, medication/anesthetic reactions, and damage to other oral structures.

4. I understand that if nothing is done, there is likely to be continuing inflammation and bone loss.

5. I understand that restoring the tooth or teeth may not be possible without crown lengthening procedures.

6. I understand that there is no method to accurately predict the healing capabilities in each patient and that there is no guarantee of success.

7. I understand that such factors as smoking, hormonal disorders, medications, and other systemic disorders may affect the overall outcome.

8. I agree to report to the doctor for postoperative examinations as instructed.

9. To my knowledge, I have given an accurate report of my physical and mental health history. I have also indicated on the health history any allergic reactions, diseases, medications, herbs, and any past problems with surgical procedures.

10. I request and authorize dental procedures for me, including crown lengthening surgery. I understand that during and following the contemplated procedure or treatment, conditions may become apparent which warrant, in the judgment of the doctor, additional or alternative treatments. I also approve any modification in design, materials, or care, if it is felt this is for my best interest.

_____

Signature of Doctor

_____

Signature of Patient
(If patient is unable to sign or is a minor, signature of parent or legal guardian)

_____

Date

_____

Relationship to Patient

_____

Witness

Form 5–1

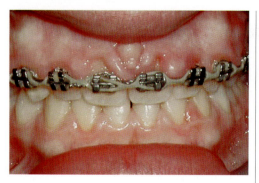

Figure 5-11. Gingival enlargement in orthodontics. The gingival enlargement in this young person is due to orthodontic braces, poor oral hygiene, and probably hormonal factors. This enlargement is a violation of the **proportional relationship** of the biologic width concept, even though the actual biologic width is intact.

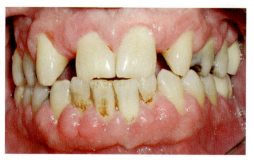

Figure 5-13. Medication-induced gingival hypertrophy. These gingival enlargements were produced by a calcium channel blocker taken for high blood pressure. Gingival hypertrophy caused by one medication is not substantially clinically different from other medication-induced enlargements, although some medications may produce more rapid growth of the gingival tissues.

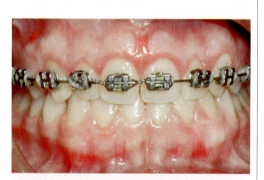

Figure 5-12. After crown lengthening procedures. This shows healthy gingiva and a return to a normal biologic width relationship, indicating that the main issue was gingival enlargement and not a vertical loss of junctional epithelium/connective tissue/bone.

Gingival Enlargement from Medications

Drug-induced gingival enlargement is now a well-known side affect of many medications. In the past only a limited number of drugs such as phenytoin (Dilantin) were known to cause gingival changes.[17] An explosion in new medications has produced a long list of drugs that can cause significant and sustained gingival hypertrophy. These include but are certainly not limited to immunosuppressants, anticonvulsants, and calcium channel blockers (see Figure 5.13).

As a class, the clinician is most likely to encounter gingival enlargement from the calcium channel blockers than other medications since they are prescribed for a wide range of cardiovascular problems.[18–20] Clinically, the appearance and treatment of the gingival enlargements does not differ from one drug category to another.

Gingival hypertrophy from drug induction poses three distinct problems for the clinician:

1. The hypertrophy may occur and enlarge even in the presence of good oral hygiene. Although good oral hygiene may reduce the speed of gingival enlargement, most studies and clinical experience indicate that good hygiene cannot prevent it. The author's clinical experience is that the patient can significantly inhibit gingival growth with good oral hygiene and frequent debridements but usually cannot totally prevent the process. This is particularly frustrating to the patient since there are few preventive measures other than to not take the medication. Alternative drugs that do not produce gingival enlargement

may be explored in consultation with the patient's physician. However the cessation of one medication and introduction of another is frequently a long process with an additional list of side affects.
2. The entire mouth may be involved. Normally, most crown lengthening needs are limited to one or two teeth. With medication-induced gingival enlargement, much of the mouth may be affected, making the surgical procedure(s) much more complex. The esthetic and function problems for the patient can be significant.
3. The surgical crown lengthening procedure may need to be repeated, sometimes frequently. As long as the patient is on the offending medication, hypertrophy is likely to continue. Cessation of medication intake may reduce the gingival size. However, this usually requires several months to a year if a reduction is to occur.

Crown lengthening procedures in patients with drug-induced gingival enlargement require a careful evaluation of the patient's medical status, the ability to heal from a surgical procedure, and an interaction between the physician and the dentist. This then becomes more complicated than the treatment of a single tooth biologic width violation.

GENETIC FACTORS IN GINGIVAL ENLARGEMENT

This section is presented only to indicate that genetics frequently is a factor in hypertrophy.[21] Some of the examples are so rare that they bear repeating only to the point that they do exist. Some of these rare gingival enlargements are connected to overall systemic issues, which may make surgical treatment difficult to manage or even dangerous to the patient. Most patients should be in the hands of skilled specialists. The role of most dental practitioners in these rare forms of gingival enlargement is to differentiate them diagnostically from other forms of hypertrophy.

For most practitioners, the role of genetics is significant only in determining why tissue regrowth occurs **after** the surgical procedure. Since these traits tend to follow a familial line, the dentist may be able to form a clinical opinion about regrowth potential before the crown lengthening by examining other family members. The presence of similar gingival enlargements in others of the same family is a good indicator of the role of genetics. Unfortunately this evaluation is usually made after the surgical healing indicates significant tissue regrowth. There are currently no clinically viable genetic tests to assist the dentist (see Figure 5.14).

Operatory Set-Up and Patient Preparation

The next step as we draw closer to the surgery is to make sure adequate attention has been given to preparing the surgical suite (operatory). The following two sections review important aspects of this phase of treatment.

STERILITY

In the past, only cursory attention was given to sterility issues in surgical procedures performed in the oral cavity. This was largely

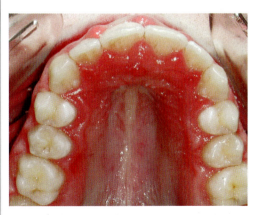

Figure 5-14. Genetic-induced gingival enlargement. Other family members have similar gingival enlargement with an absence of other factors that can produce hypertrophy.

due to the misperception that the mouth was a bacterially contaminated environment that could not or need not be controlled.

In addition it has also been argued that one cannot control the sterility of the average dental operatory to the level of a hospital surgical suite. Although these are essentially correct statements, contamination of the oral cavity by bacteria from without or contamination of deeper structures in the oral cavity during a surgical procedure, however minor, can have serious consequences. The **standard** of care is to treat the oral cavity surgically with as high a level of sterility as one can achieve in the dental operatory.

All surgical instruments should be sterilized, and the dentist should become familiar with, practice, and incorporate into the dental office strict sterile techniques. The basic tenet is that only sterile surfaces should contact sterile surfaces. Most surgeries require that an additional staff member not involved in the sterile environment be available to get instruments, charts, and other items not part of the **sterile triangle**, which is that area in the immediate vicinity of the doctor, the assistant, and the patient.

Sterile gowns for the dental staff and the patient as well as surgical packs (either launderable or single-use disposable) should be part of the normal surgical setup. The dentist and dental staff can receive training in how to create sterile surgical packs from various continuing education sources or from a local hospital.

A frequent weak link in dental office sterility is the water source. Many culinary water sources worldwide have high bacterial counts, which, when used during surgical procedures, may inject infective microorganisms directly into surgical sites.

In addition, the numerous small-diameter tubes in dental carts can concentrate bacteria and allow a significant bacterial biofilm to form in the tubes, even from culinary water sources considered to have low bacterial counts. These bacteria are then forced into the surgical site during rinsing procedures. There is mounting evidence that these contaminants may have significant infective properties, particularly in patients who have decreased immune response mechanisms. True sterile water sources should be used during oral surgical procedures.

SURGICAL INSTRUMENTS

Table 5.3 lists some the instruments commonly used in the various types of crown lengthening procedures. Since there are so many individual preferences among surgeons, the instruments are listed under six broad categories—diagnostic, debridement, incising, reflection (for flap surgeries), bone resection (where indicated), and closure—with a few examples of each category listed.

A common layout for surgical instrumentation is to place the instruments on the surgical tray in the order used. Surgeries typically require more instruments/supplies on a tray in the operatory than many other dental procedures. It may be necessary to obtain a larger tray, such as a Mayo tray, to contain them in a sterile environment. Instruments spread over many surfaces invite contamination and instrument dropping (see Figure 5.15).

Crown Lengthening–Gingival Enlargement

This type of crown lengthening is primarily a "subtraction" procedure that eliminates redundant or excessive soft tissue. The main considerations for its implementation are presented in the following sections.

SURGICAL INDICATIONS

Surgery may be indicated for the following conditions of gingival enlargement:

1. A suprabony pocket (a pocket that is caused solely by gingival enlargement):

Table 5.3 Common Surgical Instruments for Crown Lengthening

Diagnostic Instruments	Debridement Instruments	Incising Instruments	Bone Resection Instruments	Closure Instruments
Mouth mirrors	Curettes	Scalpel handle	High-speed handpiece with #4, #8 round carbide burs	Needle holder
Periodontal probe	Ultrasonic scaler	Inserts-several, such as #15, #15c, or #12		Suture (see discussion)
Furcation probes		Kirkland knife	Rhodes chisel	Suture scissor
Explorers		Orban knife	Wedelestadt chisel	
		Curved scissors	Bone files	

Flap Reflection	Anesthetic	Suction	Other
Elevators	Of choice, many available	Add a fine-tip surgical evacuator in addition to the saliva tip	2 × 2 gauze
Kirkland knife	Add some long-acting drugs such as bupivicaine and articaine		Cheek retractor such as a Bishop
			Hemostat
			Hemostatic gauze
			Ice packs

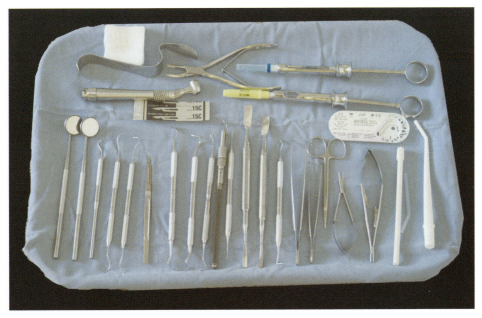

Figure 5-15. Typical surgical tray setup. Note the oversized tray to contain the instruments in one single sterile area. Tray is covered with a sterile cover. Instruments are arranged in the approximate order in which they will be used.

113

These are common during orthodontic procedures and from certain medications (see previous discussion). Although these pockets may have an intact biologic width, they still represent potential bacterial traps which can lead to bone loss.

2. A soft tissue enlargement that prohibits proper restorative/orthodontic procedures: Oftentimes these enlargements are the result of an inflammatory process associated with carious lesions or a defective restoration.

3. An esthetically unacceptable tissue enlargement, especially in the anterior areas: The so-called delayed passive eruption (actually a very active process) whereby soft tissue is significantly coronal to the CEJ (the gummy smile) is a typical example. Many of these enlargements are of a horizontal nature and do not represent a pocket or bacterial trap per se. These horizontal enlargements are sometimes known as soft tissue pearls. *Note:* All of the preceding presupposes that proper oral hygiene and nonsurgical debridement have not resolved the gingival enlargements. **Nonsurgical approaches should precede any surgery.**

SURGICAL TECHNIQUES

The gingivectomy and the flap technique are the two most commonly used surgical methods when the issue is gingival hypertrophy. Both have advantages, appropriate applications, and disadvantages, which will be detailed later in this chapter. Both should be viewed as tools, which are most appropriate or least appropriate in a given clinical situation rather than as an either/or technique. The given clinical situation and the experience of the surgeon usually dictate which technique is used. The internal thinning of gingival enlargements (internal beveled incision/flap) will be covered in the section dealing with flap surgery.

GINGIVECTOMY

The gingivectomy technique was the dominant surgical technique in periodontics prior to the introduction of the flap and osseous contouring methods. Since then it has been relegated to a minor role, that role largely being excision of gingival enlargements in the course of crown lengthening procedures.

By definition **gingivectomy** means the excision of the gingiva. Gingivectomies have or are performed via lasers (most commonly the CO_2 and Nd:YAG lasers), electrosurgery, chemicals (usually a paraformaldehyde or potassium hydroxide solution, although there are several private formulations), and the scalpel. There are enthusiastic adherents to each method, with each having a list of pros and cons. The overall outcome of each of the techniques appears to be coequal, with the final result more dependent on the clinical abilities and experience of the dentist using that method than on the method itself. Since the scalpel is a universally available item, it will be the featured instrument in this chapter.

Presurgical Considerations of the Gingivectomy Technique

A distinct advantage of the gingivectomy is its relative simplicity. Tissue is excised to the shape and contour desired or needed. However, a gingivectomy produces a fairly large surface wound that tends to produce a disproportionate amount of postoperative discomfort and hemorrhage. The lasers and electrosurgical units control well the hemorrhage.

The excision of the enlargement also removes some of the keratinized tissue in the reshaping process, which, if excessive, might lead to insufficient keratinized tissue to protect the tooth. This then may require mucogingival replacement procedures. Prior to using the gingivectomy as a technique, the clinician should ascertain whether or not sufficient keratinized tissue will remain to maintain health. If not, an alternate method should be considered, most likely a flap technique. If the gingivectomy is still deemed the most appropriate method even if protective keratinized tissue is lost, then the eventuality of soft tissue grafting should be included in the pretreatment planning.

The Gingivectomy Technique

Figure 5.16 shows the basic procedure of a gingivectomy. The following steps expand on the separate points:

1. **Anesthetic.** An anesthetic of choice is used for either local infiltration and/or block anesthesia, as the situation dictates. Generally the gingival tissues are directly injected with 1:50,000 epinephrine to better control hemorrhage.
2. **Sounding.** General pocket probing and diagnostic sounding are performed to verify the position of the alveolar bony crest (review Table 5.2 and Figure 5.4). Horizontal sounding is done at this point also to help guide the amount of buccal-lingual tissue reduction necessary.
3. **Incision.** The incision can be made with a scalpel handle containing an insert such as a #15, #15-C, or #12 blade. There are periodontal knives such as the Kirkland, Orban, and Buck knives that can also be used.

    The incision is made at the point necessary to accomplish the restorative or esthetic goals. For example, make the incision apically far enough to expose the decay in the tooth for restorative procedures or to excise enough tissue so that it esthetically matches the surrounding areas (esthetic sculpting).

    The incision most commonly used is a beveled incision at approximately a 45-degree angle to the tooth, recreating a normal festooning shape. This incision penetrates the entire gingival thickness

until the tooth surface is contacted. A similar incision at a similar beveled angle is made on adjacent teeth as needed to provide a normal contour.

An alternative method is to make the incision at the desired point with the incising instrument at a 90-degree angle to the tooth. This creates a soft tissue ledge, which can then be smoothed out with a scalpel, scissors, electrosurgery, or high-speed rotary instruments such as a course diamond or carbide bur.

With the gingivectomy technique tissue can be removed as close to the bone as necessary without removing the soft tissue covering (periosteum). If the bone needs to be exposed to accomplish the desired goal, then a full-thickness flap technique with osseous resection should have been chosen. Exposing the bone usually creates an extended healing time.

A point that we can learn about the gingivectomy technique is that the entire biologic width is oftentimes removed **without any clinical consequences**. That is to say, that the entire attachment tissues (JE, connective tissue that form the biologic width, and the sulcus) are totally removed, but they regenerate without significant hypertrophy. This means that the body re-forms this unit apically by controlled bone loss. This will be the basis for the discussion on flap techniques in crown lengthening that follows.

4. **Tissue Removal and Shaping.** The excised tissue collar is removed from the tooth, and the surgical area is shaped to match normal physiologic contours. The festooning can be done with a sharp scalpel, scissor, high-speed rotary burs, or other instruments/devices. The surrounding undisturbed areas can be used as a visual template for this process. Be certain to remove any soft tissue tags directly against the tooth surface since these irregularities produce unwanted tissue growth

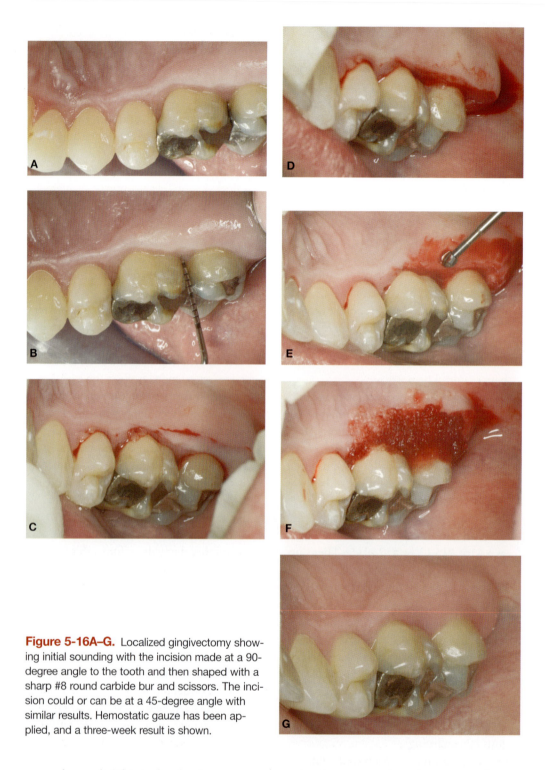

Figure 5-16A–G. Localized gingivectomy showing initial sounding with the incision made at a 90-degree angle to the tooth and then shaped with a sharp #8 round carbide bur and scissors. The incision could or can be at a 45-degree angle with similar results. Hemostatic gauze has been applied, and a three-week result is shown.

up the tooth. This is also the time to thoroughly clean the tooth surface, a process that enhances healing generally. Ultrasonics are particularly useful in the cleaning process since the water coolant acts as a lavage in the surgical area.

5. **Protecting the Site and Controlling Hemorrhage.** Since this is an open

Table 5-4. Postoperative Patient Care for Crown Lengthening Procedures

Gingivectomy Technique	Flap Procedures
• Apply a hemostatic gauze or medical-grade cyanoacrylate directly to the surgical site. Apply additional sustained positive pressure with gauze and ice packs	• Appropriate antibiotic coverage • Positive pressure with gauze and ice packs
• Patient maintains the compresses for at least two hours	• Patient maintains the compresses for at least two hours
• An alternative is to apply a periodontal dressing	• An alternative is to apply a periodontal dressing
• Patient topically applies chlorhexidine (CHX) to the area twice daily. Brushing should not touch the gingival areas (stimulates tissue regrowth)	• Patient topically applies chlorhexidine to the surgical site twice daily. No brushing or flossing in the surgical area
• Avoid chewing in the surgical site, but *do* maintain a high nutritional and fluid intake	• Avoid chewing in the surgical site, but *do* maintain a high nutritional and fluid intake
• Approriate antibiotics/analgesics	• Suture removal at one week with a continuation of CHX for an additional week

wound, the site may need to be protected with a periodontal dressing or a cyano-acrylate adhesive (which also has slight hemostatic properties). There is also a variety of hemostatic gauze strips available that effectively control bleeding and that, when combined with sustained positive pressure, can eliminate the need for bulky periodontal packings.[18]

6. **Postoperative Care.** Although postoperative care for a surgical technique rarely earns a spot equal to the technique itself, this author believes that the postoperative care given for a gingivectomy may largely determine the final result. Since this is an open wound, irritation from bacteria, oral hygiene, and chewing may cause undue hypertrophy.

   Table 5.4 summarizes typical postoperative care and instructions for a gingivectomy technique.

7. **Healing Summary.** If the excision of gingival hypertrophy was to facilitate restorative procedures or to commence or finish orthodontic procedures, then it is important to know when the surgical site will be ready for those procedures. Healing studies parallel what is seen clinically with the exception of the production of a stable sulcus. Surface epithelization and keratinization appears to be complete in about four weeks, according to research and clinical observation. The reestablishment of the biologic width is at about eight weeks.[22]

The greatest frustration for the patient and dentist trying to complete the restorative process after a gingivectomy is more likely to be the **absence** of a sulcus rather than one that is too deep. A general clinical experience is that a normal stable sulcus after a gingivectomy in which tissue was removed to the bone (the most common occurrence) may not occur for up to six months. Restoring a surgical area too soon may expose the gingival margin as the sulcus forms. This occurrence is dependant upon many factors that may be difficult to determine. Where possible restorative procedures should be delayed until there is evidence of a stable sulcus.

Gingivectomy Summary

The gingivectomy technique can be applied to the majority of the cases requiring surgical

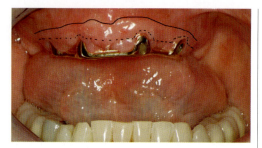

Figure 5-17. Gingival hypertrophy around dental implants caused by a combination of genetics and irritation from a removable device. Mentally plan the incision point/angle of incision and soft tissue reshaping. The dotted line shows the position of alveolar bone, and the solid line indicates the position of the mucogingival junction.

crown lengthening. By following basic surgical and postoperative guidelines, the gingivectomy can create a consistently predictable surgical result. Only those cases where the decay or a root fracture is below the bony crest, as distinguished from those that are supracrestal biologic width violations, need flap procedures. And as will be seen under the flap procedure section, the majority of the flap procedures require little or no osseous removal to provide a healthy environment. See Figure 5.17.

ESTHETIC SCULPTING

Esthetic sculpting is the term commonly applied to the removal of excessive gingival tissue largely for aesthetic rather than health or functional reasons. This so-called gummy smile problem is noted when the soft tissue is significantly coronal to the position expected for the age group, giving the appearance that the teeth are submerged into the gingival tissues. In the adult, the expected gingival position would be at or near the cementoenamel junction (CEJ). Figure 5.18 shows a clinical situation in which the gingiva covers nearly one-half of the distance between the CEJ and the incisal edge in an adult patient. The tissues are otherwise healthy.

Because the vertical dimension of the teeth is covered with gum tissue, there is the appearance that the teeth are short, square, and squatty. This appearance is most troublesome to the patient when it occurs in the anterior teeth, the upper anterior teeth in particular. Although a pseudo-pocket is present in these situations, it is uncommon for these to degenerate periodontally since oral hygiene procedures are not compromised, and a healthy attachment apparatus is generally present. The issue is mainly esthetics. This should not, however, deter the dentist from suggesting a procedure that could improve the general appearance.

Presurgical Consultation

Elective surgical procedures in dentistry usually require more explanations by the dental staff and an enhanced understanding by the patient than nonelective procedures. The fact that the impending surgery is elective means that it is the patient's option. The consequence of not having the surgery done is probably not related to oral health, just appearances.

A second consideration is that esthetic sculpting in the upper anterior may quickly and dramatically alter a patient's appearance. This sudden change is most likely a positive one, but it does nonetheless change the image that the patient may have had of themselves.

The author remembers a young patient who was excited about getting rid of her gummy smile, which she stated she had always hated. At the end of the procedure, she burst into tears when she saw the change and was inconsolable, although family members and the dental staff praised the positive changes. Two days later she contacted the office and apologized for her behavior and enthusiastically proclaimed how much she loved the new look. The rapid change to

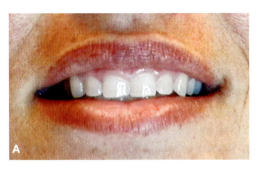
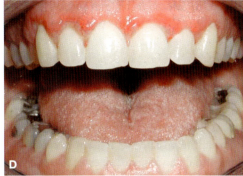
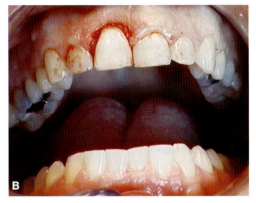
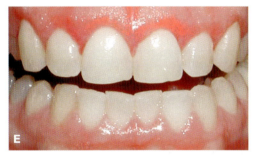
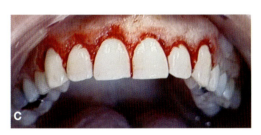
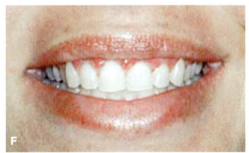

Figure 5-18A–F. Esthetic sculpting.

how she had seen herself for so many years was initially an emotional shock.

Dental models, photographs of previous patients, a potential final look as generated by computer programs, and cautious testimonials are frequently needed. Usually this should be a soft-sell approach so that the patient does not feel pressured. The other side of the equation is that the satisfied patient is frequently an enthusiastic advocate for the procedure.

Clinical Evaluations

Sounding to bone should be accomplished so that an accurate mental picture of the bone position can be made (review Figure 5.4 and Table 5.2). An evaluation of how much keratinized tissue will remain must also be determined. If the excision of the gingival tissue is likely to leave insufficient keratinized tissue to maintain health, then the need for soft tissue grafting should be part of the treatment plan or another technique chosen, such as an apically positioned flap procedure. Since this an elective surgery there is also the option not to do the procedure.

Appropriate x-rays (see the previous discussion) are cross-referenced with the soundings and other clinical observations. The position of the lip line and the extent of the smile should also be noted. A wide smile and a high lip line may necessitate extending the excision of tissue into the posterior areas for a better esthetic result. Restoration margins that might be uncovered may need to be replaced postsurgically.

Surgical Procedure

Most of the aesthetic sculpting surgical procedures are gingivectomies as previously stated. Occasionally a flap procedure is indicated when tooth structure beyond the alveolar bone needs to be exposed.

An appropriate anesthetic is administered. Since this is a gingivectomy procedure with excision of what is sometimes large amounts of surface tissue, 1:50,000 epinephrine injected directly into the tissues is a help in hemorrhage control. Dry 2 × 2 gauze should be in ready supply. Unfilled gauze more quickly absorbs blood than does the filled variety.

Since this procedure typically involves several adjacent teeth it is usually advantageous to identify the lead tooth, the one which will determine the height and shape of the others. This may be a tooth that already has a normal height or contour and to which the others must be matched, or it may be a tooth that, due to its position or rotation, is the limiting factor for the process. Figure 5.18 indicates how one tooth becomes the lead for the others.

A beveled or 90-degree incision is made midfacial at the desired apical level of the lead tooth, and the incision is carried into the mesial and distal interproximal areas.

The excised tissue is then removed. The surgeon should be careful not to extend the incision lingually beyond the contact point of the teeth since to do so usually causes vertical recession in the interproximal areas and produces an unaesthetic space devoid of tissue (the euphemistic "bullet hole" or "black triangle").

If the patient is able to view the surgical procedure, it is helpful to have them comment on the initial height of the lead tooth. Remember that one can always remove more tissue but replacing it is difficult. Therefore, a conservative approach is best until the desired result is achieved.

Similar procedures are performed on the adjacent teeth. The author has found that starting with the central incisors in the midline (unless there is a different lead tooth) and then proceeding laterally produces the best results. There are distinct advantages to facing the patient when doing the initial incisions since this gives the most realistic view of the process. Comments from staff members and others who may be in the operatory are invaluable.

Some clinicians advocate that up to 25 percent additional tissue be removed to compensate for tissue regrowth. Regrowth of this magnitude has not been routinely noted by this author. Because of this clinical observation, consider making the final tissue position at the desired height. Additional tissue removal may lead to an excessive display of tooth structure and may needlessly remove keratinized tissue.

After the apical height of all teeth is established, the tissue bulk on the labial can be thinned into the embrasures to achieve the desired scallop and shape. This can be done with scissors and rotary burs, at the surgeon's discretion. Electrosurgical units and lasers should be used with great caution since they can inadvertently cause recession or bone necrosis.

Remember the caution stated previously about removing tissue beyond the contact point. This rule is violated only if restorative procedures, such as veneers or crowns, are to be placed since they need additional lateral width and additional space to the lingual.

Postoperative Care

Refer once again to Table 5.3 for a summary of postoperative procedures. Uncontrolled hemorrhage can lead to clot organization and an irregular surface. Use of hemostatic gauzes, sustained positive pressure (normal gauze rolled up like a pencil over the hemostatic gauze), and an ice pack with applied pressure for 1–2 hours is quite effective.

Chlorhexidine is topically applied to the area twice daily to control the oral bacteria. The patient should be instructed not to directly brush the gingival areas for two weeks since this irritation delays healing, increases discomfort, and may cause irregular gingival growth.

Systemic antibiotics are not routinely used, being common only where antibiotic prophylaxis for systemic purposes is indicated. The chlorhexidine applied to the area controls the bacterial population until normal oral hygiene procedures can be resumed.

The patient is typically seen in one week for reevaluation. Any small tissue regrowths can be removed at this time if necessary with a minimum of discomfort since nerve endings are not fully established. The patient is seen again at three weeks, at which time normal oral hygiene is reinstituted. Another evaluation is made at six weeks, assuming that a normal healing course has occurred. Maintenance for gingivectomies should include a three-month recall prophylaxis with tissue evaluations in the surgical area for the first year postoperatively and then as indicated.

Esthetic Sculpting Summary

Esthetic sculpting is a predictable procedure that can produce enhanced esthetics for pa-

tients exhibiting a smile with excessive tissue. Dentistry is much more than a technical discipline concerned only with oral health. It is well-established that a portion of the mental psyche revolves around physical appearance, either real or perceived. The teeth and gum relationships contribute greatly to that overall personal perception. Although listed as an elective procedure, more and more patients are requesting it for personal reasons.

A Conservative Flap Procedure for Crown Lengthening

The majority of cases requiring surgical crown lengthening can be handled by the gingivectomy techniques as previously described. The limited numbers requiring a flap procedure can be done with less bone removal and better esthetics by understanding and applying the actual necessities of the biologic width rather than the perceived requirements as dictated by studies of the past. This approach also takes into account changes in restorative methods and materials that do not require extensive exposure of the tooth surface.

REVISITING THE BIOLOGIC WIDTH ISSUES

Clinical crown lengthening procedures are guided by research on the proportional relationships among the sulcus, junctional epithelium, and the connective tissue overlying the alveolar bone. Traditionally, clinicians have been instructed to allow between 3 and 5.5 mm of vertical height between the restorative margin and the alveolar bone for the preceding clinical structures.[1–4] This represents a significant problem in that most surgical procedures must remove supporting bone to fulfill these objectives. This may compromise tooth support and/or alter facial esthetics (see Figure 5.19).

Although the following represents the author's personal clinical experiences, the con-

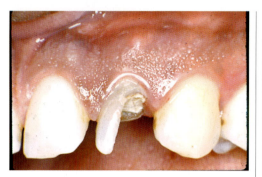

Figure 5-19A. Reviewing the suitability of a tooth for crown lengthening. There is adequate attached gingiva in this case. If crown lengthening is performed, the tooth will most likely end up with a longer clinical crown, which, depending on the patient's smile line, could have adverse esthetic consequences.

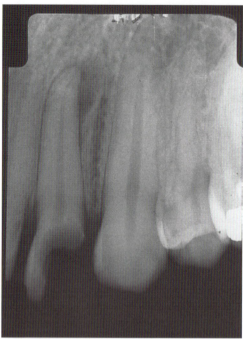

Figure 5-19B. The radiograph shows good osseous support for the proposed crown lengthening. However, the tooth should be provisionalized until after the endodontic treatment has proved to be successful, and then the periodontal surgery can be performed.

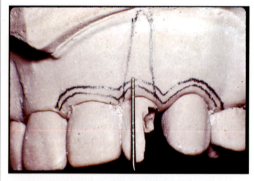

Figure 5-19C. Model of this case, with vertical measurements denoting the biologic width.

clusions have been universally the same. This is less a challenge to established studies and more a support for clinical realities for achieving the proportional relationships established by that research. Basic premises are given here:

1. The total amount of sound tooth structure that needs to be exposed is substantially less today due to improved restorative techniques and materials. Most restorative dentists need only a couple of millimeters of sound tooth above the gingival margin in order to complete the restorative procedure.
2. Bone removal is necessary only when there is a restorative need **below the bony crest** or a need to esthetically expose more tooth than is allowed by an excision of soft tissue only (gingivectomy). Both of the preceding are relatively uncommon occurrences. After flap reflection (excepting the preceding two examples), there is usually enough space between the tooth margin and the bone to apically position the flap without bone removal. This represents either an inflammatory degeneration or the natural space occupied by the biologic width. See Figure 5.17.
3. If the soft tissue flap is placed at the bony crest, the body will automatically provide the height necessary for the biologic width, presumably by biologic resorption of enough bone to accommodate it. Clinical experience verifies this phenome-

non. Consider the gingivectomy case in which the soft tissue is removed to the bone. A stable final healing result without coronal soft tissue regrowth shows a normal sulcus and normal attachment (as revealed via sounding techniques), again presumably due to physiologic resorption of bone to allow such. The summary point is that if a soft tissue flap is placed at or coronal to the crest of bone, the body will resorb adequate bone to establish a sulcus and biologic attachment without the bone removal advocated by traditional means. So rather than removing bone to allow space for the 3-mm biologic width, place the flap directly at the bony crest and let the body form the requisite space below the flap. This can preserve at least 3 mm of bone, improve tooth stability, and provide enhanced esthetics (see Figure 5.20).

Surgical Indications for a Flap Procedure

Flap procedures in crown lengthening may be indicated over the gingivectomy techniques in the following cases:

1. When only a limited amount of attached keratinized tissue is present in the proposed surgical site. In those cases in which removal of keratinized tissue by the gingivectomy would likely create mucogingival defects and/or create the need for soft tissue replacement procedures, a flap procedure might be the indicated method. A reflected flap with apical positioning can preserve and actually enhance the amount of keratinized tissue available by secondary intention healing.
2. When restorative needs are apical to the osseous crest and there is an obvious need to remove bone. This may be deep caries, resorption, or fracture of the clinical crown or root. This represents a severe condition and may necessitate tooth removal if too far apical to the bony crest.
3. When the alveolar bone is healthy and at the normal height but procedures require the soft tissue height to be more apical than is possible with tissue excision (gingivectomy). This is the case when restora-

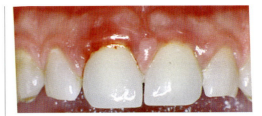

Figure 5-20A. Crowns on teeth numbers 8 and 9 with overextended margins into the biologic width and accompanying chronic inflammation.

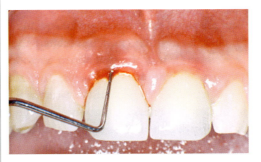

Figure 5-20B. Probing reveals the pocket depth.

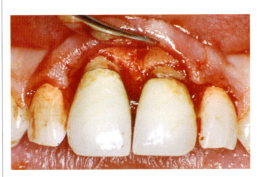

Figure 5-20C. It is not uncommon with cases such as this for the body to physiologically (via inflammation) resorb bone in an attempt to regain the needed biologic width.

tive or esthetic needs must extend beyond the CEJ. This is found when the clinical crown height is genetically short and/or the esthetic needs require crown height beyond the CEJ, such as in preparation for veneers or crowns.

Flap Presurgical Evaluations

Flap procedures are decidedly more complex than gingivectomies. They introduce the need for suture and suturing techniques to maintain a moveable flap in position. Thus, the clinician must know and understand the varieties and merits of each suturing technique. In addition there may be the need to remove bone, which demands knowledge about alveolar bone, tooth support, and the physiology of bone healing.[23]

Since crown lengthening is a localized procedure surrounded by normal and usually healthy tissues, any flap procedure must take into account the potential effect flap displacement may have on these tissues and the overall esthetic impact. Decisions must also be made regarding flap design and the extension into healthy areas.

Bone removal may be necessary in order to accomplish the final goal. Tooth stability issues must, therefore, be addressed—that is, how much bone to remove, how much bone can be removed, and the impact on the integrity of the tooth. Radiographic analysis, thus, becomes important. Localized bone removal generally requires more decisions, surgical skill, and presurgical evaluation than a flap procedure that encompasses much of a quadrant.

It is at this point that the clinician should make the decision to treat or refer to a specialist. The decision to refer or not is usually made on the basis of perceived clinical factors, potential complicating issues, and the skill and experience of the treating dentist.

As with the other crown lengthening procedures, the target area should be made as healthy as possible via proper oral hygiene

and debridement procedures well before the surgical procedure is performed. Healthy tissues heal more predictably during surgical healing than do those that are inflamed.

The Flap Technique in Surgical Crown Lengthening

This section details the more complicated, serious, and aggressive type of crown lengthening. It requires more knowledge and experience to diagnose and treat successfully.

ANESTHESIA

Since flap procedures generally require more time to perform than the gingivectomy and may be perceived by the patient as a **major** surgery, sedative techniques may be indicated. Local anesthetic is administered into the surgical site and also to an area distant from the actual flap since reflection techniques produce some pressure to the surrounding tissues. It is generally useful to inject anesthetic containing 1:50,000 epinephrine directly into the tissues to help control any hemorrhage.

SOUNDING TECHNIQUES

These are performed with a periodontal probe to determine the topography of the underlying bone. This should also be performed laterally into adjacent nonsurgical areas. The intent of sounding in flap crown lengthening procedures is to help produce a mental image of the bony topography. A knowledge of the shape and position of the bony crest is even more important in flap procedures than it is in gingivectomies.

FLAP DESIGN

See Figure 5.21. Flap design is the intended path of the incision. For crown lengthening there are three elements that determine the

CONSERVATIVE SURGICAL CROWN LENGTHENING 125

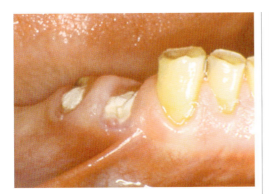

Figure 5-21A. Preoperative view from the buccal.

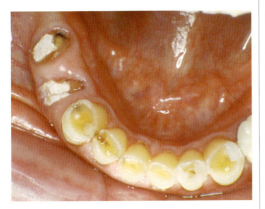

Figure 5-21B. Preoperative view from the occlusal.

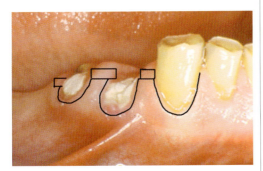

Figure 5-21C. Flap design (proposed flap incisions). The flap design is as such to allow full closure of interproximal soft tissue.

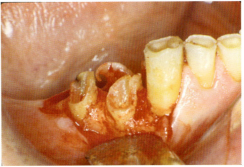

Figure 5-21D. Flap reflected away from bone to allow visualization, debridement, and apical repositioning of soft tissue.

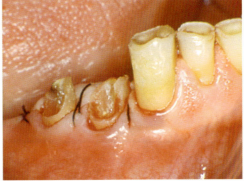

Figure 5-21E. Flap apically repositioned and sutured in place. No bone was removed and yet there is adequate tooth structure above the gingival margin for restorative purposes.

overall path of the incision(s). These are presented in the following paragraphs.

The first consideration is to choose an incision path that will help maintain the maximum amount of the keratinized tissue. If there is only a minimal amount of keratinized tissue available, then the incision should be in the sulcus or no greater than 0.5–1.0 mm below the free gingival margin. This maintains the maximum amount of keratinized tissue and at the same time allows the flap to be elevated.

A second guiding principle is the need to thin bulky tissues. If the need is to just detach thin soft tissue from the bone, then the blade angle ranges from 45 degrees to almost parallel with the long axis of the tooth, either in the sulcus or slightly apical to the gingival margin. If the tissue is bulky and needs to be thinned internally, then an internal bevel incision can largely accomplish this at the same

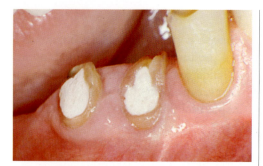

Figure 5-21F. Buccal view of healing at four weeks.

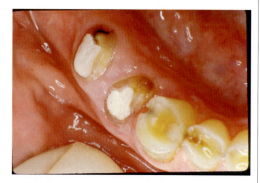

Figure 5-21G. Occlusal view of healing at four weeks.

time that the tissue is released from the underlying bone.

The third element in flap design is to create a flap that will cover the maximum amount of bone but at the same time allow the flap to be placed where needed. Each clinical situation requires its own unique flap design. Since it is not possible to describe or diagram every case, the principles as stated previously become the guides for the clinician.

Internal Bevel Incision

The internal beveled incision is a basic part of most flap surgeries.[24] The intent of the internal bevel incision in crown lengthening is to thin the tissue of the flap so that it forms a flap margin that will adapt to the tooth and bone in a normal relationship.

It consists of three separate incisions (see Figure 5.22). The first incision (also called a reverse-bevel incision since the blade-to-tissue angle is the reverse of the gingivectomy) is designed to thin the tissues **internally**, leaving the surface keratinization intact—just the opposite of the gingivectomy. The blade, which can be a #15, #15-c, #11, or one of the #12 series blades, is inserted into the tissue until bone is contacted. This is at an angle that will leave the external tissue flap at the desired thickness. This is then carried into the interproximal areas. Since this path of incision usually leaves thicker tissue interproximally than on the labial surfaces, a second incision is required to internally thin the interproximal tissues before flap reflection.

The final incision is used to detach the remaining tissue from the tooth. The point of the scalpel blade or other thin surgical instrument is placed in the sulcus vertically along the long axis of the tooth. This incision is forced to the alveolar bone crest, effectively detaching the collar of tissue next to the tooth.

This technique is best understood from diagrams since written descriptions tend to make it more complex than it really is. Study Figure 5.22 for a visual approach to understanding.

The internal-bevel incision approach can also be used to thin gingival hyperplasia rather than using the gingivectomy technique described previously. This miniflap procedure retains the surface tissue intact and may allow the flap to be collapsed onto the bony crest and the surface of the tooth in a manner that may produce a better esthetic/functional result than excision of the surface tissue. The dental practitioner should have the knowledge and ability to perform both where indicated.

Restated, the flap design (incision) should allow coverage of as much bone as possible with the soft tissue flap, allow the flap to be placed where needed, provide an appropriate

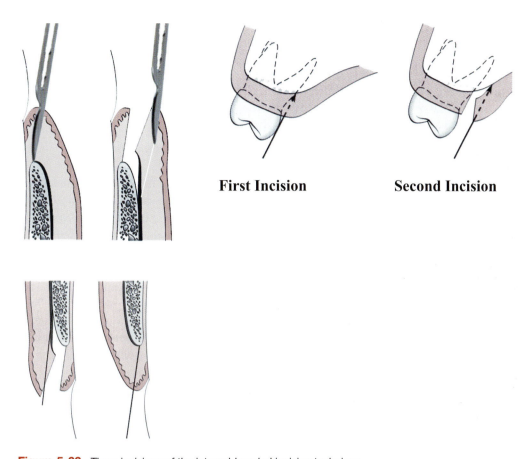

Figure 5-22. Three incisions of the internal-beveled incision technique.

thickness of soft tissue, and preserve keratinized tissue. It is well to mentally review the preceding principles in each clinical case before the initial incision. The final flap design usually determines many elements in the final product.

The previously described incisions and flap design produce a flap that when elevated is called an envelope flap. Although this may be sufficient to expose adequate tooth structure for minor violations of the biologic width, deep caries and/or a deep coronal fractures require that the flap be positioned more apical than is possible with a envelope flap. This may require vertical incisions, also called vertical releasing incisions.

These incisions can be made at one or both ends of the flap as the situation demands. They allow the entire flap to be placed apically without loss of keratinized tissue. These vertical incisions are usually made at the line angles of teeth so that closure of the vertical incisions is not over the radicular surface of a tooth and so that the papillae are retained. Incisions are made to bone, extending apically beyond the mucogingival junction into the vestibule far enough that the flap can be elevated and positioned apically without excessive muscle tension. See Figure 5.23.

Flap Elevation

Flap elevation can be accomplished via two methods or a combination of both:

1. Split-thickness flaps are created at the same time as the flap design incisions are

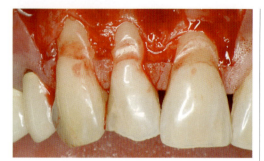

Figure 5-23. Vertical releasing incisions with a full mucoperiosteal flap. Note how the interproximal tissue and the position of the alveolar bone have been retained (**no** bone has been surgically removed).

done, as indicated previously. All or a portion of the keratinized attached tissue is elevated to the mucogingival junction using blunt dissection (a periosteal elevator, Kirkland knife, or similar instrument) producing a full-thickness mucoperiosteal flap. This miniflap is gently retracted and with a scalpel or similar sharp surgical blade placed parallel with the underlying bone; the tissue is incised vertically into the vestibule, leaving a portion of the connective tissue on the bony surface. Split-thickness flaps may offer the ability to tightly suture the mobile portion of the flap against the alveolar bone.

2. Full-thickness flaps are created by blunt dissection, separating the mucoperiosteum from the bone. This full-thickness flap is necessary when bone removal is needed to expose an additional amount of the tooth. An incision is made intra- or subsulcular to bone. The entire mucoperiosteum is reflected with a periosteal elevator or similar instrument. This full-thickness reflection is extended into the vestibule far enough to allow the flap to be positioned where desired without undo muscle tension. Review Figure 5.23.

3. A combination of the preceding two methods (partial thickness and full thickness) is useful when bone must be removed and yet the flap rigidly held in position. Initially a full-thickness mucoperiostial flap is elevated by blunt dissection apically, exposing the requisite amount of tooth or bone. The incision is then continued into the vestibule, creating a split-thickness flap, as described previously.

Surgical Site Evaluation

When the flap has been elevated, the tooth and bone interface should be examined. This is the important time to determine whether the tooth is restorable. Occasionally the extent of carious destruction or amount of resorption is such that the tooth cannot be restored. There may be also an undetected root fracture not visible by clinical methods. Flap entry with direct visualization is frequently the only method to determine these things. Alternative methods may then be needed such as extraction.

A thorough evaluation of the bony support should also be accomplished. Does any bone need to be removed to accomplish the objectives? If so, how much needs to be removed, and what are the consequences for the tooth support and general esthetics? Does the flap need to be elevated an additional distance laterally or apically? In summary, should alternative techniques be considered?

Debridement

Debridement is the term that covers all techniques used to clean the tooth and remove inflammatory products. These can be mechanical instruments such as ultrasonics and rotary burs or hand instruments such as curettes and surgical tools. All can be used coequally at the individual dentist's discretion. A bacteria- and inflammation-free environment heals quickly, predictably, and with reduced postoperative pain.

The tooth should be cleaned free of all plaque and calculus deposits. The end-point determination (when the process is complete) is the same as with scaling and root planing.

Granulation tissue (a combination of bacteria, their inflammatory products, and partially destroyed soft tissue and bone) is now removed from the alveolar bone. This is especially important at the bone-tooth interface.

Some granulation tissue is usually present on the underneath side of the soft tissue flap. This can be removed with a pair of sharp curved scissors or a carefully placed scalpel.

These procedures have now replaced an inflammatory wound having a diminished capacity to heal with a surgically created wound that has an enhanced healing ability. The entire surgical site should now be thoroughly flushed with a sterile solution such as sterile water or sterile saline. This flushing action can greatly reduce postoperative infections and should be a part of all surgeries.

Bone Removal

The vast majority of crown lengthening cases need little or no bone resection/removal. In those cases that do need some bone removed, this can be accomplished by a variety of burs and hand instruments.[25] Review Figures 5.19–5.21, and 5.23.

Rotary burs, in either high-speed or low-speed handpieces, can be used to remove the majority of the bone. Most commonly #4 and #8 carbide or diamond round burs are used. Most studies indicate that the sharp carbide bur produces less heat and trauma when applied to the bone than a diamond bur. In any case there should be a **copious water stream** applied to cool the bur/bone and flush the debris away.

Round rotary burs are initially and carefully used to remove the requisite amount of bone immediately adjacent to the tooth. Only enough bone needs be removed from around the tooth to allow the restorative procedures to be performed or to allow adequate tooth height for esthetic needs. As

mentioned several times already, there only need to be 1–2 mm of tooth above the gingival margin to accomplish most restorative tasks.

There is also a class of end-cutting burs available that can remove the bone next to the tooth.[24] These burs have some advantages over the round burs in that they are less likely to nick the tooth during bone resection.

The round burs are then used to create and shape natural physiologic contours around the tooth and into the interproximal areas (sometimes called **sluicing**). The intent of this osseous shaping is to create a form to which the soft tissue flap can adapt. A general principle is that the shape of the bone determines the form of the soft tissue.

Hand instruments are typically used to refine and remove small amounts of bone immediately adjacent to the tooth. These hand instruments are generally kinder to the root surface than the burs. These can be sharp curettes or specialized-for-the-process instruments such as the Rhodes back action chisel.

Flap Stabilization

The flap can now be manually placed to verify that the flap design/incisions will allow the soft tissue to be placed where intended. Any minor reshaping of the flap can be done with curved scissors, scalpel, or other devices.

Stabilizing the flap in the intended position throughout the healing phase is one of the mandatory principles of surgical crown lengthening. Most of the stabilization is accomplished via sutures, the next topic. Suturing is commonly presented as a short statement—"and the flap is sutured in position"—giving the impression that it is a minor procedure all in dentistry intuitively know and understand. The realities are that the suturing techniques and to a lesser degree the type of suture used may determine the success and failure of the entire procedure.

Typically, the coronal portion of the flap is positioned and sutured first, and then any vertical incisions are closed. The reader should always remember that there is also an infinite variety of ways to accomplish the desired goal.

Suture Types

Dentists the world over have and do successfully use a wide variety of suture materials. What is used seems to be determined by availability and/or personal experience. The successful use of a specific suture material seems to be related more to technique than specific type. An explosion of different sutures made from many different materials make strict cataloging of sutures less precise than before. The categories presented in this section have many suture types that fit almost as neatly in one category as another. The following is presented as a guide more than a specific recommendation.

Absorbable (resorbable) sutures are either from synthetic or biologic sources. They offer the advantage of not needing to be removed and as a class show less irritation where they contact the tissue. They also show little tendency to wick bacteria into the surgical site. They may suffer from a dissolution either more or less rapid than wanted. A secure knot usually requires several reversing ties and sustained tension on the suture ends to prohibit the knot from unraveling (known as suture memory).

Nonresorbable sutures, of course, are those that require removal. This group includes such diverse materials as silk (perhaps the most used material worldwide), stainless steel, and a large group of synthetic formulations. Sutures such as silk are easy to tie and maintain the knot well without multiple ties. However, silk wicks significant bacteria into the suture penetration site, which can be a concern in thin tissues. The foregoing is meant to stimulate investigation into the various sutures available, how to use them in

clinical situations, and the relative merits of each. This, as with oral hygiene procedures, is an area that can enhance general surgical treatment when the proper choices are made.

Suturing Techniques

The gingival flap, whether split-thickness or full-thickness mucoperiosteal, must be held in an immobile position until it is biologically anchored to the underlying connective tissues or bone. This is the role of the suturing. As with the sutures themselves, several techniques can nicely accomplish this task. An experienced surgeon may use several different suturing methods in a single surgical site, thus emphasizing that there is likely no single universal method; only the proper application of techniques. The suturing methods that follow are those most likely to surface in a discussion of how to immobilize a soft tissue flap in crown lengthening procedures.

Single Interrupted

These are the simplest to use, consisting of a single penetration of the flap on the buccal surface, through the flap on the lingual, and then a single tie. They can nicely appose two flaps together or a flap to unreflected tissue for a full and tight closure. The single interrupted suture is also the most commonly used method to close any vertical releasing incision. The sutures may, however, cause bunching of the flap if pulled too tightly.

Vertical Mattress Suturing Technique

The vertical mattress suturing technique is a modification of a technique used in wound closure in medicine. In dentistry the presence of teeth necessitates modifying a medical technique that is designed solely for apposition of soft tissue. For most cases of crown lengthening, this is an invaluable suturing method because it apposes the mobile flaps toward each other and pulls the flap(s) downward toward the bone without bunching. This anchors the flap tightly against both the tooth and the underlying bone, thus minimizing excess tissue at the tissue-tooth interface. The vertical mattress suturing technique is likely the preferred method in suturing the areas immediately adjacent to a tooth.

It is slightly more difficult to learn than the single interrupted method but is well worth the learning. The accompanying diagram shows the basics visually (see Figure 5.24A and B).

A teaching dictum that the author has developed to go along with the visual diagram is stated as, "The suture goes from the 'outside to the inside' and from the 'inside to the outside' of the buccal flap, over the bone (which is interproximal if teeth are present), then from the 'outside to the inside' and then the 'inside to the outside' of the palatal/lingual flap. It then backtracks over the bone to tie at the starting point." If the tie is made close to the initial suture penetration point, then the flap is compressed to the bone without bunching the tissue up the tooth coronally.

Sling Suture

The sling suturing technique is used by many to allow the flap some vertical movement during normal functional healing. The theory is that the flap will assume a natural position relative to the muscle pull.

The flap is manually positioned, and then the suture from the outside flap is sutured to the inside flap, and a tie is made so that the suture itself limits the vertical extent of flap movement. This then allows both flaps some back-and-forth movement but is restricted by the suture.

A variation to the preceding is to place the suture through the flap, around the tooth, through the flap, around the tooth again, with a tie at the starting point (a true sling). In order to hold a flap in position

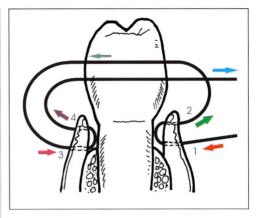

Figure 5-24A. Diagram of the author's vertical mattress suture technique to apically reposition buccal and lingual flaps used for surgical crown lengthening. This suture anchors the flaps tightly against both the tooth and the underlying bone.

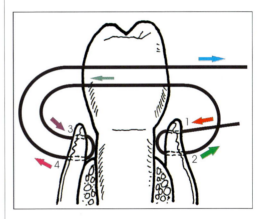

Figure 5-24B. Diagram of a vertical mattress suture that shows a variant of the one illustrated in Figure 5-24A.

with the sling methods, a periodontal dressing is frequently necessary.

Suture of Vertical Incisions

Generally the last areas of a flap to be closed are the vertical incisions (if created). Slight apical tension is placed in the area of the vertical incisions by pulling the lip or cheek apically with the same tension on either side of the incision. This then will bring the soft tissue lateral to the incision into a proper relation. While holding this position (either the doctor or an assistant), single interrupted sutures are placed along the length of the incision. Enough tension is placed on the suture during knot tying to appose the two halves of the flap so that they close tightly but without significant overlap or bunching. If the knot is tied without apical tension on the flap, then the tissues bunch together, forming scar tissue at maturity, which is at the same time a weakness in healing and an esthetic defect.

After the suturing is complete, the flap should be compressed against the tooth and underlying bone. Compression can be done with sustained digital pressure, gauze compresses, and/or ice packs. The intent of this compression is to express out excess blood and allow a fibrin clot to form with the bone. Failure to adequately compress the surgical site may lead to clot formation, delayed healing, and increased postoperative pain and infection.

POSTOPERATIVE CARE

Most flap surgeries should have antibiotic coverage. There is ample research and clinical evidence of the positive healing effects of antibiotics to justify its common usage.[25]

The most commonly used antibiotics that are backed by credible research are the penicillins and the tetracycline compound doxycycline. Whatever is prescribed is most effective when taken from one day to one hour prior to the procedure. This allows adequate time for the antibiotic to reach needed therapeutic blood levels before the surgical procedure. The amount prescribed should be sufficient for a minimum of five days, which matches healing studies and normal maturation of the flap procedure.[26]

Antimicrobial oral rinses can effectively control the bacteria on the exposed surface areas of the surgical site and should be considered postoperatively. Chlorhexidine (CHX) in all its formulations is considered as the most effective of oral rinses. At this writing it is considered the standard against which other rinses are compared.[27]

Calculus formation on hard surfaces and tooth staining are two worrying negative side effects of chlorhexidine (CHX) use. The author has long advocated the use of chlorhexidine postoperatively not as a full mouth rinse but as a topical application to the immediate surgical site only. CHX is topically applied with a cotton swab to the surgical area only twice daily. This puts the solution where it is needed and minimizes staining and calculus formation generally.

Periodontal dressings are used much less frequently now than in the past. Developed primarily to cover the large denuded surface areas of gingivectomies, periodontal dressings initially became a common part of the flap procedures. The bulk of the dressing, esthetic concerns, the clinical observation that the dressings attract bacterial plaque, and an overall feeling that they are not necessary have greatly reduced usage.[28] Most practitioners rely on suture stabilization to hold the flap in place and prefer to have the surgical area cleansed by oral rinses than to cover them with a surgical dressing.

Ice packs can be applied to the surgical site to reduce overall swelling and also lessen postoperative pain. The ice packs should be applied as much as possible in a sustained manner for the first 24 to 48 hours. The cold from the pack not only reduces edema as indicated previously but also allows the patient to apply sustained positive pressure over the surgical area.

Food intake should be altered as the surgery dictates. For localized crown lengthenings the patient may not have to change much in the dietary intake; simply be careful during chewing. For more extensive surgeries, a softer diet and counseling about diet may be appropriate. It is well established that an increase in fluid intake is a necessity postsurgically.

Suture Removal

Sutures are removed in one or two weeks, dependant upon the overall healing and the technique performed. The most common time is at one week. After suture removal, CXH can be continued for one additional week, and then normal oral hygiene methods are initiated, or if healing is advanced, normal brushing and flossing immediately follows. The important point is to control the bacteria postsurgically for optimum healing.

Postsurgical Complications

The well-known adage "the best cure is prevention" applies particularly well to surgical procedures of all types in the oral cavity. It is well documented that the more experienced one is surgically, the fewer are the complications. Nevertheless, a small percentage of the cases do have some complications. Some of the most common are presented in this section with preventive methods listed and management for when they do occur.

Hemorrhage

A small amount of bleeding occurs in most flap procedures. It is best prevented by precise surgical incisions and suture techniques designed to tightly close the vertical releasing incisions (perhaps the most common site of prolonged hemorrhage) and sustained positive pressure immediately after the surgery. Gauze compresses can be placed in the surgical area and the patient instructed to compress the site with ice packs for the first few hours.

If there is a recurrence of bleeding in spite of the preceding, then the patient should be seen, and blood clots that may have formed under the flap removed with gentle suction and positive pressure reapplied. Infrequently the area may need to be resutured.

Infections

As a prevention, antibiotics should be initiated before the surgical procedure. When infections do occur in spite of the above, the dentist should ascertain as much as possible the underlying cause(s) and initiate corrective procedures. Surgical debris left under the flap, prolonged hemorrhage with clot formation and infection, and reduced patient systemic healing capacities are the most frequent issues.

Most of these can be managed by gentle irrigation of the surgical site and either continued antibiotic usage or changing to an antibiotic better suited to controlling the bacteria. The goal should be not only to correct the problem but also to prevent cellulitis, which is an infection that enters normal body cavities and spaces and that may require a regimen of intravenous antibiotics.

Pain

Several studies in medicine and dentistry have demonstrated the effectiveness of analgesics taken prior to the surgery, usually one hour prior. The modus operandi is that it is easier to prevent pain than to play catch up.

This subject requires an intimate understanding of the various analgesics and how to use them. Each patient is likely to be distinctly different in their reaction to pain. Some insight into this can be learned by questioning the patient before the surgery about what they have used for other surgeries.

Healing Time before Restorative Procedures

How long one should wait after a flap surgery before initiating restorative procedures is an oft-debated topic. There are several considerations, all dependent on actual clinical healing and on research studies. Most histologic studies have noted the presence of a mature epithelial surface and a well-defined biologic width at four weeks postsurgery (assuming normal healing).[19] Bone remodeling after osseous contouring or resection in crown lengthening can continue for up to six months postoperatively.

The most frequent time table for healing after flap surgery and before restorative procedures is six weeks or greater.[26] However, Kois indicated that it may take nearly three years in some patients for a stable gingival environment to form.[27]

The realities for the restorative dentist are the formation and maturation of a stable sulcus. Unless there is adequate sulcus depth, impression techniques and tooth preparation may once again impinge on the biologic width, thus negating the effect of the crown lengthening. Restorative procedures beginning before the gingival site is healthy and mature may lead to gingival recession in thin tissue or inflammatory pocketing in thick tissue. A mature surgical site after flap procedures can take additional time beyond that described previously and is very case dependant. The best guide is to wait as long beyond six weeks (mandatory minimum) as the situation will allow. The considerations listed previously are for a flap procedure only, the gingivectomy having a generally shorter healing time frame.

Surgical Crown Lengthening Summary

This chapter has dealt with both diagnostic and treatment fundamentals of surgical crown lengthening. The intent has been to provide a clinically practical background that will allow the practitioner to use the fundamentals and modify them for the individual cases. The assumption has been that the more complex things are, the more important are the basics. An almost infinite variety of treatment methods is available to the dental practitioner who understands the underlining principles.

As one explores the relationship between the tooth and the biologic width, one discovers many individual variations. These variations then require the dentist to modify the surgical approach.[28]

Surgical crown lengthening is still one of the underutilized procedures in dentistry. Granted that new dental materials and techniques have reduced the number of teeth requiring crown lengthening before restorative procedures, there are still many teeth that are compromised for lack of crown lengthening. By indicating the relative simplicity and predictability of crown lengthening, this is a call to use the procedures more frequently where indicated.

Finally, a more conservative crown lengthening procedure has been presented. This is one that uses the body's natural resorption of bone in most cases to provide the needed vertical height for the attachment fibers. This then allows a bone conservative/preservative approach to crown lengthening surgeries.

Bibliography

1. H. Sicher. Changing concepts of the supporting dental structures. *Oral Surgery Oral Medicine Oral Pathology* 12: 31–35. 1959.

2. A. Gargiulo, F. Wentz, B. Orban. Dimensions and relations of the dentogingival junction in humans. *Journal of Periodontology* 32: 261. 1961.

3. J. S. Vacek, M. E. Gher, D. A. Assad, et al. The dimensions of the human dentogingival junction. *International Journal of Periodontology and Restorative Dentistry* 14(2): 155. 1994.

4. B. D. Wagenberg. Surgical tooth lengthening: Biologic variables and esthetic concerns. *Journal of Esthetic Dentistry* 10(1): 30–36. 1998.

5. A. B. Wade. The relation between the pocket base, the epithelial attachment and the alveolar process. *Les Parodontopathies*. 16th ARPA Congress, Vienna, 1960.

6. G. C. Armitage. Periodontal diseases: Diagnosis. *Annual of Periodontology* 1: 37. 1996.

7. J. M. Goodson, A. D. Haffajee, S. S. Socransky. The relationship between attachment level loss and alveolar bone loss. *Journal of Clinical Periodontology* 11: 348. 1984.

8. M. K. Jeffcoat, I. C. Wang, M. S. Reddy. Radiographic diagnosis in periodontics. *Periodontology* 7: 54. 2000, 1995.

9. G. Dahlen, J. Lindhe, K. Sato, H. Hanamura, H. Okamoto. The effect of supragingival plaque control on the subgingival microbiota in subjects with periodontal disease. *Journal of Clinical Periodontology* 19: 802–809. 1992.

10. T. Katsanoulas, I. Renee, R. Allstrom. The effect of supragingival plaque control on the composition of the subgingival flora in periodontal pockets. *Journal of Clinical Periodontology* 19: 760.

11. E. F. Corbet, W. I. Davies. The role of supragingival plaque in the control of progressive periodontal disease: A review. *Journal of Clinical Periodontology* 20: 307. 1993

12. N. P. Lang, B. R. Cumming, H. Low. Toothbrushing frequency as it relates to plaque development and gingival health. *Journal of Periodontology* 44: 396–405. 1973.

13. H. Loe, E. Theilade, S. B. Jensen. Experimental gingivitis in man. *Journal of Periodontology* 177. 1965.

14. H. C. Sullivan, J. H. Atkins. Autogenous gingival grafts. *Periodontics* 6: 5–13. 1968.

15. A. Diamanti-Kipioti, F. Gusberti, N. Lang. Clinical and microbiological effects of fixed orthodontic appliances. *Journal of Clinical Periodontology* 14: 326. 1987.

16. M. Paolantonio, G. Girolamo, V. Pedrazzoli, et al. Occurrence of actinobaccillus actinomycetem comitans in patients wearing orthodontic appliances: A cross-sectional study. *Journal of Clinical Periodontology* 23: 112. 1996

17. I. Glickman, M. Lewitus. Hyperplasia of the gingiva associated with Dilantin (sodium dipheryl hydantoinate) therapy. *Journal of the American Dental Association* 28. 1941, 1991

18. T. D. Daley, G. P. Wysocki, C. Day. Clinical and pharmacologic correlations in cyclosporine-induced gingival hyperplasia. *Oral Surgery* 62: 417. 1986

19. D. Lederman, H. Lummerman, S. Reuben, et al. Gingival hyperplasia associated with nifedipine therapy. *Oral Surgery* 57: 620. 1984.

20. B. J. Russel, L. M. Bay. Oral use of chlorhexidine gluconate toothpaste in epileptic children. *Scandinavian Journal of Dental Research* 86: 52. 1978.

21. F. A. Carranza, E. L. Hogan. Gingival enlargement. M. G. Newman (ed.). *Clinical Periodontology,* ed. 9. Philadelphia, PA: Saunders. 2002.

22. G. Stanton, M. Levy, S. S. Stahl. Collagen restoration in healing human gingiva. *Journal of Dental Restorations* 48: 27. 1969.

23. T. N. Sims, W. Ammons. Resective osseous surgery. M. G. Newman MG (ed.). *Clinical Periodontology,* ed. 9. Philadelphia, PA: Saunders. 2002.

24. R. G. Caffesse, S. P. Ramfjord, C. E. Nasjleti. Reverse bevel periodontal flaps in monkeys. *Journal of Periodontology* 39: 219. 1968.

25. J. Kois. Altering gingival levels: The restorative connection. Part 1: Biologic variables. *Journal of Esthetic Dentistry* 6: 3. 1994.

26. J. M. Goodson, A. D. Haffajee, S. S. Socransky. The relationship between attachment level loss and alveolar bone loss. *Journal of Clinical Periodontology* 11: 348. 1984

27. W. Becker, C. Ochsenbein, E. Becker. Crown lengthening: The periodontal-restorative connection. *Complete Continuing Education in Dentistry* 19: 239–254. 1998.

28. A. B. Wade. The relation between the pocket base, the epithelial attachment and the alveolar process. *Les Parodontopathies,* 16th ARPA Congress, Vienna, 1960.

Chapter 6

Endodontic Periradicular Microsurgery

Dr. Louay Abrass

Introduction

In the past decade the field of endodontics has seen numerous advances, the scope of which have reached all facets of endodontic treatment in both conventional and surgical aspects. These technological advances have introduced new instruments and materials that did not exist before and revolutionized the way endodontic treatment is performed. This change could not be more evident than in the field of surgical endodontics, where both theoretical and practical aspects have completely transformed. The purpose of this chapter is to present to the surgical-minded general dentist the current standards and techniques in performing apical surgery with evidence-based rationales.

Problems with Traditional Endodontic Surgery

Traditional apical surgery is viewed as an invasive, difficult, and less successful procedure than conventional endodontic treatment. Many reasons contribute to this, examples of which include working on a conscious patient in an area with restricted access, limitations in visibility, and operating on minuscule microstructures that are often obscured by bleeding. To manage these challenges, operators had to prepare large osteotomies to gain sufficient access that would accommodate the large surgical instruments that were traditionally utilized. This unnecessary removal of healthy buccal bone structure sometimes resulted in incomplete healing. The root apex was routinely resected with a 45-degree bevel angle with no biological or clinical imperative. Such a practice was performed merely to allow visualization of root canal anatomy and to facilitate retropreparation and retrofilling. This steep-bevel angle root resection created more problems than solutions. It exposed more dentinal tubules, which translated into an increase in apical leakage.[1, 2] In addition, this method sacrificed more periodontal support of the buccal root surface, shortening the distance between the base of the gingival sulcus and the osteotomy site. This further predisposed the tooth for an endodontic-periodontal communication. This resection technique also frequently resulted in an incomplete root resection in which the root apex was merely beveled rather than excised and in which the lingual aspect of the root was never resected. Surgeons thus neglected to eliminate apical ramifications and lateral canals and failed to identify more lingually situated additional canals.[3,4] Finally, it produced a distorted and elongated view of the internal root canal anatomy that makes it harder to clearly and accurately identify and treat the apical anatomy. Figure 6.1 illustrates most of the common problems associated with conventional apical surgery and how microsurgical techniques can address and correct these deficiencies.

Comparison of Traditional Surgery to Microsurgery

Introduction of the surgical operating microscope and ultrasonics paved the way in changing how endodontic surgery is per-

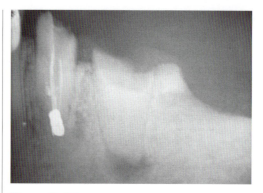

Figure 6-1B. Due to failure of previous treatment and restorability issues extraction was recommended.

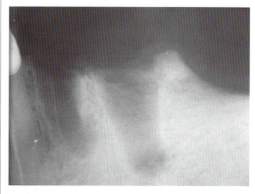

Figure 6-1C. Socket after extraction.

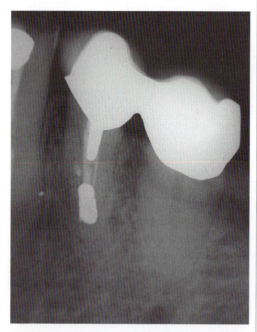

Figure 6-1A. Radiograph of tooth #21 with conventional apicoectomy and amalgam retrograde filling that appears to be well centered within the root parameter. (All figures in 6–1 are of tooth #21).

formed (see Figures 6.2 and 6.3). The microscope provides illumination and magnification of the surgical site where it is most needed. The ultrasonic tips allow a coaxial preparation of the root canal system to a depth of 3 mm that provides an optimum apical seal.[1] These two advances led to the miniaturization of surgical instruments. The net result of all the previously mentioned developments revolutionalized the traditional technique into a more precise method—an apical surgery with minimal healthy bone removal and a conservative shallow-bevel angle root resection. This transformation allows periradicular surgery to be performed on a solid biological and clinical basis.

ENDODONTIC PERIRADICULAR MICROSURGERY

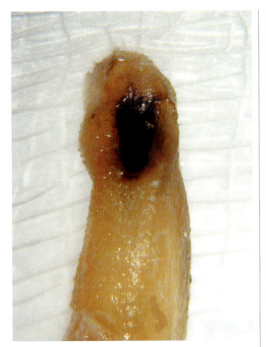

Figure 6-1D. Buccal view of extracted tooth. Amalgam retrograde is visible.

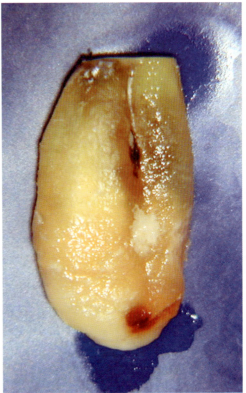

Figure 6-1F. Shows 0-degree bevel root resection that eliminates the apical 3mm of the root.

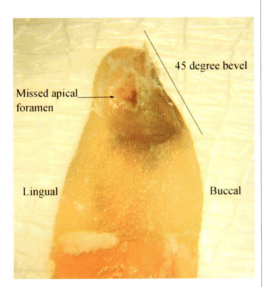

Figure 6-1E. Proximal view that shows the 45-degree bevel with incomplete root resection and failure to eliminate apical ramifications.

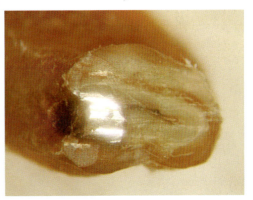

Figure 6-1G. Microscopic inspection of the resected root surface reveals the buccally situated amalgam, the untreated lingual canal, and the missed isthmus.

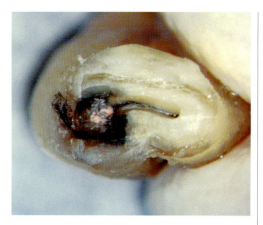

Figure 6-1H. Ultrasonic retropreparation of 3 mm depth that includes buccal and lingual canals and the connecting isthmus.

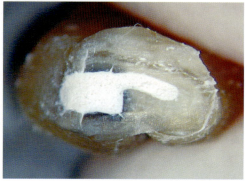

Figure 6-1I. Super EBA retrograde filling.

The Need for Endodontic Surgery

The success rate of endodontic treatment varies and has been reported to be as high as 94.8 percent or as low as 53 percent (see Figure 6.4). This variability stems from many factors, such as the type of study, sample size, pulpal and periapical status, follow-up period, and number of treatment visits. Conventional retreatment has a lower success rate that ranges between 48 percent and 84 percent (see Figure 6.5). One important fact remains—a certain percentage of failures will be encountered even when the root canal treatment has been carried out to the highest quality. The following etiological factors explain why some conventional endodontic treatments fail and eventually necessitate surgical intervention.

ANATOMICAL FACTORS

Careful examination of the root canal system reveals enormous complexities such as accessory canals, C-shaped canals, fins, and isth-

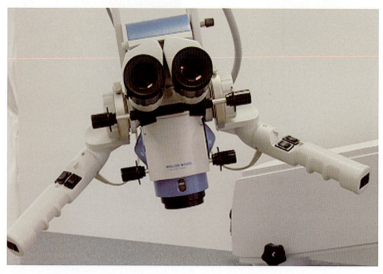

Figure 6-2. The surgical operating microscope.

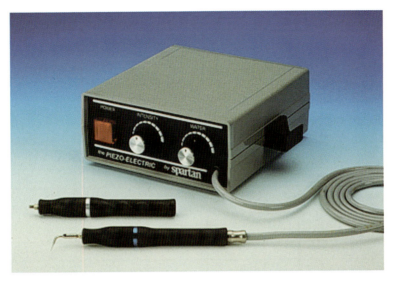

Figure 6-3A. The ultrasonic unit by Spartan.

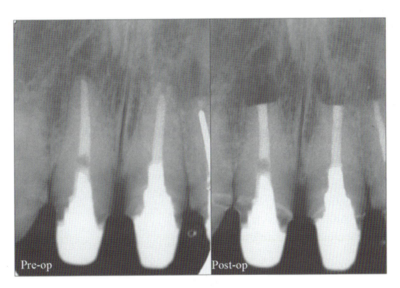

Figure 6-3B. An ideal case of periradicualr microsurgery; note the 0-degree bevel angle root resection and the coaxial retropreparation.

muses (see Figure 6.6). These microstructures are more abundant in the apical one-third of the root[5, 6] and are farthest away from the operator's control. By providing a safe haven for bacteria from biomechanical instrumentation, these anatomical complexities can impair the treatment outcome in cases in which the pulp space is infected. This contributes to the lower success rate of endodontic treatment in infected cases.

BACTERIOLOGICAL FACTORS

Posttreatment apical periodontitis is caused by microbial infection that persists either in the intraradicular space or in the extraradicular area. Certain bacteria, such as *E. faecalis*, can withstand antibacterial measures, survive a restricted nutritional environment, and exist in the root canal as a single type of bacteria.[7] Although extraradicular infection has

Conventional Endodontic Success Rate

Author/Year	# of cases	Follow-up (yr)	Success %
Strindberg 1956	529	4	87
Seltzer et al 1963	2921	0.5	80
Bender et al 1964	706	2	82
Grossman et al 1964	432	1-5	90
Ingle 1965	1229	2	91.5
Jokinen et al 1978	1304	2-7	53
Pekruhn 1986	925	1	94.8
Ray et al 1995	1010	1 and up	61.1

Figure 6-4. This table presents a summary and a comparison of multiple studies of conventional endodontic success rates. It clearly demonstrates that a 100 percent success rate is not achievable.

a lower prevalence than that of root canal infection, it could, nonetheless, be the etiological factor behind therapy-resistant apical periodontitis.[8] Additional studies have shown that bacteria such as actinomyces israelii[9, 10] and arachnia propionica[11] can survive in the periapical tissue. Some can even invade periapical cementum.[12]

HISTOLOGICAL FACTORS

A nonmicrobial source of endodontic failure is the presence of periapical cysts, which represent up to 15 percent of all periupical lesions.[13, 14] Periapical cysts exist in two structurally distinct classes: periapical true cysts and pocket cysts.[15] Pocket cysts contain epithelium-lined cavities that are open to the root canals. These can heal following nonsurgical root canal therapy. On the other hand, true cysts are less likely to heal without surgical intervention.

Case Selection

When an endodontic treatment fails, clinicians ought to carefully investigate to reveal the true etiology behind the failure. It is of great importance to reach a sound diagnosis, leading to a treatment plan that would address the disease rather than just the symptoms (see Figure 6.7).

In assessing a previously root canal–treated tooth, the following three factors should be evaluated: 1) quality of previous endodontic treatment, 2) quality of coronal restoration, and 3) accessibility to the canals. Conventional retreatment should always be considered first. Surgical retreatment should be considered when access to canals is impossible or when the current endodontic treatment and coronal restoration seem to be of an adequate quality (see Figure 6.8).

Failures associated with silver points pose another challenging situation. Failing silver points usually present with gross leakage and

Conventional Retreatment Success Rate

Study	Follow-up (yr)	Success rate (%)
Strindberg (1956)	4	66
	7	84
Molven & Halse (1988)	10-17	71
Bergenholtz et al (1979)	2	48
Allen et al (1989)	0.5-1	73
Sjogren et al (1990)	8-10	62
Sundqvist et al (1998)	5	74

Figure 6-5. This table summarizes the results of different studies in regard to conventional endodontic retreatment success rates. It clearly demonstrates the lower success rate associated with endodontic retreatment cases.

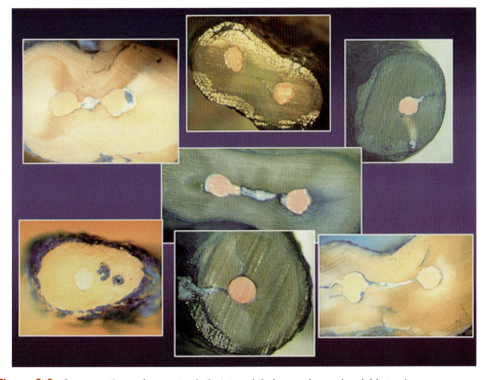

Figure 6-6. Cross sections of some teeth that reveal their complex and variable anatomy.

143

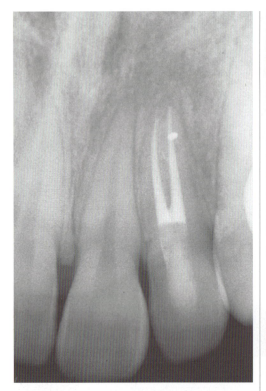

Figure 6-7A. A radiograph of a rare two-rooted maxillary lateral incisor with previous endodontic treatment. Patient presented with severe spontaneous pain and tenderness to percussion.

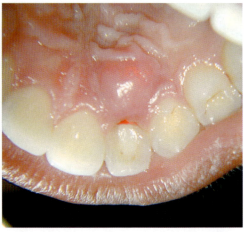

Figure 6-7B. Clinical examination reveals localized palatal swelling.

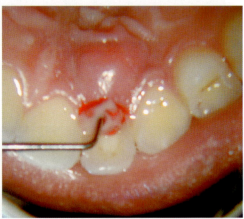

Figure 6-7C. Periodontal examination shows a 12-mm probing on the palatal surface associated with a purulent discharge; the diagnosis is periodontal abscess associated with a palatal developmental groove.

corrosion byproducts. Surgical treatment can only marginally address these problems. Since it is extremely difficult to adequately retroprepare and retrofill the canals to provide a good apical seal, every effort should be made to re-treat these cases and to avoid surgery at any cost (see Figure 6.9).

INDICATIONS

There are several reasons why this surgery should be performed. The operator should consider these indications and then either perform the surgery or refer the patient to someone who will perform the procedure according to current accepted standards.

Failure of Previous Endodontic Therapy

When previous endodontic treatment seems to be of an adequate quality and/or retreatment has already been attempted without further success, periradicular surgery becomes rightly indicated (see Figure 6.10).

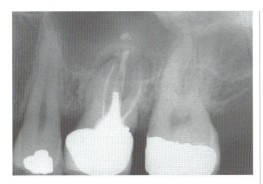

Figure 6-8A. A preoperative radiograph of tooth #14 that has a failing inadequate endodontic treatment. Close examination reveals the untreated second mesiobuccal (MB) root and an ill-fitting crown.

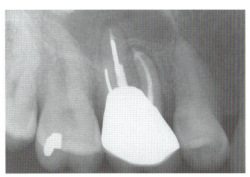

Figure 6-9B. Localized conventional retreatment of the MB root is performed to address the pathology without compromising the crown.

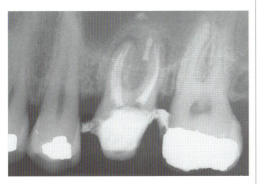

Figure 6-8B. Crown removal and conventional retreatment are performed; the second mesiobuccal and second distiobuccal canals are localized and treated.

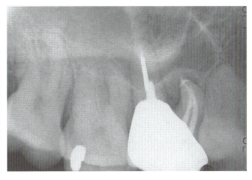

Figure 6-9C. An angulated radiograph showing the two treated mesiobuccal canals.

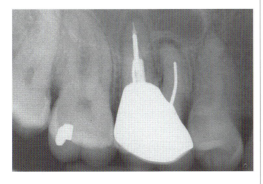

Figure 6-9A. Tooth #3 that has a previous endodontic treatment with silver points and has a new crown of good quality. A symptomatic periapical lesion is limited to the MB root only.

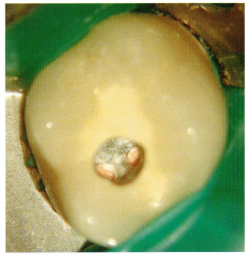

Figure 6-9D. The microscopic access needed to perform the retreatment.

145

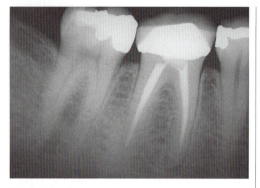

Figure 6-10A. Failing inadequate root canal treatment.

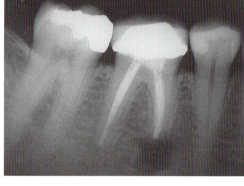

Figure 6-10D. Apical surgery performed.

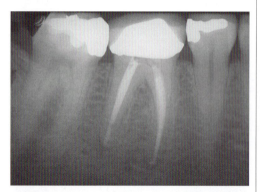

Figure 6-10B. Conventional retreatment performed.

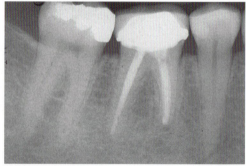

Figure 6-10E. Two-year recall demonstrates complete healing.

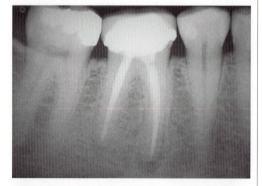

Figure 6-10C. Retreatment failed again after two years.

Failure of Previous Apical Surgery

Clinicians should not hesitate to perform apical microsurgery on previously failed apicoectomies. This is especially true when it is evident that the previous surgery was inadequate or not performed according to the current standards of care (see Figure 6.11). In these cases, it is common to discover an incompletely resected apex with malpositioned retrofilling material that is mostly placed outside the root canal parameter. Thorough presentation of such deficiencies was covered in a previous section of this chapter.

Iatrogenic Factors

Procedural mishaps can occur during the course of endodontic treatment. Examples include canal transportation, perforation, ledge formation, blockage, or separated instruments (see Figure 6.12). These complications are likely to result in incomplete

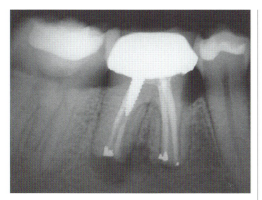

Figure 6-11A. Failed previous surgery where both mesiolingual (ML) and distolingual (DL) roots were not resected nor retroprepared.

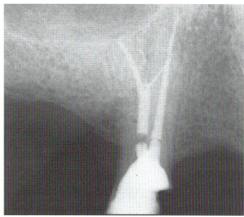

Figure 6-12A. Separated file in the MB root of tooth 12.

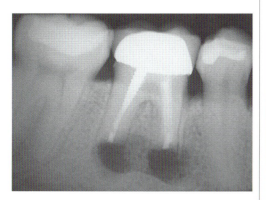

Figure 6-11B. Complete root resection with minimum bevel angle and 3 mm retrofilling.

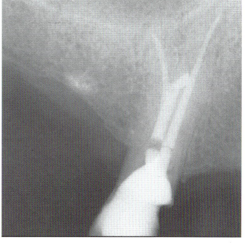

Figure 6-12B. Instrument removed and canal retrofilled.

biomechanical debridement and a compromised apical seal. Cases involving mishaps in the apical one-third of the canal are good candidates for apical surgery. However, if the error is located in the middle to coronal one-third of the root canal, then alternative approaches should be considered.

Anatomical Deviations

Teeth can present with challenging root anatomy that complicates endodontic therapy and compromises complete debridement. Common examples include canal calcifications, blunderbuss apices, S- and C-shaped canals, and severe root curvatures.

The case illustrated in Figure 6.13 shows a maxillary lateral incisor that presents with dens-in-dente, canal calcification, and a blunderbuss apex. Conventional endodontic therapy was initially performed. Despite the fact that the canal was localized and treated, it was still difficult to establish an apical seal due to the large, divergent, and irregular apical foramen. Microsurgery was performed to remove the gross overfill and to establish a precise apical seal.

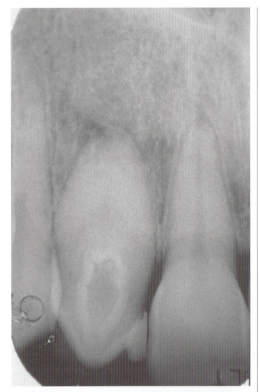

Figure 6-13A. Tooth #7 presented with dens-in-dente, canal calcification, and a blunderbuss apex.

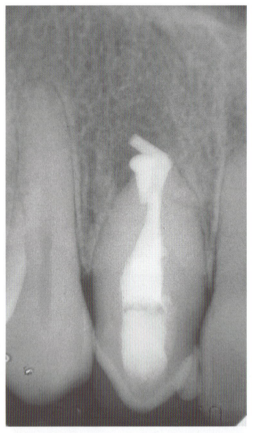

Figure 6-13B. A gross overfill of gutta-percha was difficult to avoid due to the large, irregular, and divergent walls of this blunderbuss apex.

Contraindications

Of the few contraindications to endodontic surgery, only some are absolute. The majority of these conditions are only temporary and can either be corrected or managed by a knowledgeable surgeon. These contraindications can be categorized as dental, anatomical, and medical. The following sections will present each category in detail.

Tooth-Specific Factors

The restorability and the periodontal health of a tooth are important factors in planning treatment and determining a prognosis. Probing depth and mobility should be carefully assessed before surgery. Another concern is the clinical crown-root ratio the tooth exhibits. Apical surgery on a short-rooted tooth with significant attachment loss will further compromise the crown-root ratio (see Figure 6.14). Moreover, such a course of treatment could result in an endodontic/periodontic communication, compromising the overall outcome of the surgery and leading to eventual tooth loss. In these situations, conventional retreatment should be considered if it is feasible. Otherwise, extraction may be the best solution.

Anatomical Factors

The Inferior Alveolar Nerve

The location of the mandibular canal and the mental foramen should be carefully as-

ENDODONTIC PERIRADICULAR MICROSURGERY   149

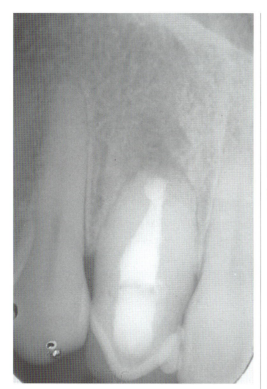

Figure 6-13C. Surgical correction of the overfill and the establishment of a precise apical seal using microsurgical techniques. The canal was retroprepared using surgical ultrasonic tip and then retrofilled with super EBA.

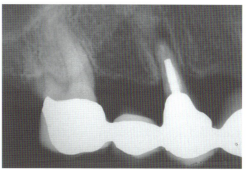

Figure 6-14. A radiograph of tooth #4 that has a poor crown-root ratio and a moderate attachment loss. Apical surgery is contraindicated.

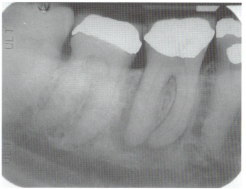

Figure 6-15. A radiograph that reveals the close proximity of the mandibular nerve and the mental foramen to the apices of teeth #29, 30, and 31. Apical surgery can be risky, and therefore, it might be contraindicated in certain cases to avoid permanent paresthesia.

sessed prior to surgery in the posterior mandible. The use of a microscope facilitates easy identification of the neurovascular bundle. The added magnification also assists in the preparation of the groove technique (a shallow horizontal groove in bone), a measure that prevents unintentional instrument slippage and avoids permanent nerve damage. However, in certain cases the extreme proximity of the neurovascular bundle could render the procedure risky and, therefore, contraindicated (see Figure 6.15).

The Maxillary Sinus

The apices of maxillary molar and premolar teeth can be in close proximity to the floor of the sinus (see Figure 6.16). In some in-

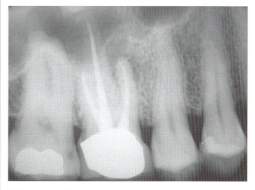

Figure 6-16. This radiograph demonstrates the close proximity of the maxillary sinus to the apices of the teeth in that quadrant.

stances, the apices are located inside the sinus. A watchful examination of preoperative radiographs, coupled with careful surgical dissection under magnification, will minimize the chances of sinus membrane perforation.

When sinus membrane is inadvertently perforated, if meticulous surgical techniques and proper postoperative care were employed, the outcome of apical surgery will not be compromised and complications are usually minimal.[16]

Barrier placement is recommended to block the perforation area during the surgery and to ensure that foreign material or even a resected apex does not enter the sinus.[17] Telfa pads (Kendall Company, Mansfield, MA) are excellent materials to use as a sinus barrier (see Figure 6.17). They can be cut to fit the perforation size, and they contain no cotton fibers that could contaminate the surgical field. To prevent the Telfa pad from getting dislodged into the sinus cavity, a suture is tied through its center, which will keep the barrier in place throughout the surgery and will allow the operator to easily pull the barrier out at the end of the surgery. In addition, patients should be prescribed an antibiotic (1 g amoxicillin immediately following the perforation, continued with 500 mg tid for 24 hours) and a nasal decongestant for five days.

The Second Mandibular Molar Area

The mandibular second molar presents many difficult obstacles for apical surgery. Due to a thick buccal cortex of bone, lingually inclined roots, and close proximity of the apices to the mandibular canal, these teeth are usually poor candidates for surgery. In addition, as the far distal location in the dental arch impedes easy access, surgery becomes nearly impossible. For mandibular second molars, an alternative approach to surgery should be considered, such as retreatment or replantation.

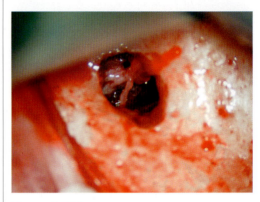

Figure 6-17A. Sinus perforation.

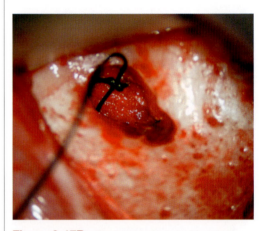

Figure 6-17B. Barrier placement with suture.

Medical Factors

A thorough review of a patient's medical history is of paramount importance. All medical concerns and questions should be answered prior to surgery. There are a few medical conditions that contraindicate endodontic surgery, such as clotting deficiencies, brittle diabetes, dialysis, and compromised immune system. With certain other medical conditions, endodontic surgery should be postponed until the condition is treated or stabilized and no longer presents any risk to the patient. Good examples include recent myocardial infarction, radiation therapy, anticoagulant medications, and first

ENDODONTIC PERIRADICULAR MICROSURGERY

and third trimesters of pregnancy. The decision for surgery should be evaluated on a case-by-case basis and in consultation with the patient's physician.

The Surgeon's Skill and Ability

One very important factor in case selection is the surgeon's level of knowledge and experience. Clinicians should carefully assess the difficulty of each case and decide who is best suited to perform the procedure. Challenging cases should be referred to

endodontists or oral surgeons with microsurgical expertise.

Armamentarium

A basic endodontic surgery kit should contain the most commonly used instruments to perform periradicular surgical procedures. Key instruments and materials with their general use are listed in Table 6.1. The surgical kit should be supplemented with the following instruments and devices to perform apical microsurgery.

Table 6-1. Surgical Kit

Examination Instruments
Mirror, endodontic explorer, and periodontal probe

Soft Tissue Incision, Elevation, and Reflection
15C blade
Microblades
Periosteal elevators (Howard, #9 Molt, and #149)
Kim/Pecora retractors 1 through 4 (Hartzell & Sons, Inc.)
Tissue forceps

Osteotomy and Root Resection Instruments
Impact Air 45 handpiece
H 161 Lindemann bone cutting bur (Brasseler, Inc.)
Surgical-length round burs

Curettage Instruments
Small endodontic spoon curette
Periodontal curette (Columbia 13/14)
34/35 Jaquette and Mini-Jaquette scalers
#2/4 Molt curette

Inspection Instruments
Micromirrors (5 mm round and modified rectangular)

Root-end Preparation Instruments
Ultrasonic unit (Spartan or Miniendo)
Surgical ultrasonic tips (KiS 1 through 6, BK3-R and BK3-L, or CT tips)

Root-end Filling/Finishing Instruments
Retrofilling carrier (West carrier)
MTA pellet forming block with KM-3/Km-4 placement instruments (Hartzell & Son, Inc.)
Micropluggers and ball burnishers
Polishing burs

Suturing and Soft Tissue Closure
Castroviejo needle holder
Surgical scissors
Various suture types and sizes (5-0 and 6-0)
Sterile gauze for soft tissue compression

Miscellaneous Instruments and Materials
Surgical aspirator
Irrigation syringes and needles
Stropko irrigator/drier with disposable micortip (Ultradent, Inc.) Cut-Trol (50% ferric sulfate)
Super EBA (Bosworth,Inc.)
MTA (ProRoot by Dentsply/Tulsa, Inc.)
Racellet #3 epinephrine cotton pellet (Pascal Company, Inc.)
Methylene blue stain (Fisher Scientific, Inc.)
Microapplicator tips (Quick Tips by Worldwide Dental, Inc.)

Surgical Operating Microscope

The microscope is defined as an instrument that gives an enlarged image of an object or substance that is minute or not visible with the naked eye. The incorporation of the operating microscope into apical surgery carries great benefits simply by providing illumination and magnification to a small surgical field. This will translate clinically into a more precise and conservative surgical procedure with minimal guesswork. It will also allow accurate assessment and excision of all pathological changes with very conservative removal of healthy structures. For the first time, the resected root surface can be clearly inspected for any anatomical complexities or microfractures.

Every microscope contains the following components: eyepieces, binoculars, objective lens, and the magnification changer (see Figure 6.18). Magnification is determined by the power of the eyepieces (M_e), the focal length of the binoculars (f_t), the magnification changer factor (M_c), and the focal length of the objective length (f_0). Total magnification can be calculated using the following equation:

$$\text{Total Magnification } M_t = f_t/f_0 + M_e + M_c$$

Recommended settings for surgical operating microscope in endodontics are ×12.5 eyepieces, five-step magnification changer, 200–250 mm objective length, and 60 degrees or more inclinable binoculars.

Incorporating the microscope into general dentistry practice is costly and initially will slow the operator's speed due to the nature of the learning curve. However, it is the single most important element in performing apical surgery up to the current standards. The use of magnifying loupes with an added fiber optic headlamp is helpful, but it is only the minimum requirement in performing apical surgery. Loupes can only provide a 2×

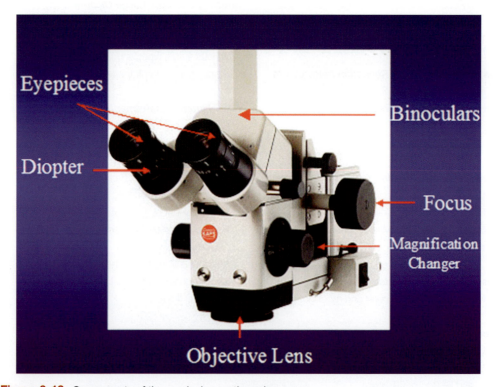

Figure 6-18. Components of the surgical operating microscope.

to 6× range of magnification, which is marginally useful in anterior surgery. In surgeries involving posterior teeth, the microscope is absolutely essential due to restricted access, limited visibility, and far more complicated root anatomy.

The surgical microscope, in contrast to loupes, provides a wide range of magnification from ×3 to ×30. The lower range of magnification (×3 to ×8) provides a wider field of view and a high focal depth, which is practical for orientation. The middle range of magnification (×10 to ×16) is the working range, which provides adequate enlargement of the surgical field to perform most of the surgical steps. The highest range of magnification (×20 to ×30) is only used for fine inspection of the resected root surface. It has a shallow focal depth, and the focus can easily be affected by the slightest movement, such as the breathing of the patient.

MICROSURGICAL INSTRUMENTS

Many microsurgical instruments are miniaturized versions of traditional surgical instruments. Other instruments are specifically invented and designed to perform apical microsurgery.

The following is a list of microsurgical instruments and their general uses:

Microblades. A 15C blade is the blade of choice in most surgical procedures. However, when the interproximal spaces are tight, such as the anterior mandibular area, a microblade becomes more useful and will precisely incise the flap without any tissue damage.

Micromirrors. A large variety of micromirrors are available on the market in different materials, shapes, and sizes. Only two micromirrors are needed, a round shape (5 mm in diameter), and a modified rectangular (see Figure 6.19). Both can be purchased in stainless steel, sapphire, or diamond mirror surfaces. The sapphire and

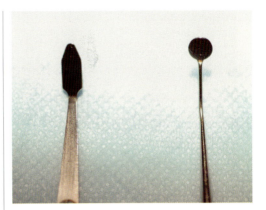

Figure 6-19. Modified rectangular and round micromirrors.

diamond micromirrors have scratch-free surfaces and are brighter than stainless ones. They are also more costly.

Ultrasonic units and tips. The introduction of the ultrasonic units and tips has replaced the traditional use of microhandpieces. The two most widely used ultrasonic units are the Miniendo II (Analytic/SybronEndo) and the Spartan (Spartan/Obtura) (see Figure 6.3).

There are many different ultrasonic tips available on the market, but the three most popular are the KiS, CT, and BK3 (see Figures 6.20–6.22). All three types are very effective and precise; however, they vary in material, tip angulation, and design. The size of these tips is 1/10 the size of a conventional microhead handpiece. CT and BK3 tips are made of stainless steel, and they are also available with a diamond coating that improves their cutting efficiency.

The BK3 tips come in a set of two (BK3-R right, BK3-L left), and each tip has three bends that facilitate easy access to any preparation. BK3 right is designed for use in the upper right and lower left, and BK3 left is designed for use in the upper left and lower right.

The KiS ultrasonic tips come in a set of six different tips, all of which are coated with

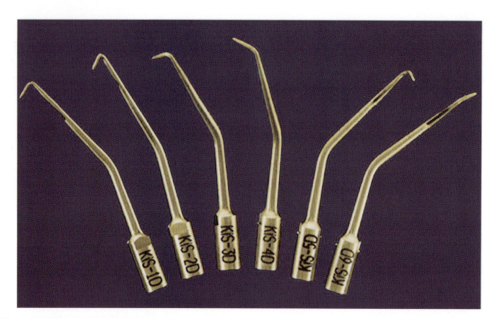

Figure 6-20. KiS ultrasonic tips.

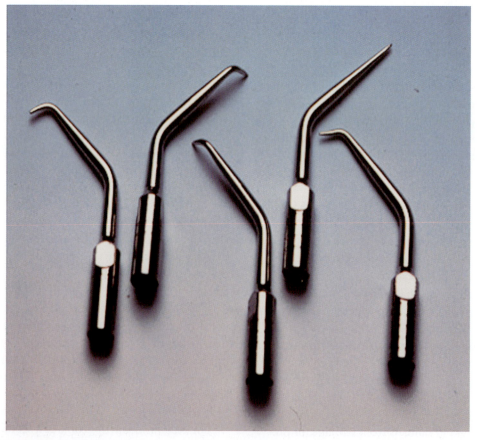

Figure 6-21. CT ultrasonic tips.

ENDODONTIC PERIRADICULAR MICROSURGERY

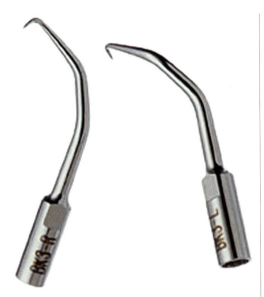

Figure 6-22. BK3 tips.

zirconium nitride for smoother and more efficient cutting. The irrigation port is located close to the 3-mm cutting tip. The KiS 1 tip has an 80-degree angled tip and is 0.24 mm in diameter. This thin-diameter tip is ideal for apical preparation on mandibular anteriors and premolars. The KiS 2 tip has a wider diameter and is ideal for wider preparation such as with maxillary anteriors. The KiS 3 tip has a double bend and a 70-degree angled tip. It is helpful in reaching the maxillary left and mandibular right posteriors. The KiS 4 tip is similar to the KiS 3 tip except that the tip angle is 110 degrees, which is designed to reach the lingual apex of molar. The KiS 5 tip is the counterpart of the KiS 3 tip. The Kis 6 tip is the counterpart of the KiS 4 tip.

Stropko irrigator/drier. This device fits on a standard air/water syringe and uses a microtip needle (Ultradent, Inc.) to effectively irrigate and dry retropreparations. However, it should be used cautiously and only inside the retropreparation to reduce the chance of emphysema. It is recommended to change the pre-existing obtuse angle bend on the microtip needle to a 90-degree bend that is 3 mm in length (see Figure 6.23). This manipulation will facilitate direct insertion of the tip into the retropreparation for a thorough drying with min-

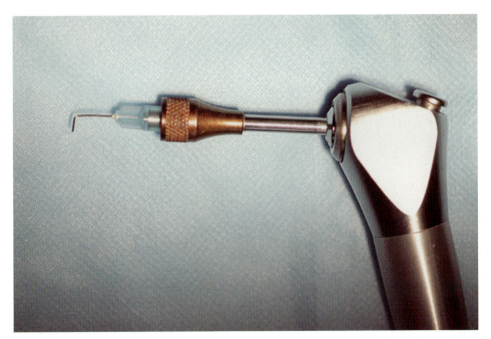

Figure 6-23. Stropko irrigator/drier. Note the microtip needle with the correct 90-degree bend that is 3 mm in length.

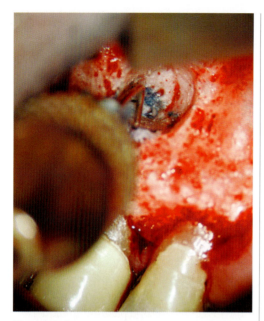

Figure 6-24. The 90-degree bend of the microtip needle will facilitate direct insertion of the needle tip into the retropreparation for a thorough drying with minimal disturbance of the delicate hemostasis of the crypt.

imal disturbance of the delicate hemostasis of the crypt (see Figure 6.24).

Retrofilling instruments. Micropluggers, retrofilling carriers, and ball burnishers (see Figure 6.25) are retrofilling instruments. Micropluggers come in ball ends ranging from 0.25 to 0.75 mm. They can be either straight-handled or double-angled. The straight-handled micropluggers come in two different angles: a 90-degree tip for universal use and a 65-degree tip helpful for the lingual apex (see Figure 6.26). The double-angled microplugger tips are offset by 65 degrees—one left and one right for left and right molar surgeries.

The Super EBA retrofilling carrier has a flat surface that is designed to carry the retrofilling material into the retropreparation. Figure 6.27 shows the West carriers with straight and offset angles.

Burnishers are ball shaped and are available in different sizes. They are used immediately following retrofilling material placement to

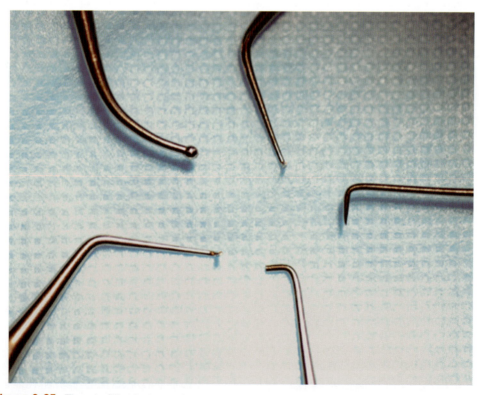

Figure 6-25. The retrofilling instruments.

ENDODONTIC PERIRADICULAR MICROSURGERY

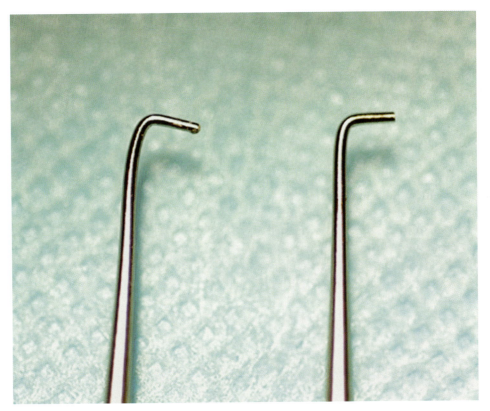

Figure 6-26. The straight-handled micropluggers come in two different angles: a 90-degree tip that is for universal use and a 65-degree tip that is helpful for the lingual apex.

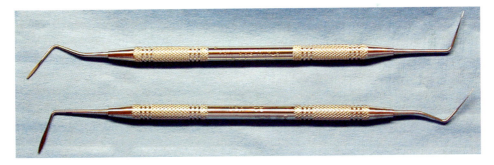

Figure 6-27. The West carriers.

adapt the retrofilling material into the retropreparation and to seal all the margins.

If mineral trioxide aggregate (MTA) will be used as retrofilling material, then a carrier system is needed to transport this delicate material into the retropreparation. A variety of Messing gun systems are available and can be used for this purpose. More recently, a MTA pellet-forming block has become available (Hartzell & Son, Concord, CA) and has proven to be more effective and less complicated than other systems. Directions for using this block will be provided later in the retrofilling section of this chapter.

Preoperative Assessment

The prognosis following surgery is dependent on thorough preoperative medical, intra-oral, periodontic, and radiographic evaluations—along with good surgical technique and proper postoperative instruction.

MEDICAL EVALUATION

A routine review of the patient's medical history and current medications should be performed, and when necessary, additional medical consultations should be requested. As a general rule, no special precautions need to be taken when surgery is planned other than those that normally apply to routine dental procedures.[18]

A special emphasis should be placed, however, on noting any blood-thinning medications, especially aspirin. They are so commonly prescribed that patients often forget to include it in their medical history. Aspirin should be discontinued at least 10 days prior to surgery.

Another consideration is the need to prescribe prophylactic premedication. The American Heart Association recommends prophylactic premedication for patients with a history of rheumatic heart fever, endocarditis, abnormal or damaged heart valves, organ transplantation, and placement of an implant prosthesis such as hip joint or knee replacement within the past two years.[19] Table 6.2 represents the currently recommended regimens.

INTRA-ORAL EVALUATION

A thorough oral examination should comprise all of the following:

- Patient's chief complaint
- Chronological history of the problem tooth
- Presence of swelling
- Tracing of existing sinus tract with a gutta-percha point (see Figure 6.28)

Table 6-2. Recommended Prophylaxis Regimen for Dental Procedures in High-risk Patients

Standard Regimen

Amoxicillin
- Adults: 2 g orally (PO)
- Children: 50 mg/kg (PO) 1 hour before procedure

If the patient cannot take oral medications, the regimen is:

Ampicillin
- Adults: 2 g intramuscularly (IM) or intravenously (IV)
- Children: 50 mg/kg IM or IV within 30 minutes before procedure

Regimen for Patients Allergic to Penicillin

Clindamycin
- Adults: 600 mg PO
- Children: 20 mg/kg PO 1 hour before procedure

or

Cephalexin or Cefadroxil
- Adults: 2 g PO
- Children: 50 mg/kg PO 1 hour before procedure

or

Azithromycin or Clarithromycin
- Adults: 500 mg PO
- Children: 15 mg/kg PO 1 hour before procedure

Regimen for Patients Allergic to Penicillin and Unable to Take Oral Medications

Clindamycin
- Adults: 600 mg
- Children: 20 mg/kg IV within 30 minutes before procedure

or

Cefazolin
- Adults: 1 g
- Children: 20 mg/kg IM or IV within 30 minutes before procedure

PERIODONTAL EVALUATION

The periodontal examination should include mobility, probing depth, and requests for preoperative scaling and/or root planning if needed. Probing depth measurements are an

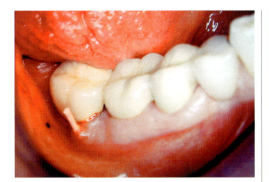

Figure 6-28A. Sinus tract opening buccal to tooth #31.

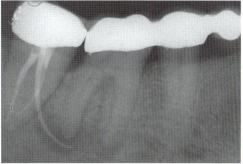

Figure 6-28B. Radiograph of gutta-percha (GP) point traced to apex of tooth #30.

essential part of the consultation that aides in the diagnosis of vertical root fracture or combined perio-endo lesions. Detections of such periodontal involvements could drastically alter the treatment plan and save patients from undergoing unnecessary surgical procedures. If patient sensitivity prevents accurate probing, administration of a local anesthetic is recommended.

RADIOGRAPHIC EVALUATION

A radiological examination is essential and should include prior radiographs if available. Two radiographs taken from two different angles (straight on and mesially angulated) can uncover concealed anatomical structures by adding a third dimension to an otherwise two-dimensional image.

Preoperative radiographs should be assessed in a systemic manner for the following:

- Approximate root length
- Number of roots and their configuration
- Degree of root curvature (see Figure 6.30)
- Proximity of adjacent root tips, especially in anterior teeth (see Figure 6.31)
- Proximity of anatomical structures including mandibular canal, mental foramen, external oblique ridge, zygomatic process, and the maxillary sinus
- Approximate size, location, and type of lesion

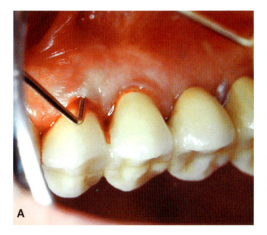
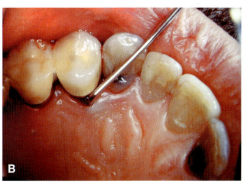

Figure 6-29A–B. Bilateral deep pockets on buccal and palatal—suggestive of a vertical root fracture.

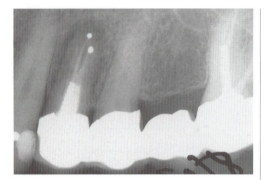

Figure 6-29C. J-shaped radiolucency commonly associated with root fracture.

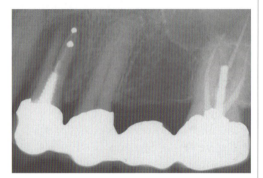

Figure 6-29D. Radiograph taken at slightly different angulation clearly shows the fracture.

- Vertical root fracture or radiographic signs most commonly associated with it such as thickening of the periodontal ligament (PDL) surrounding lateral root surfaces, J-shaped lesions, or possible endodontic/periodontal lesions

PREOPERATIVE MEDICATIONS

The following preoperative regimens are recommended:

- 0.12 percent chlorhexidine mouth rinse starting the day before surgery and continuing for up to a week after surgery to reduce the oral microflora.
- Ibuprofen 800 mg one hour before surgery, which is effective in reducing the inflammatory response and postoperative pain.[20]
- Tranquilizers for anxious patients such as Valium (5 mg) one hour before the surgery. If a tranquilizer is used, another persn must accompany the patient on the trip to the office and then back home after the procedure.
- Patients should be advised to refrain from smoking.

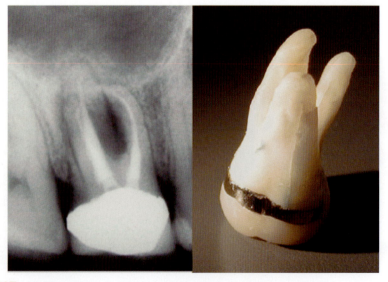

Figure 6-29E. Radiographic and clinical views of a vertical root fracture case.

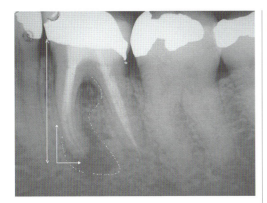

Figure 6-30. Preoperative radiographs provide valuable information such as the approximate root length, the number of roots and their configuration, and the degree of root curvature. The approximate size, location, and type of lesion can also be assessed.

- As discussed previously, antibiotic prophylaxis premedication should be prescribed when indicated.

Surgical Technique

ANESTHESIA AND HEMOSTASIS

The ability to achieve profound anesthesia and hemostasis in the surgical site is crucial in microsurgery. Profound anesthesia will eliminate patient discomfort and anxiety during, and for a significant time following, the procedure. Excellent hemostasis will improve visibility of the surgical site, allow microscopic inspection of the resected root surface, and minimize the surgery time.

Hemostatic control can be divided into preoperative, intraoperative, and postoperative phases. These phases are interrelated and dependent on each other.

Preoperative Phase

An anesthetic solution containing a vasoconstrictor is indicated to achieve anesthesia and hemostasis.[21] While 2 percent lidocaine with 1:100,000 concentrations of epinephrine is

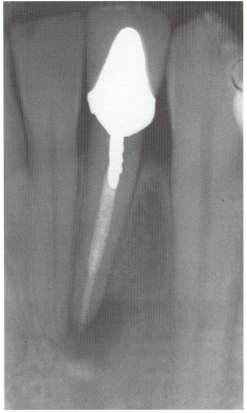

Figure 6-31. Note the close proximity of the apices of these two mandibular incisors. Patient should be made aware of the possible loss of vitality of the adjacent tooth after apical surgery.

recognized as an excellent anesthetic agent, clinical evidence suggests that 1:50,000 concentration offers better hemostasis.[22, 23] The amount of the anesthetic solution containing 1:50,000 epinephrine that is necessary to achieve anesthesia and hemostasis is dependent on the size of the surgical site; however, 2.0 to 4.0 ml is usually sufficient. This amount of local anesthetic should be slowly infiltrated using multiple injections. Solution should be deposited throughout the entire submucosa superficial to the periosteum at the level of the root apices in the surgical site. It is worth mentioning that there is a narrow margin of error in delivering local infiltration. Skeletal muscles respond to epinephrine with vasodilation

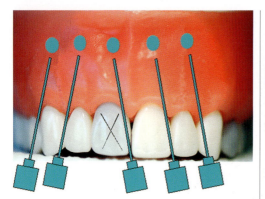

Figure 6-32. Local infiltration for surgery on tooth #8 should extend from tooth #6 to #10 at the level of the root apices.

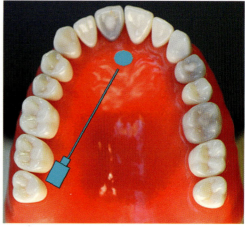

Figure 6-33. Incisive foramen block injection.

instead of vasoconstriction as they contain blood vessels that are mostly innervated with β-2 adrenergic receptors. Thus, great care should be taken to avoid infiltrating into deeper skeletal tissue beyond the root apices and over basal bone instead of alveolar bone.

In the maxilla, anesthesia and hemostasis are usually accomplished simultaneously by local infiltration in the mucobuccal fold over the apices of the tooth in question and two adjacent teeth both mesial and distal to that tooth (5 teeth total). This should be supplemented with a nerve block near the incisive foramen to block the nasopalatine nerve for surgery on maxillary anterior teeth, or near the greater palatine foramen to block the greater palatine nerve for surgery on the maxillary posterior teeth (see Figures 6.32 and 6.33).

In the mandible, anesthesia and hemostasis are usually achieved separately. Anesthesia is established by a regional nerve block of the inferior alveolar nerve, using 1.5 cartridges of 2 percent lidocaine with 1:100,000 epinephrine. Hemostasis is established with two cartridges of 2 percent lidocaine with 1:50,000 epinephrine at the surgical site via multiple supraperiosteal injections into the mucobuccal fold. An additional supplement of 0.5 cartridge is also injected into the lingual aspect of the tooth.

The rate of injection will relate to the degree of hemostasis and anesthesia obtained. A rate of 1–2 ml/min is recommended.[24] Injecting at a faster rate results in localized pooling of the solution, delayed and limited diffusion, and less than optimal anesthesia and hemostasis. It is essential to allow the deposited solution sufficient time to diffuse and reach the targeted area to produce the desired effects before any incision is made. The recommended wait time is usually 10–15 minutes, until the soft tissue throughout the surgical site has blanched (see Figure 6.35).

Intraoperative Phase

The most important measure in achieving hemostasis is effective local vasoconstriction. Following osteotomy, curettage, and root resection, hemostasis needs to be established *again* as newly ruptured blood vessels emerse the bone crypt and the buccal plate with blood. The use of a topical hemostatic agent is frequently needed at this point of surgery to control bleeding. Such an agent maintains a dry surgical field that will allow microscopic inspection of the resected root surface,

ENDODONTIC PERIRADICULAR MICROSURGERY 163

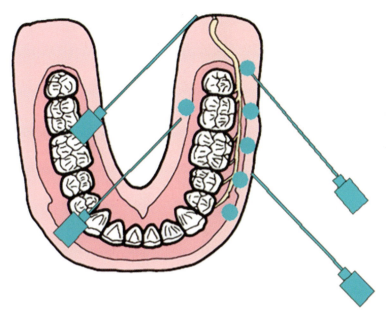

Figure 6-34. In the mandible, anesthesia is established by a regional nerve block of the inferior alveolar nerve, using 1.5 cartridges of 2% lidocaine with 1:100,000 epinephrine. Hemostasis is established with 2 cartridges of 2% lidocaine with 1:50,000 epinephrine at the surgical site via multiple supraperiosteal injections into the mucobuccal fold. An additional supplement of 0.5 cartridge (also mainly for hemostasis) can be injected at the lingual aspect of the root.

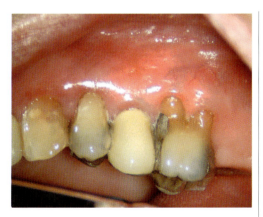

Figure 6-35A. Before anesthesia.

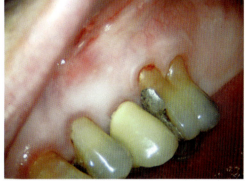

Figure 6-35B. 10 minutes following local infiltration.

adequate visibility during ultrasonic retro-preparation, and good isolation during retrofilling material placement.

Many topical hemostatic agents are available. The two most widely used by endodontists are epinephrine cotton pellets and ferric sulfate solution. The following is a presentation of the properties of these two chemical agents and their mechanisms of action.

Epinephrine pellets. Racellets are cotton pellets containing racemic epinephrine HCl (Pascal Company, Inc., Bellvue, WA). The amount of epinephrine in each varies depending on the number on the label (see Figure 6.36). Racellet #3 pellet contains an

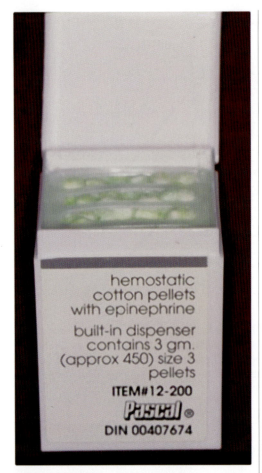

Figure 6-36. Epinephrine pellets.

very acidic solution (pH 0.21). The agglutinated proteins form plugs that occlude the capillary orifices to achieve hemostasis.

Ferric sulfate is commercially available in different solutions with different concentrations. The recommended solution for endodontic surgery is Cutrol, which contains 50 percent ferric sulfate (see Figure 6.37). Cutrol is an excellent surface hemostatic agent on the buccal plate of bone and inside the bone crypt. It should be applied directly to the bleeding point with a microapplicator tip or a cotton pellet (see Figure 6.38A). Upon contact with blood, this yellowish solution immediately turns dark brown. This color change is helpful in identifying any remaining bleeders that need to be addressed in the same manner (see Figure 6.38B).

Ferric sulfate is a very effective hemostatic agent that works instantly, but it is also cyto-

average of 0.55 mg of racemic epinephrine and is usually recommended for apical surgery. The racellet pellets are inexpensive and highly effective in achieving hemostasis in the bone crypt via the vasoconstriction effects of epinephrine coupled with the pressure applied on these pellets.[25] It has been shown that one to seven pellets of Racellets #3 can be applied directly to the bone crypt and left for two to four minutes with no evident cardiovascular changes.[26]

Ferric sulfate. This is another chemical hemostatic agent that has been used for a long time in restorative dentistry. Its mechanism of action is not completely clear, but it is believed to be due to agglutination of blood proteins when in contact with this

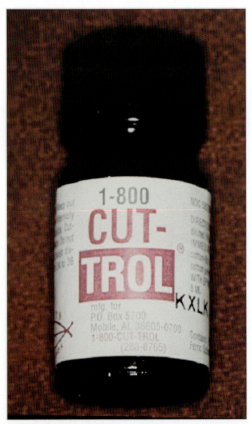

Figure 6-37. Cutrol (50 percent ferric sulfate).

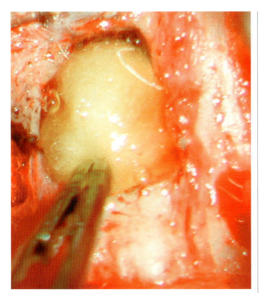

Figure 6-38A. Cutrol application to bone.

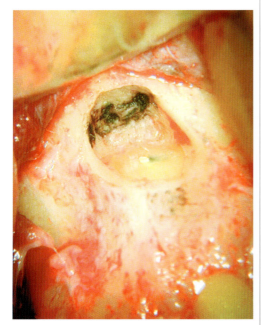

Figure 6-38B. Bone color change.

toxic and causes tissue necrosis. For this reason, it should not come in contact with the flap tissue. The use of this agent should be limited as an adjunct to other hemostatic measures. For example, if bleeding persists after using the epinephrine cotton pellet technique. When used correctly as described in the previous paragraph, systemic absorption is unlikely since the coagulum stops the solution from reaching the blood stream.

Ferric sulfate also has been proved to damage bone and delay healing when used in large amounts and left in situ after surgery (Lemon 1993). It should therefore only be used in small amounts and should be immediately and gently irrigated with saline after application. If the coagulum is thoroughly removed and irrigated before closure, there is no adverse reaction.[27]

The following steps outline the most effective method to achieve local hemostasis quickly during apical surgery:

1. Complete all the cutting necessary (osteotomy and root resection) and then thoroughly remove all granulation tissue from the bone crypt.
2. Place a small Racellet #3 cotton pellet in the bone crypt and firmly pack it against the lingual wall (see Figure 6.39A).

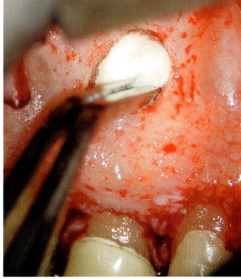

Figure 6-39A. Initial Racellet pellet placed inside the crypt.

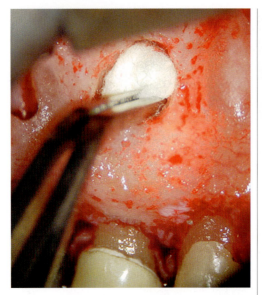

Figure 6-39B. Bone crypt filled with pellets.

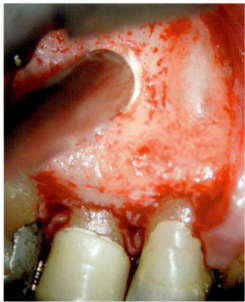

Figure 6-39C. Pressure application on top of the pellets.

3. In quick succession, additional Racellet pellets are packed in against the first pellet, until the entire crypt is filled with pellets (see Figure 6.39B). Depending on the size of the crypt, this can take a variable number of pellets. A study by Vickers[26] has shown that up to seven Racellets #3 pellets can be safely used to fill the crypt. If more are needed due to the large size of the crypt, then some sterile cotton pellets should be added until the crypt is completely filled.
4. Pressure is applied on these pellets with a blunt instrument (for example, back of a micromirror handle) for 2–4 minutes until no further bleeding is observed (see Fig 6.39C).
5. All pellets are removed one by one, except the last epinephrine pellet, which is left inside the crypt to avoid reopening of the ruptured vessels (see Figure 6.39D). This pellet should only be removed at the end of the surgical procedure before final irrigation and flap closure.
6. If small bleeders are still present on the buccal plate or inside the crypt, then

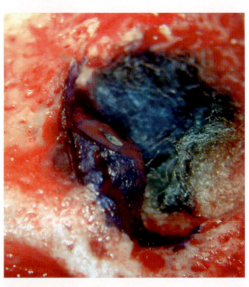

Figure 6-39D. Racellet pellets removed until resected root is exposed leaving at least one pellet against the crypt wall.

Cutrol should be applied directly to the bleeding areas. Without disrupting the coagulum, the solution is quickly rinsed with saline to remove any excess. The coagulum formed should be left intact during the surgical procedure but must be thoroughly curetted and the corresponding area rinsed before closure.

Postoperative Phase

Periradicular surgery should be performed within a reasonable amount of time so that complicated and hemostasis-dependent steps are completed before reactive hyperemia occurs. As restricted blood flow returns to normal, it rapidly increases to a rate well beyond normal to compensate for localized tissue hypoxia and acidosis. Reactive hyperemia is clinically variable and unpredictable. It can be prevented or reduced by compressing the flap tissue for three minutes and applying firm finger pressure with saline-soaked gauze pads placed over the surgical site. This is done to induce hemostasis, prevent hematoma formation, and enhance good tissue reapproximation.[28] Flap compressions should be followed immediately with postsurgical cold compressions to the cheek.

FLAP DESIGNS

The semilunar flap used to be the flap of choice for apical surgery (see Figure 6.40). It is not advocated today for a number of reasons. The semilunar flap provides a restricted surgical access and has limited potential for further extension if deemed necessary. It also carries the danger of postsurgical defects by incising through tissues that are not supported by underlying bone.[29] Furthermore, this type of incision results in maximum severage of periosteal blood vessels. This compromises the blood supply, which could lead to shrinkage, gapping, and secondary healing. Another disadvantage to the semilunar flap is the close proximity of the incision to the osteotomy site, which makes hemostatic control more challenging.

The following are flap designs recommended for periradicular surgery.

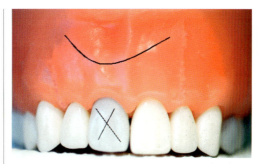

Figure 6-40. Semilunar flap design.

Full Mucoperiosteal Tissue Flap

There are strong biological reasons to use this kind of flap whenever possible.[18, 30] It maintains intact vertical blood supply and minimizes hemorrhage while providing adequate access. It allows a survey of bone and root structures, which facilitates excellent surgical orientation. However, since this flap involves the gingival papilla and exposes the crestal bone, it can carry a few potential risks including loss of tissue attachment, loss of crestal bone height, and possible loss of interdental papilla integrity.

The two recommended designs of full mucoperiosteal tissue flaps for periradicular surgery are the triangular and rectangular (trapezoidal) designs.

The **triangular** flap design is the most widely used flap design in periradicular surgery, and it is indicated in the anterior and posterior regions of both the mandible and the maxilla. It requires a horizontal intrasulcular incision and a single vertical releasing incision (see Figure 6.41).

The horizontal incision is made with the scalpel held near a vertical position, extending through the gingival sulcus and the gingival fibers down to the level of the crestal bone. When passing through the interdental region, care should be taken to ensure that the incision is separating the buccal and lingual papillae in the midcol area. A microblade will ease this separation if the embra-

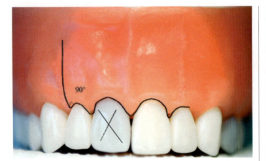

Figure 6-41A. Anterior triangular flap design.

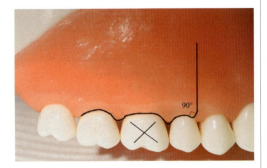

Figure 6-41B. Posterior triangular flap design.

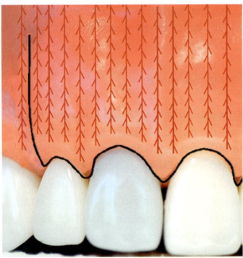

Figure 6-42. Vertical releasing incision is parallel to microvasculature.

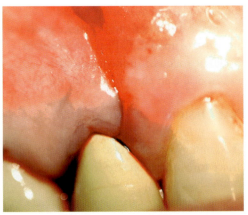

Figure 6-43. Vertical releasing incision terminating at the tooth line angle. It is perpendicular to the free gingival margin.

sure space is narrow (for example, mandibular anterior area). A clean incision located exactly midcol is vital to prevent sloughing of the papillae due to a compromised blood supply and to prevent the unaesthetic look of double papillae.[18]

The vertical releasing incision is prepared between the root eminences parallel to the long access of the roots. In anterior surgery, the vertical incision is prepared in the flap perimeter closest to the surgeon. In posterior surgery, it always constitutes the mesial perimeter of the flap. It is important to keep the base of the flap as wide as the top so that the vertical incision is kept parallel to the vertically positioned supraperiosteal microvasculature and tissue-supportive collagen fibers.[31] In this manner, the least number of vessels and fibers are severed, which will translate into faster healing without scarring (see Figure 6.42). Vertical incisions should terminate at the mesial or distal line angles of teeth and never in the papillae or the midroot area. It also should meet the tooth at the free gingival margin with a 90-degree angle (see Figures 6.41 and 6.43).

The advantages of the triangular flap design are simplicity, rapid wound healing, ease of flap reapproximation, and ease of suturing. A disadvantage, on the other hand, is the limited surgical access. In situations where more access is warranted, either the horizontal or the vertical incisions can be extended to allow some additional mobilization of the flap.

Alternatively, a rectangular flap design should be considered if maximum access is required.

The **rectangular** flap design is very similar to the triangular design except for the addition of a second vertical releasing incision (see Figure 6.44). The rectangular flap design is indicated for anterior surgery when more access is needed. It is also used when multiple teeth will be operated on or when the roots are long (for example, cuspid). Potential disadvantages associated with this flap design include technique sensitive wound closure and a higher chance for flap dislodgment.

Limited Mucoperiosteal Tissue Flap (Scalloped Flap)

This limited tissue flap does not include the marginal and interdental gingival within its perimeter. It is indicated in teeth with existing fixed restorations and in cases where aesthetics are a major concern. The limited tissue flap can be used in both the maxillary anterior or posterior regions but only when sufficient width of attached gingiva is available. It is usually contraindicated in the mandible since the attached gingiva is narrow in that region and aesthetics are not a major concern.

An absolute minimum of 2 mm of attached gingiva from the depth of the gingival sulcus must be present before this flap design is selected[32] (see Figure 6.45). This submarginal flap design is formed by a scalloped horizontal incision and one or two vertical releasing incisions depending on the surgical access needed (see Figure 6.46). The scalloped incision reflects the contours of the marginal gingiva and provides an adequate distance from the depth of the gingival sulci.[18] It also serves as a guide for correctly repositioning the elevated flap for suturing.[25]

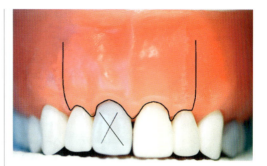

Figure 6-44. Rectangular flap design.

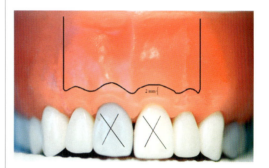

Figure 6-45. Rectangular submarginal flap design.

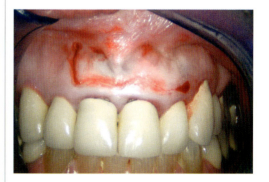

Figure 6-46. Triangular submarginal flap design.

All the flap corners, either at the scalloping or at the junction of horizontal and vertical incisions, should be rounded to promote smoother healing and minimize scar formation. The angle of the incision in relation to the cortical plate is 45 degrees to allow the widest cut surface as well as better adaptation when the flap is repositioned (see

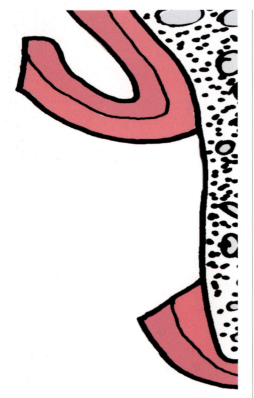

Figure 6-47. 45-degree bevel incision angle.

Figure 6.47). This 45-degree bevel at the scalloped horizontal incision is made with the tip of the scalpel pointing away from the gingival sulcus. This adds an additional safety measure to protect the minimum 2 mm of attached gingiva.

The submarginal flap has the advantage of leaving the marginal and interdental gingiva intact in addition to leaving the crestal bone unexposed. The major disadvantage is the severance of supraperiosteal vessels, which could leave the unreflected tissue without blood supply. This can be prevented by preserving an adequate width of unreflected gingival tissue, which will derive secondary blood supplies from the PDL and intraosseous blood vessels. The healing of this flap seems to be quite similar to the full mucoperiosteal flap.[30]

ELEVATION AND RETRACTION

Tissue elevation always starts in the attached gingiva of the vertical incision (see Figure 6.48A and 6.48B). This allows the periosteal elevator to apply reflective forces against the cortical bone and not the root surface while elevating the tougher fibrous tissue of the gingiva. Special attention should be directed to ensure that the periosteum is entirely lifted from the cortical plate with the elevated flap (see Figure 6.49). The elevator should then be moved more coronally to elevate the marginal and interdental papilla atraumatically using the undermining elevation technique.[18] In this technique, all reflective forces should be applied to the bone and periosteum, with minimal forces on the gingival tissue (see Figures 6.50A and 6.50B). Subsequently, the elevation continues in a more apical direction into the submucosa to expose the root tip area and to render the flap more flexible and movable.

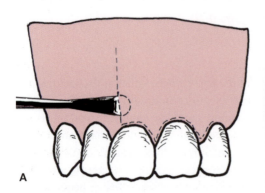
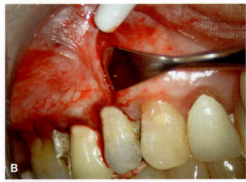

Figure 6-48A–B. Elevation starts at the middle portion of the vertical incision.

ENDODONTIC PERIRADICULAR MICROSURGERY

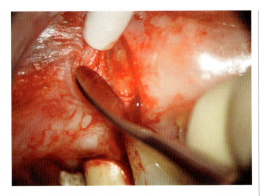

Figure 6-49. Visual inspection to ensure that the periosteum is included within the flap elevation and is completely lifted off the cortical plate.

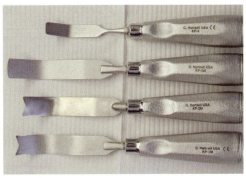

Figure 6-51A. The Kim/Pecora (KP) retractors 1 through 4 (Hartzell & Sons Co.).

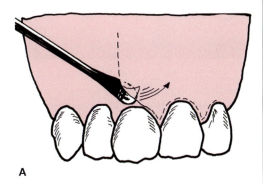

A

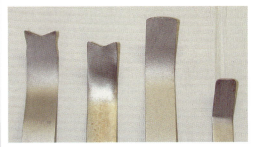

Figure 6-51B. A closer view of the different shapes of the KP retractor tips.

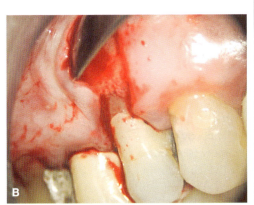

Figure 6-50A–B. The undermining elevation technique.

At this point a retractor should be used to provide access to the periradicular tissue. The retractor tip should rest on bone with light but firm pressure and without any trauma to the flap soft tissue. The surgeon must ensure that minimal tension exists at all perimeters of the flap before the osteotomy. If tension exists, then one or both of the releasing incisions should be extended or the reflected tissue should be elevated further. It is important to evaluate the cortical plate bone topography (flat, convex, or concave) to choose the right retractor tip—a shape that will fit the anatomy to maximize stable anchorage (see Figure 6.51A and 6.51B). For example, if the cortical bone anatomy is convex such as the area of the canine eminence or the zygoma, then a retractor with a concave or V-shaped tip will best fit this anatomy (see Figure 6.52). An appropriate retractor tip will allow maximum surface contact between the retractor and bone to prevent unintentional retractor slippage and possible flap impingement.

For posterior mandibular surgery, the

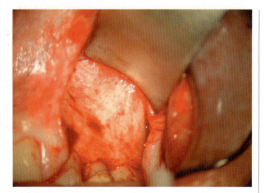

Figure 6-52. KP 2 retractor with a v-shape tip perfectly fits against the zygoma and provide maximum retention.

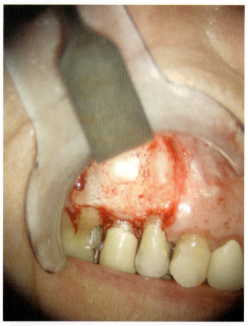

Figure 6-53. The use of the cheek retractor underneath the surgical retractor improves surgical access and provides added safety to patient's soft tissue.

groove technique should be used to provide a stable anchor for the retractor. In this technique, a 15 mm shallow horizontal groove is prepared using the Lindemann bur. This groove is prepared beyond the apex for molar surgery and above the mental foramen for premolar surgery.

The use of a plastic cheek retractor underneath the surgical retractor provides better access and visibility to the surgical site while protecting the patient's lips at the same time (see Figure 6.53).

The amount of time that the tissue is retracted is an essential factor in the speed of healing. Although related literature does not give a specific answer, it seems logical to keep this time to a minimum. On the other hand, operators should take sufficient time to solve the clinical goals of the surgical procedure.[29] By keeping the surgical site well hydrated with sterile saline, there seems to be no specific time limit to the procedure.

OSTEOTOMY

The purpose of the osteotomy in endodontic surgery is to deliberately and precisely prepare a small window through the cortical plate of bone to gain direct visual and instrumental access to the periapical area. The osteotomy should allow identification of the root apex and thorough enucleation of the periapical lesion.

The osteotomy size should be as small as possible but as large as necessary.[33] However, a minimum diameter of 4 mm is absolutely essential. This is very important in order to allow a 3-mm root resection and to accommodate free manipulation of microsurgical instruments inside the bone crypt. An ultrasonic tip can be used to verify if the osteotomy is adequate. Ideally, the ultrasonic tip (which is 3 mm long) should fit freely inside the crypt without any contact on bone (see Figure 6.54). When a larger lesion is encountered, the osteotomy might have to be further extended to ensure complete curettage of the lesion.

The osteotomy should be accurately prepared over the root apex to prevent any unnecessary overextension. This is an easy task when fenestration through the cortical plate is present. On the other hand, when the buccal cortical plate is intact and the lesion is

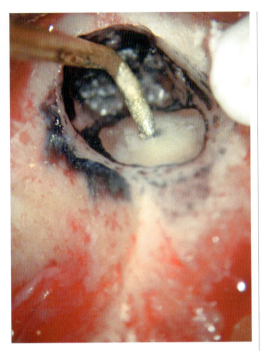

Figure 6-54. Ideal osteotomy size of 4 mm is confirmed with the use of an ultrasonic tip. It allows free manipulation of the microsurgical instruments inside the bone crypt.

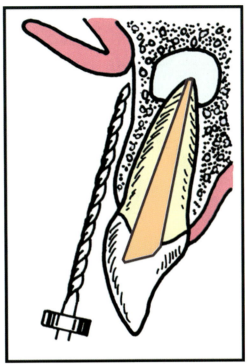

Figure 6-55A. Transferring the estimated root length measurement to the buccal plate using an endodontic file (adapted from *Practical Lessons in Endodontic Surgery* by D.E. Arens).

limited to the medullary bone space, a careful assessment should precede any osteotomy preparation.

An important clinical clue in finding the apex is the estimated root length, which can be measured from a preoperative radiograph or simply be obtained from working length recorded in the patient's chart. The length measurement is then transformed to the buccal plate using a file or periodontal probe (see Figure 6.55A and 6.55B). In addition to the length, the radiograph should be carefully examined for root curvature, position of the apex in relation to the cusp tip, and proximity of the apex to the adjacent apices or anatomical structures (mental foramen, mandibular nerve, and maxillary sinus). In most cases, a visual inspection of the buccal bone topography will reveal the root location and direct the surgeon to the root apex. In other cases, osseous palpation using an endodontic explorer is recommended in an attempt to

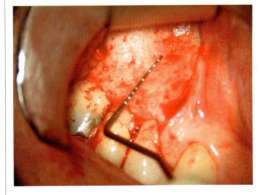

Figure 6-55B. Measuring with a periodontal probe.

penetrate through the thinned cortical plate into the lesion to confirm the exact location of the apex (see Figure 6.56A and 6.56B).

If the operator is still unsure about the exact location of the apex, the following procedure can provide better orientation. Using

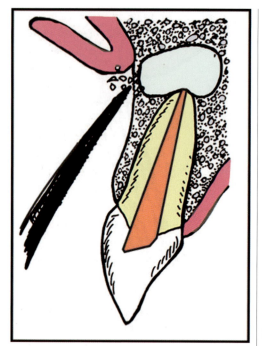

Figure 6-56A. Apical osseous palpation with endodontic explorer to locate exact location of the lesion (adapted from *Practical Lessons in Endodontic Surgery* by D.E. Arens).

a surgical #1 round bur, an indentation is prepared on the cortical plate over the estimated location of the apex. The indentation is then filled with a radio-opaque material such as gutta-percha or tin foil. A radiograph is taken with the marker in place to ascertain the location of the apex in relation to the marker (see Figure 6.57A and 6.57B).

The osteotomy is usually accomplished with a Lindemann bone cutter bur mounted on a surgical high-speed handpiece such as the Impact Air 45. It is used in a brush-stroke fashion coupled with copious saline irrigation (see Figure 6.58). The Lindemann bur has fewer flutes than conventional burs, which results in less clogging and more efficient cutting with minimal frictional heat

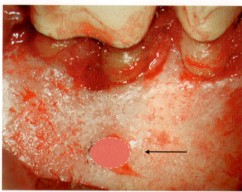

Figure 6-57A. Gutta-percha (arrow) placed into the indentation prepared over the estimated location of the apex.

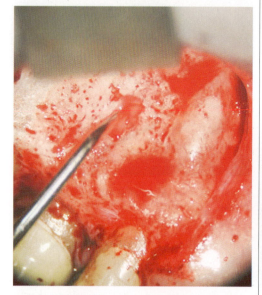

Figure 6-56B. Endodontic explorer breaking through the thin buccal plate and confirming the exact location of the lesion and the apex.

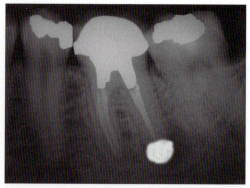

Figure 6-57B. The marker location is verified radiographically.

ENDODONTIC PERIRADICULAR MICROSURGERY

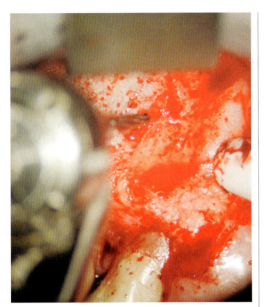

Figure 6-58. Lindemann bone cutter bur mounted on an Impact Air 45 handpiece.

produced. The Lindemann bur also produces a smoother bone surface with divergent walls and fewer undercuts in comparison to a round bur. The advantage of the Impact Air 45 handpiece is that water is directed along the bur shaft while air is ejected out of the back of the handpiece, thus minimizing the chance of emphysema.

During the osteotomy preparation, it is essential to use the microscope at a lower magnification (4× to 8×) in order to make the distinction between bone and root tip. The root structure can be identified apart from bone by texture (smooth and hard), color (darker yellowish), lack of bleeding upon probing, and the presence of an outline (PDL). When the root tip cannot be distinguished, the osteotomy site is stained with methylene blue dye, which preferentially stains the periodontal ligament (see Figure 6.59) and identifies the root apex.[25, 33, 34]

PERIRADICULAR CURETTAGE

It is important to emphasize that periradicular curettage alone does not eliminate the origin of the lesion but, rather, temporarily relieves the symptoms. The purpose of the curettage is only to remove the reactive tissue, whether it is a periapical granuloma or cyst. It is usually performed prior to or in conjunction with root-end resection.

Curettage is accomplished with bone curettes (#2/4 Molt), with the concave surface of the instrument facing the bony wall first[18] (see Figure 6.59). Pressure is applied only against the bony crypt until the tissue is freed along the lateral margins (see Figure 6.60A–E). Then, the bone curette can be rotated around and used in a scraping motion. Once loosened, tissue forceps are used to grasp the tissue and transfer it directly to the biopsy bottle. Periodontal curettes (Columbia 13/14, Jaquette 34/35, and mini-Jaquette) can be used to remove any remaining lesion tissue or tags, especially in the region lingual to the apex.

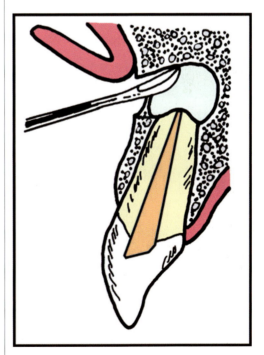

Figure 6-59. Apical curettage (adapted from *Practical Lessons in Endodontic Surgery* by D.E. Arens).

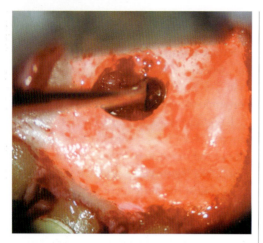

Figure 6-60A. Apical curettage using the back action of the spoon excavator.

Apical Root Resection

This is also referred to as apicoectomy. Apical root resection is performed to ensure the removal of aberrant root entities and to allow microscopic inspection of the resected root surface. Similar to the osteotomy, it is usually accomplished with the Lindemann bur in an Impact Air 45 handpiece using copious saline spray and under low range of magnification (4× to 8×) (see Figure 6.61). The smooth resected root surface produced by the Lindemann bur facilitates and eases microinspection (see Figure 6.62).

There are two important factors to con-

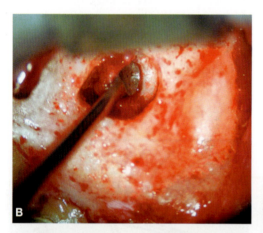

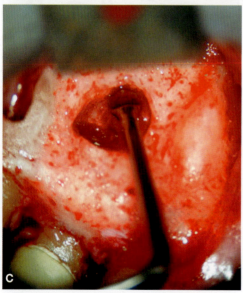

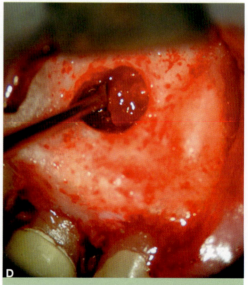

Figure 6-60B–D. The spoon is used circumferentially around the granulation tissue until the lesion is completely separated from the wall of the bone crypt.

ENDODONTIC PERIRADICULAR MICROSURGERY

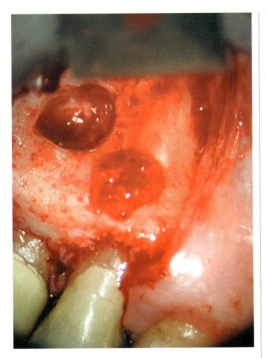

Figure 6-60E. Lesion removed in one piece.

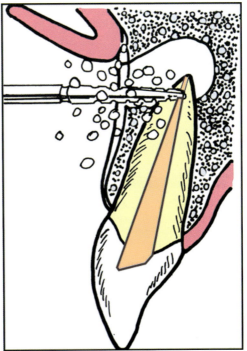

Figure 6-61. Apical root resection (adapted from *Practical Lessons in Endodontic Surgery* by D.E. Arens).

sider with this procedure: the extent of apical resection and the bevel angle.

Extent of Apical Resection

The amount of root resection depends on the incidence of lateral canals and apical ramifications. Apical resection of 3 mm at a 0-degree bevel has been shown to reduce lateral canals by 93 percent and apical ramifications of lateral canals, deltas, and isthmi by 98 percent[25] (see Figure 6.63). Additional resection does not reduce this percentage significantly.

The level of root resection may need to be modified due to the presence of the following factors:

- Presence and position of additional roots (for example, a mesiopalatal root of a maxillary molar that is shorter than the mesiobuccal root).
- Presence of a lateral canal at the root resection level (see Figure 6.64).

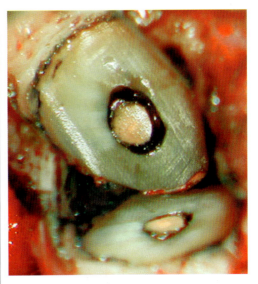

Figure 6-62A. The smooth and flat resected root surface produced with the Lindemann bur as viewed with the help of a micromirror following methylene blue staining. This picture shows gross apical leakage. All pictures in Figure 6-62 (A–D) are courtesy of Dr. Syngcuk Kim.

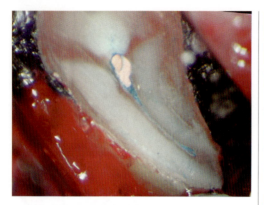

Figure 6-62B. MB root of a maxillary molar revealing a missed MB2 canal and an isthmus.

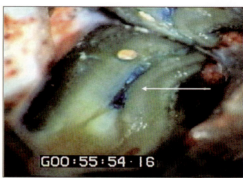

Figure 6-62D. Apical transportation. Note the off-center location of the GP fill in comparison to the original canals that are stained in blue (arrow).

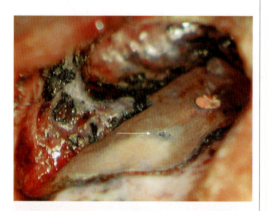

Figure 6-62C. Untreated canal space (arrow).

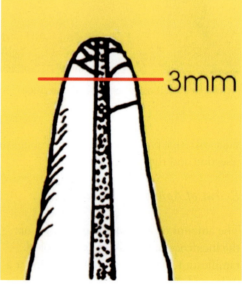

Figure 6-63. Three-millimeter apical root resection eliminates 93 percent of lateral canals.

- Presence of a long post and the need to place a root-end filling (see Figure 6.65A and 6.65B).
- Presence and location of a perforation.
- Presence of an apical root fracture.
- Amount of remaining buccal crestal bone (a minimum of 2 mm should remain to prevent periodontic-endodontic communication).
- Presence of an apical root curvature (see Figure 6.65C and 6.65D)

Bevel Angle

Apical root resection should be performed perpendicular to the long axis of the root (see Figure 6.66). This 0-degree bevel will ensure equal resection of the root apex on both buccal and lingual aspects.[35]

In some situations, a 0-degree bevel might not be possible (for example, severe lingual inclination of an anterior tooth, wide roots in a buccolingual dimension). In these cases, the operator should use a small bevel angle (up to 10 degrees). This bevel should be kept to the smallest angle possible, since the real bevel angle is almost always greater than

ENDODONTIC PERIRADICULAR MICROSURGERY

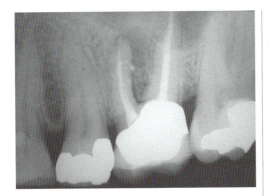

Figure 6-64A. Radiograph of a maxillary first molar revealing an obvious lateral canal.

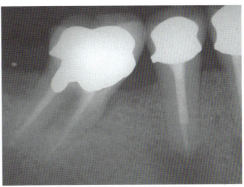

Figure 6-65A. 3mm root resection in this case will leave limited room for an adequate retropreparation and retrofilling.

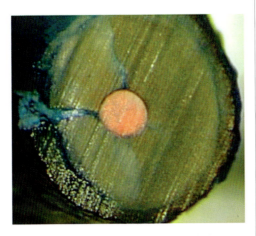

Figure 6-64B. Some resection has been accomplished but additional resection is necessary to eliminate the lateral canal as a possible avenue for leakage.

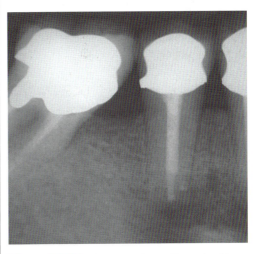

Figure 6-65B. Postoperative radiograph with a more conservative root resection.

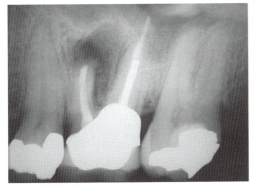

Figure 6-64C. Radiograph of completed resection, retropreparation, and retrofill.

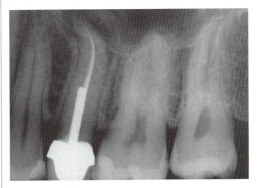

Figure 6-65C. Presence of apical curvature.

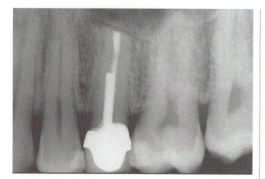

Figure 6-65D. Root resection extended to eliminate the apical curvature so that retropreparation to a depth of 3 mm could be performed.

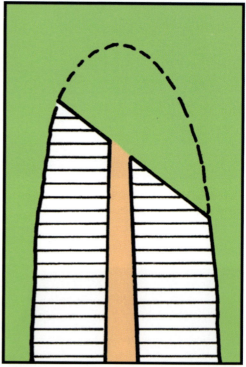

Figure 6-67. 45-degree bevel angle will expose a large number of dentinal tubules and will barely resect the lingual aspect of the root.

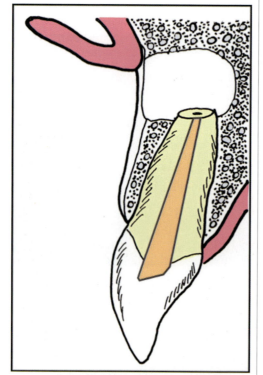

Figure 6-66. 0-degree bevel angle. (Adapted from *Practical Lessons in Endodontic Surgery* by D.E. Arens).

what it appears to be depending on the angle at which the tooth is proclined in the alveolus. For example, mandibular and maxillary anterior teeth have lingual inclinations. Surgeons might resect the root at what seems to be a 10-degree bevel, but in reality the root is being resected with a bevel of 20 degrees or more. The surgeon should compensate for this distortion of perspective by minimizing the angle of the bevel, keeping it as close to 0 degrees as possible.[3, 35]

An important advantage of the perpendicular root resection is the minimal exposure of dentinal tubules, which results in a reduction in apical leakage[1] (see Figure 6.67). In addition, the root canal anatomy is no longer elongated in a buccolingual direction as it is by traditional wide-angled methods (see Figure 6.68A–B), thus facilitating retropreparation and retrofilling procedures.

Figure 6.69 shows apical root resection being performed on tooth #4. An adequate osteotomy is prepared to expose the apical 3 mm of the root prior to resection (see Figure 6.69A). Root resection is performed at a 0–10-degree bevel angle (see Figure

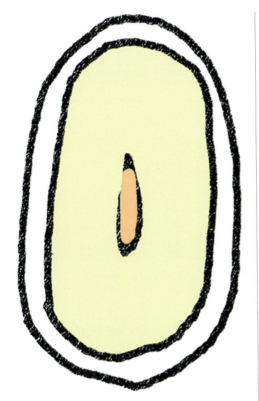

Figure 6-68A. 45-degree bevel will produce a distorted elongated view of the canal in a buccolingual direction.

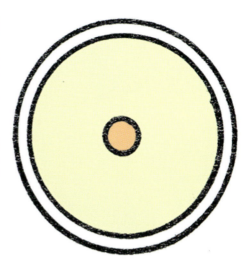

Figure 6-68B. 0-degree bevel will produce a more accurate and centered view of the canal shape.

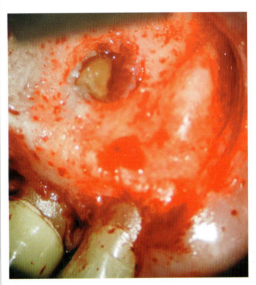

Figure 6-69A. An osteotomy has been prepared to expose the apical 3 mm of the root of tooth #4 prior to resection.

6.69B). The root tip is completely separated and is removed (see Figure 6.69C and 6.69D)

MICROSCOPIC INSPECTION OF THE RESECTED ROOT SURFACE

The smooth surface of a perpendicular root resection will best prepare the root to reveal its hidden anatomy to microscopic inspection. This is usually accomplished under high magnification (16× to 25×) and after staining with methylene blue dye. Without the added clarity provided by the dye, magnification alone is insufficient for an accurate inspection. Like adding colors to a black-and-white film, the dye adds borders and contrasts to an otherwise monochromatic surgical field, revealing a surprising degree of additional detailed anatomy.

Methylene Blue Staining Technique

The resected root surface has to be thoroughly dried using the Stropko drier prior to the application of the dye with a microapplicator tip (see Figure 6.70A–B). After waiting a few seconds, the excess dye is rinsed with

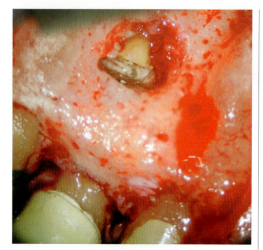

Figure 6-69B. Root resection performed at a 0–10-degree bevel angle.

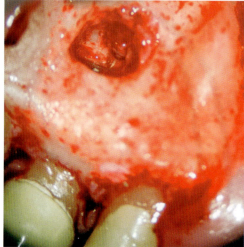

Figure 6-69D. Root tip removed.

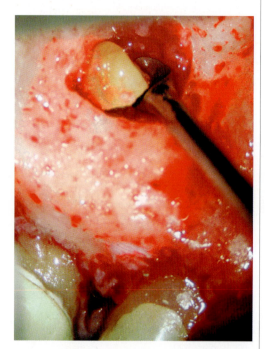

Figure 6-69C. The root tip has been separated from the root.

saline and the root surface is dried again in final preparation for microinspection. At this time, the periodontal ligament and leaky areas are clearly defined by the blue stain. If the entire root tip has been resected, the PDL can be identified as a continuous line around the root surface (see Figure 6.70B). A partial line indicates that only part of the root has been resected.

Microscopic Inspection

Microinspection of the resected root surface is the single most important step in the entire surgical procedure. This novel method was not available during the period when traditional surgical techniques were employed. Only when it is performed accurately can a definite diagnosis be made to identify the true etiology of the disease.

The appropriate size and shape micromirror is used to reflect a clear and direct view of the resected root surface (see Figure 6.71). Potentially leaky anatomy or suspicious microfractures can be confirmed by probing with the CX-1 microexplorer.

At this point, the resected root surface should be checked for the following anatomical and pathological details:

- Missed canals
- Isthmuses, fins, C-shaped canals, and accessory canals
- Leaky canals
- Microfractures

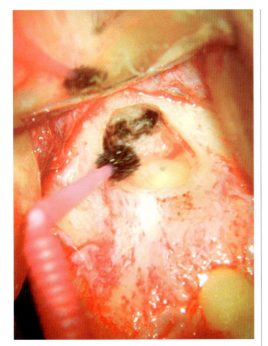

Figure 6-70A. Methylene blue dye application.

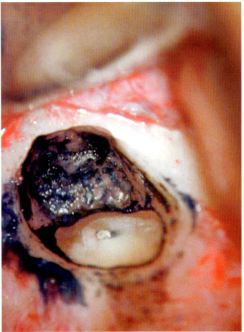

Figure 6-70C. After rinsing the excess dye with saline the PDL and any leakage around the GP are clearly stained in blue.

- Apical canal transportation
- Separated instruments

After all of these structures and defects are identified, the operator can proceed with their treatments and corrections (see Figure 6.72).

If an apical microfracture is discovered, further root resection and staining is performed until the fracture line is completely eliminated. If the fracture line persists, then either root amputation or extraction should be considered.

All anatomical variations (such as isthmuses and fins) should be included in the retropreparation to eliminate them as avenues for leakage.

Separated instruments in the apical third of the canal can be effectively removed with the combination of the 3 mm root resection and retropreparation.

The majority of apical perforations and transportations can simply be corrected with

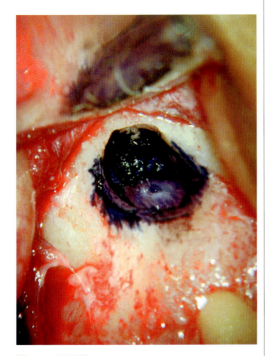

Figure 6-70B. Dye generously applied over the root surface.

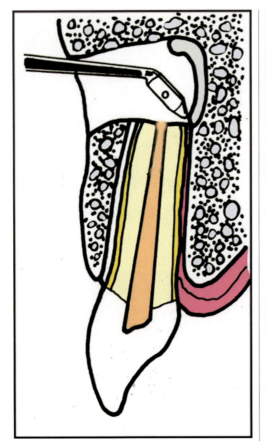

Figure 6-71. The micromirror is appropriately positioned to reflect a direct view of the resected root surface.

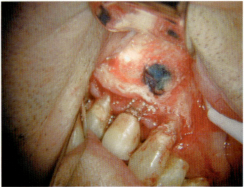

Figure 6-72A. Resected root viewed at 4× magnification.

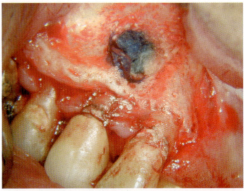

Figure 6-72B. 10× magnification.

root resection. When resection alone is inadequate in correcting the problem, the transported canal will look off-center while the original untreated canal space will be more centered and stained in blue (as shown in Figure 6.62D). If further resection cannot be performed, then emphasis should be placed on treating the untreated canal rather then the deviated gutta-percha fill.

ULTRASONIC RETROPREPARATION

The objective of retropreparation is to clean and shape the apical canal while providing at the same time a retentive cavity preparation to receive the root end filling material and secure an apical seal.

An ideal retropreparation is best described as: "a class one preparation that is at least three millimeters into root dentin with walls parallel to and coincident with the anatomic outline of the pulpal space"[4] (see Figure 6.73).

The outline of the preparation depends mainly on the anatomy of the exposed canal space in cross-section. For example, in the maxillary central incisor, the shape of the preparation will be round. In premolars and molars, the outline of the preparation will be more oval and narrow.

A preparation depth of 3 mm with 0–10 degrees root resection bevel angle is generally recommended[1] (see Figure 6.74). This depth has been shown to significantly

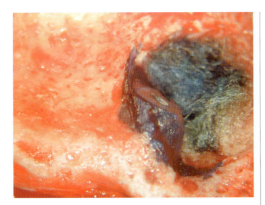

Figure 6-72C. 16× magnification.

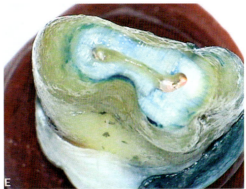

Figure 6-73. Ideal retropreparation outline that follows and includes the anatomic outline of the pulpal space. This is a case of a maxillary molar with fused roots and an isthmus that connects the buccal roots to the palatal root.

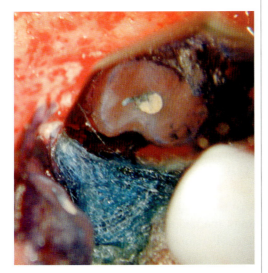

Figure 6-72D. Microinspection of the resected root surface at 20× magnification with the use of the micromirror. The missed second canal and isthmus are clearly identified.

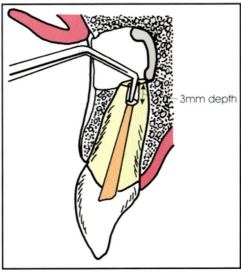

Figure 6-74. Adapted from *Practical Lessons in Endodontic Surgery* by D.E. Arens.

reduce apical dentin permeability and apical microleakage.

Apical dentin permeability is directly related to the number of open dentinal tubules at the resected root end. Tidmarsh and Arrowsmith suggested that the angle of the bevel should be kept to a minimum to reduce the number of exposed dentinal tubules. They also recommended the canal to be retrofilled at least to the level of the coronal end of the beveled root to internally seal any exposed tubules (see Figure 6.75).

Apical microleakage is the leakage along the interface between the filling material and the canal wall. Microleakage is dictated by two interconnected factors: the retrograde filling depth and the root resection bevel angle.

Increasing the depth of the retrograde fill-

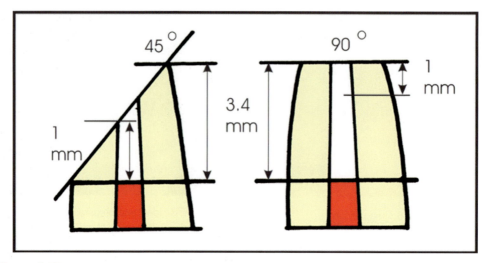

Figure 6-75. Increasing the depth of the retrograde filling significantly decreases apical leakage. If teeth are resected at 0 degrees to the long access, a retrograde filling with a depth of 1 mm is sufficient to prevent apical microleakage. A steeper-beveled apex will require a deeper retrofilling. As the bevel angle increases to 30 and 45 degrees, the depth of the retrograde filling should be increased to 2.1 and 2.5 mm, respectively, to achieve a similar apical seal. This is due to the shorter buccal wall of the retroprepared canal space of a beveled resected apex.

ing significantly decreases apical leakage.[1] If teeth are resected at 0 degrees to the long access, a retrograde filling with a depth of 1 mm is sufficient to prevent apical microleakage. But a steeper-beveled apex will require a deeper retrofilling. As the bevel angle increases to 30 and 45 degrees, the depth of the retrograde filling should be increased to 2.1 and 2.5 mm, respectively, to achieve a similar apical seal. This is due to the shorter buccal wall of the retroprepared canal space of a beveled resected apex (see Figure 6.75).

Because a small bevel angle is sometimes necessary for good surgical access as opposed to the ideal 0-degree bevel angle, and because it is difficult to accurately assess the extent of the bevel angle clinically, retrograde filling with a depth of 3 mm is recommended to minimize apical microleakage.

Using traditional endodontic surgery instruments and techniques, the objectives mentioned above are rarely achieved. Most traditional preparations are performed with a miniature contra-angle handpiece using small round or inverted-cone carbide burs. These obsolete approaches often fail to execute retropreparation with adequate depth that is parallel with the long axis of the root, and frequently result in unintentional lingual perforation. The net result is retrofilling that fails to achieve a hermatic seal due to its large size, shallow depth, and deviated location.

The use of ultrasonic tips in apical microsurgery eliminate most of the major inadequacies and complications associated with bur-type root-end preparations. The ultrasonic tips are 1/10 the size of a microhandpiece and have a diameter that is as small as 0.25 mm. When performed correctly and accurately, the ultrasonic technique provides the following advantages:

- Conservative preparations coaxial with the long axis of the root and of an adequate depth of 3 mm.
- Preparations that are confined to internal root canal anatomy.

- Precise isthmus preparations.
- Better access with unrestricted visibility.
- Thorough debridement of tissue debris.
- Smoother and more parallel walls.

The Ultrasonic Technique

After completing osteotomy preparation, apical root resection, crypt hemostasis, methylene blue staining, and microscopic root inspection, the ultrasonic retropreparation should be methodically performed. The technique is performed in the following steps:

1. Selection of an ultrasonic tip with the appropriate tip angulations and/or diameter.
2. Thorough examination of the stained resected root surface for all microanatomy at high magnification (16× to 25×).
3. Developing a mental image of the necessary retropreparation outline needed to include all anatomy (see Figure 6.76).
4. The selected ultrasonic tip is positioned at the apex parallel with the long axis of the root (see Figure 6.77). This can only be achieved at a lower magnification (4× to 6×), which has a wider field of view that enables the surgeon to observe the crown, the cervical root area, the root eminence, and the apical area—all at the same time.

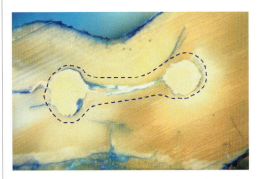

Figure 6-76B. Ideal retropreparation outline of a mandibular molar mesial root. The outline includes both mesial canals and the connecting isthmus.

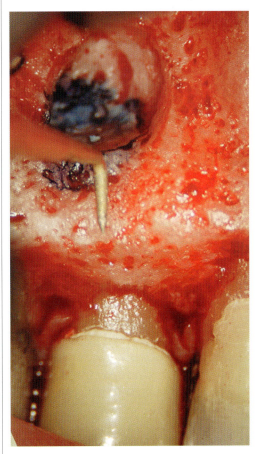

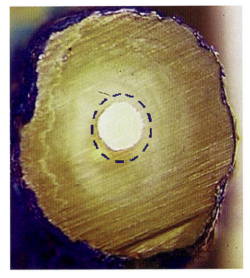

Figure 6-76A. The dotted line represents the ideal retropreparation outline for this round canal.

Figure 6-77A. Ultrasonic tip aligned along the long access of the root.

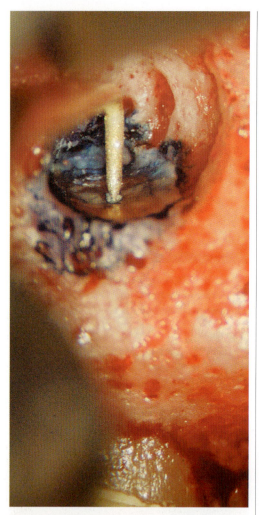

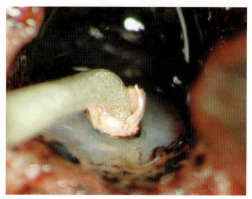

Figure 6-78. Tip is activated, and the canal is prepared to a depth of 3 mm (which is the length of the ultrasonic tip).

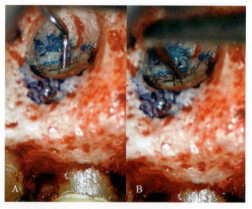

Figure 6-79. Microplugger is used to verify preparation depth and to condense down the GP.

Figure 6-77B. Tip transferred into the canal keeping the exact orientation.

This is important to prevent off-angle retropreparation and possible perforation.

5. While maintaining the same orientation, the ultrasonic tip is activated and the apical canal is retroprepared with copious saline coolant to a 3 mm depth. This should be an easy task if the tip is parallel to the gutta-percha-filled canal (see Figure 6.78). If resistance is encountered, then angulation of the tip should be slightly modified.
6. A microplugger is used to check the 3-mm depth of the preparation (see Figure 6.79).

It is important to maneuver the ultrasonic tip in a gentle up-and-down brushing movement in order to cut effectively. Application of pressure that is too firm will dampen its movement and render it ineffective.

If an isthmus is present between canals, the canals on the ends are prepared first without the connecting isthmus. The isthmus is then scored with the tip of a microexplorer (C×1) producing a tracking groove.[35] This groove will act as a guide to the ultrasonic tip and will help in keeping it centered during isthmus preparation. A narrow ultrasonic tip (such as KiS-1 or CT-1) is needed

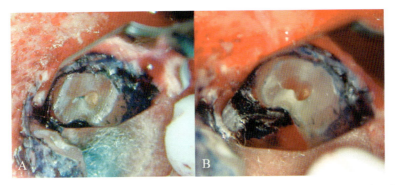

Figure 6-80A,B. Isthmus retropreparation. **A.** The resection of the root has been completed. **B.** The two canals on each end of the isthmus are prepared first, followed by scoring of the isthmus with a tracking groove. Finally, the isthmus is prepared to the same depth as the two canals.

in this area since the isthmus is located in the thinner portion of the root, which can be perforated easily. The isthmus is prepared using a light sweeping motion in a forward and backward direction connecting the two canals. The isthmus also has to be prepared to a 3-mm depth (see Figure 6.80).

After the retropreparation is completed, the cavity is inspected with the micromirror at high magnification (16× to 25×). The surgeon should confirm that the walls are smooth and parallel and that the retroprepared cavity outline has included all the microanatomy (see Figure 6.81).

Gutta-percha remaining on the walls needs to either be condensed with a microplugger or removed with a microexplorer. The use of an activated ultrasonic tip in chasing small pieces of gutta-percha is not only ineffective but possibly results in widened preparation and unnecessary weakening of the walls.

Retrograde Filling

The purpose of retrograde filling is to provide an adequate apical seal that will prevent the leakage of remaining bacteria and their by-products from the root canal system into the periradicular tissue.

Ideal properties for retrograde filling ma-

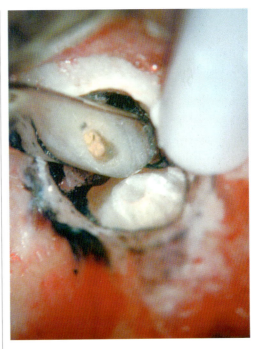

Figure 6-81. Microinspection of the retroprepared canal.

terial as proposed by Grossman are summarized in Table 6.3.

Amalgam has previously been the most widely used root-end filling material. It is easily manipulated and readily available and seems to provide a good initial seal. Amalgam use is no longer recommended due to its corrosion, leakage, staining of soft

190 CHAPTER 6

Table 6-3. Ideal Properties for Retrograde Filling Materials

1. Readily available and easy to handle.
2. Well-tolerated by periapical tissues.
3. Adheres to tooth structure.
4. Dimensionally stable.
5. Bacteriocidal or bacteriostatic.
6. Resistant to dissolution.
7. Promotes cementogenesis.
8. Noncorrosive.
9. Does not stain tooth or periradicular tissue.
10. Electrochemically inactive.
11. Allows adequate working time, then sets quickly.
12. Radiopaque.

Table 6-4. Bosworth's Super EBA retrofilling material composition

Powder
   Zinc oxide—60%
   Alumina—37%
   Natural resin—3%
Liquid
   Eugenol—37.5%
   Orthoethoxybenzoic acid—62.5%

tissue, persistent apical inflammation, and lack of long-term success.[36, 37]

The two retrograde filling materials currently recommended are Super EBA and MTA.

Super EBA

In 1978, Oynick and Oynick[38] suggested the use of Stailine (later marketed as Super EBA) as a retrograde filling material. They reported that Super EBA is unresorbable and radiopaque. Histological evaluation showed a chronic inflammatory reaction, which is considered normal in the presence of a foreign body, but it also showed the possibility of collagen fibers growing over the material.

Super EBA is a modified zinc oxide eugenol cement (see Table 6.4). The eugenol is partially substituted with orthoethoxybenzoic acid to shorten the setting time. Alumina is added to the zinc oxide powder to make the cement stronger.

Super EBA has a neutral pH, low solubility, and high tensile and compressive strength.[39] Several in vitro studies demonstrated that Super EBA has less leakage than amalgam and IRM.[39–41]

Advantages of Super EBA include fast setting time, dimensional stability, good adap-

tation to canal walls, and the ability to polish. However, it is a difficult material to manipulate because the setting time is greatly affected by temperature and humidity.

Preparation and Placement of Super EBA

The liquid and powder are mixed in 1:4 ratio over a glass slab. Small increments of powder are incorporated into the liquid until the mixture loses its shine and the tip of EBA does not droop when picked up with an EBA carrier.

When the right consistency is reached, the EBA mix is shaped into a thin roll over the glass slab. A 3-mm-long segment is picked up by the carrier and placed directly into the dried retroprepared cavity under midrange magnification ($10\times$ to $16\times$) (see Figure 6.82). Using a microplugger of appropriate tip size and angulation, the EBA is gently condensed into the cavity (see Figure 6.83). Placement and packing are repeated until the entire retroprepared cavity is filled. At this point, a microball burnisher is used to further condense the material and to seal the margins while at the same time pushing aside any extra filling material (see Figure 6.84). A periodontal curette can be used to carve away excess Super EBA (see Figure 6.85). A dry field is maintained from the start of the retrofilling process until the Super EBA is completely set. Once the material sets, it can be polished with a composite finishing bur to a smooth finish (see Figure 6.86).

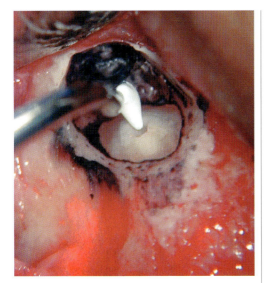

Figure 6-82. A 3-mm-long segment is picked up by the carrier and placed directly into the dried retroprepared cavity under midrange magnification.

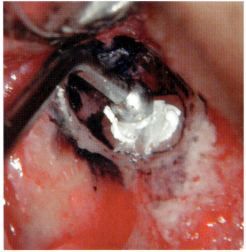

Figure 6-84. A microball burnisher is used to further condense the material and to seal the margins while pushing aside any extra filling material.

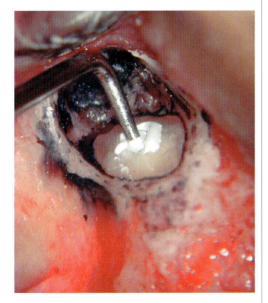

Figure 6-83. The EBA is condensed into the cavity.

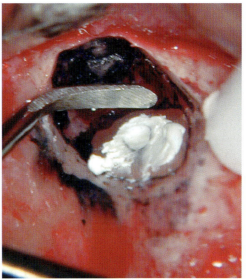

Figure 6-85. A periodontal curette can be used to carve away excess Super EBA.

Although polishing the Super EBA will remove extra filling material and produce an esthetically pleasing image of the retrofilled root-end, a recent study suggests that burnishing the EBA without polishing provides a better seal.[42]

Mineral Trioxide Aggregate (MTA)

This relatively new material was developed by Torabinejad and coworkers in 1995[43]

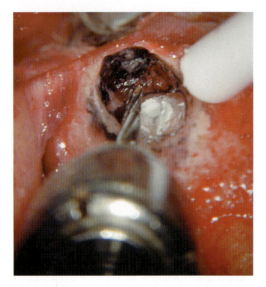

Figure 6-86. The material can be polished with a composite finishing bur to a smooth finish.

and has proven to be superior to other retrofilling materials. MTA is mainly composed of tricalcium silicate, tricalcium aluminate, and tricalcium oxide in addition to small amounts of other mineral oxides (see Figure 6.87). Bismuth oxide is added to render the mix radiopaque.

MTA is biocompatible and hydrophilic and seems to provide excellent sealing properties that are not affected by contamination with blood.[43–45] MTA has a high pH, similar to calcium hydroxide. It is the only material with the ability to promote regeneration of the periodontal apparatus where new cementum is formed directly over MTA.

The two disadvantages of MTA are long setting time (48 hours) and the difficult handling of the material. Due to the long setting time and solubility, the bone crypt area cannot be flushed with saline. Otherwise, the material would be washed out. The difficulty in the handling of MTA is due to its loose granular characteristics; it sticks very well neither to itself nor to any instrument. Fortunately, the handling problem has been solved with the introduction of the MTA pellet-forming block.

To use a system of MTA placement utiliz-

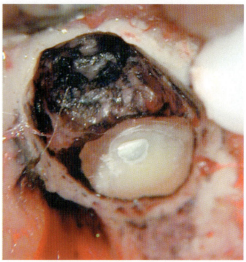

Figure 6-87. ProRoot MTA (by Dentsply/Tulsa Dental).

ing the pellet-forming block, the MTA should be mixed to the proper consistency. If the MTA mix is too wet, the pellet will not form. If it is too dry it will be crumbly and unmanageable. A proper mix should have a matte finish and not a watery gloss. This system is simply composed of a block and a placement instrument (see Figure 6.88). The block has precision grooves into which properly mixed MTA can be loaded using a spatula[46]; then any excess material outside the groove should be wiped off using

ENDODONTIC PERIRADICULAR MICROSURGERY

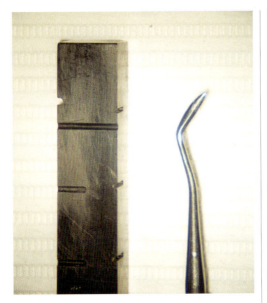

Figure 6-88. Pellet forming block and placement instrument.

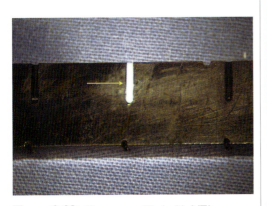

Figure 6-89. The groove filled with MTA.

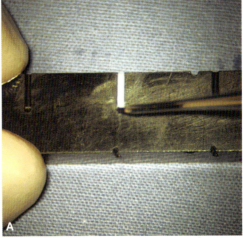

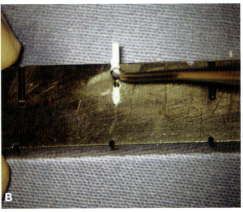

Figure 6-90A and B. The MTA pellet is carried out of the groove using the placement instrument.

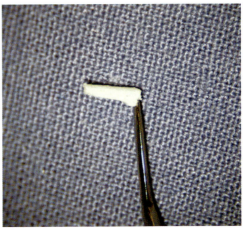

Figure 6-91. The MTA pellet on the placement instrument.

a cotton swab (see Figure 6.89). Finally the placement instrument, which perfectly fits the groove, should be used to gently slide out the MTA (see Figure 6.90). This forms a small pellet—shaped like the groove—that should stick to the tip of the placement instrument (see Figure 6.91). This MTA pellet can be precisely inserted into the root end preparation and condensed with a microplugger and a ball burnisher. The excess material can be simply removed using a wet cotton pellet (see Figure 6.92A–E).

194 CHAPTER 6

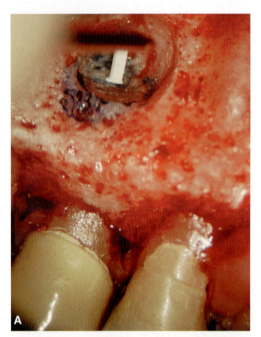
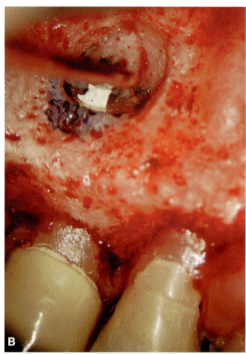

Figure 6-92A and B. MTA transferred into the retropreparation.

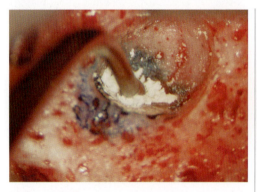

Figure 6-92C. Packing MTA with a ball burnisher.

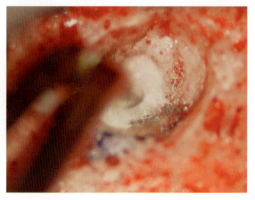

Figure 6-92D. A wet cotton pellet is used to wipe off excess cement.

Wound Closure

Wound closure after surgical procedure has three stages: reapproximation and compression, stabilization with sutures, and suture removal.

Reapproximation and Compression

After surgery, the surgical site is thoroughly rinsed with copious saline to ensure the removal of any debris or blood clots. This should apply to the entire surgical field, including the surrounding buccal plate of bone, the periradicular bone cavity (except where MTA has been used), and the underside of the reflected flap.

If ferric sulfate was used, it should be curetted and rinsed until fresh bleeding is observed. When epinephrine Racellet cotton

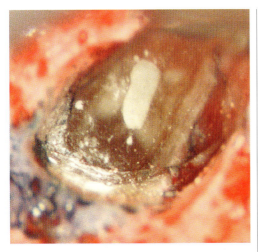

Figure 6-92E. Microinspection of MTA filling.

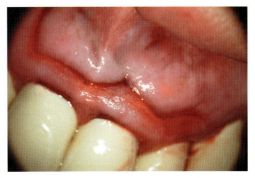

Figure 6-93. The flap is nicely reapproximated following saline wet gauze compression of three minutes.

pellets are used they should be removed before final irrigation. Any loose cotton fibers should be removed from the bone crypt with the aid of microscopic inspection. Undetected cotton fibers left in situ will induce inflammation and retard healing.[35]

Accurate reapproximation of the tissue aids in the initiation of healing by primary intention. After the flap is repositioned, saline-soaked gauze is used to compress the wound site, using firm finger pressure for three to five minutes. This is essential for the creation of a thin fibrin clot between the flap and the bone and between the wound edges[18, 47] (see Figure 6.93).

Stabilization with Sutures and Suture Removal

A variety of suture materials are available, each demonstrating advantages and disadvantages. Suture materials are divided into absorbable and nonabsorbable. They can also be monofilament or multifilament.

Silk sutures have been used for years. They are easy to handle and inexpensive. Unfortunately, since silk sutures are braided, they exhibit a wicking effect in which they attract fluid and bacteria in as early as 24 hours postoperatively, making them highly inflammatory to the wound.[48, 49] However, with smaller suture sizes (5-0 or 6-0), proper suture placement, use of chlorhexidine rinse, and timely suture removal in 48–72 hours, this problem can be minimized.[18]

Chromic gut sutures are resorbable. The treatment of this type of suture with chromic acid prolongs its retention in tissues. Nevertheless, they are difficult to handle.

The use of synthetic monofilament sutures such as nylon is desirable. They are nonresorbable and available in small sizes and cause minimal tissue reaction. They are the sutures of choice in areas with higher esthetic demand. The only disadvantage is their high cost.

Of the many suturing techniques available, the interrupted and sling suturing techniques seem to be the ones most commonly used because they are simple and effective. The interrupted suturing can be used for the vertical releasing incision, while the sling suture technique can be used for the sulcular incision.

Suture knots should always be placed away from the incision line to minimize microbial colonization in that area (see Figure 6.94). The minimal number of sutures that provide adequate flap reapproximation should be used. All sutures should be removed in 48–72 hours.

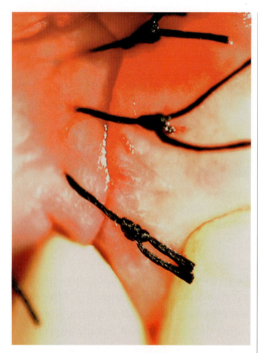

Figure 6-94. Interrupted suturing of the vertical incision; note the placement of the suture knots away from incision line.

Postsurgical Care

Postoperative patient instructions should include the following:

1. Intermittent application of ice pack to the surgical site (30 minutes on, 30 minutes off) starting immediately after the surgery and continuing for six to eight hours.
2. Strenuous activity, smoking, and alcohol should be avoided.
3. Normal food is permitted with emphasis on the avoidance of hard, sticky, and chewy food.
4. Do not pull the lip or facial tissues.
5. Continue the use of analgesics given presurgically (600 mg ibuprofen every 6 hours as needed). Slight to moderate discomfort is expected for the first 24–48 hours. Narcotic analgesics are provided and used only as an adjunct to ibuprofen if needed.
6. Oozing of blood from the surgical site is normal for the first 24 hours. It can be managed with application of a wet gauze pack to the site, pressed in place with an ice pack.
7. The day following the surgery, chlorhexidine rinses should be used twice a day, continuing for three to four days. Warm salt water rinses can be used every two hours.
8. Brushing of the surgical site is not recommended until the sutures are removed. Cotton swabs can be used to clean the surgical site.

Surgical Sequelae and Complications

Oral and written postoperative instructions will minimize the occurrence and severity of surgical sequelae and will reduce patients' anxiety when and if problems develop.

Pain, swelling, and hemorrhage are the most common postsurgical complications. They can be easily managed with NSAIDs, pressure, and ice application.

After two to three days, if signs of infection are present (for example, fever, pain, and progressive swelling with pus drainage), antibiotics should be considered. If patients develop a serious facial space infection, they should be immediately referred for emergency medical care and intravenous antibiotics.

Rarely, ecchymosis can develop. It is characterized by a discoloration of the facial and oral soft tissue due to the extravasation and subsequent breakdown of blood in the interstitial subcutaneous tissue. Usually it occurs below the surgical site due to gravity. It can also develop in a higher site like the infraorbital area (see Figure 6.95).

Paresthesia can develop when surgery is performed near the mental foramen even when the surgical site is far from the nerve. It is usually transient in nature and is mainly caused by the inflammatory swelling of the

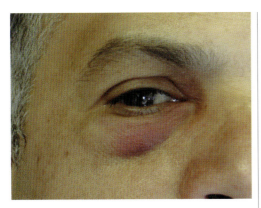

Figure 6-95. Ecchymosis in the infraorbital area following apical surgery in the maxilla.

surgical site that impinges on the mandibular nerve. If the nerve has not been severed, normal sensations usually return in few weeks, but it can take up to a few months. On rare occasions paresthesia can be permanent.

Microsurgery Success Rate

Periradicular microsurgery is a predictable and successful treatment of endodontic failure when the previous root canal treatment and coronal restoration are of adequate quality. (The reasons for an endodontic failure are not obvious.)

Surgical treatment is, however, not always successful. Possible etiological factors for failure are as follows:

- Poor case selection
- Incomplete root canal space debridement
- Incomplete debridement of the canal isthmus
- Inadequate apical seal
- Missed canals
- Failure to manage the root-end or retrofilling material properly
- Vertical root fracture
- Endodontic periodontic communication
- Recurrent cystic lesion

Other uncertain factors can also play a role such as infected dentinal tubules, type of root canal filling, more coronally located lateral canals, and failure to use antibiotics.

When appropriate case selection criteria are used, endodontic microsurgery seems to have great success. One study showed a success rate of 96.8 percent after a one-year follow-up.[50] With longer follow-up periods of up to 8 years of the same surgical cases, a success rate of 91.5 percent was achieved.[51] Similar results are reported with other long-term prospective studies.[52]

Conclusion

Periradicular surgery in the hands of operators who can perform the procedure accurately can be a great service for patients. With the presentation of this chapter, the author would like to bring a more thorough understanding of contemporary endodontic surgical techniques to general dentists who have an interest in incorporating this procedure into their practices. Needless to say, materials and methods in dentistry are changing constantly. It is the author's hope that readers will continuously enrich themselves with evidence-based literature relating to the study of endodontics in the grand scheme of providing better patient care.

References

1. P. A. Gilheany. Apical dentin permeability and microleakage associated with root end resection and retrograde filling. *J Endod* 20(1): 22–26. 1994.
2. B. G. Tidmarsh. Dentinal tubules at the root ends of apicected teeth: a scanning electron microscopic study. *Int Endod J* 22: 184–189. 1989.
3. G. B. Carr. Common errors in periradicular surgery. *Endod Rep* 8: 12. 1993.
4. G. B. Carr. Ultrasonic root-end preparation. *Dent Clin North Am* 41(3): 541–554. 1997.
5. W. Hess. Formation of root canal in human teeth. *J Nat Dent Assoc* 3: 704–734. 1921.
6. W. Hess, E. Zurcher. The anatomy of the root canals of the permanent dentition. New York: William Wood & Co. 1925.

7. G. Sundqvist. Microbiological analysis of teeth with failed endodontic treatment and the outcome of conservative re-treatment. *Oral Surg Oral Med Oral Pathol* 85(1): 86–93. 1998.

8. B. E. Wayman. A bacteriological and histological evaluation of 58 Periapical lesions. *J endod* 18: 152–155. 1992.

9. G. Sundqvist. Isolation of actinomyces israelii from periapical lesion. *J Endod* 6: 602–606. 1980.

10. P. N. R. Nair. Periapical Actinomycosis. *J Endod* 10: 567–570. 1984.

11. U. Sjögren. Survival of arachnia propionica in periapical tissue. *Int Endod J* 21: 277–282. 1988.

12. T. Kiryu. Bacteria invading periapical cementum. *J Endod* 20: 169–172. 1994.

13. P. N. R. Nair. Types and incidence of human periapical lesions obtained with extracted teeth. *Oral Surg Oral Med Oral Pathol* 81: 93–102. 1996.

14. P. N. R. Nair. Non-microbial etiology: periapical cysts sustain post-treatment apical periodontitis. *Endod Topics* 6: 96–13. 2003.

15. J. H. S. Simon. Incidence of periapical cysts in relation to the root canal. *J Endod* 6: 845–848. 1980.

16. A. Freedman. Complications after apicoectomy in maxillary premolar and molar teeth. *Int J Oral Maxillofacial Surg* 28: 192–194. 1999.

17. C. E. Jerome. Preventing root tip loss in the maxillary sinus during endodontic surgery. *J Endod* 21: 422–424. 1995.

18. J. L. Gutmann, J. W. Harrison. Surgical Endodontics. St Louis, MO: Ishiyaku EuroAmeria. 1994.

19. A. S. Dajani. Prevention of bacterial endocarditis, recommendations by the American Heart Association. *J Am Med Assoc* 277: 1794. 1997.

20. D. Jackson. Preoperative non-steroidal anti-inflammatory drugs for the prevention of postoperative pain. *J Am Dent Assoc* 119: 641–647. 1989.

21. J. T. Jastak. Vasoconstrictors and local anesthesia: a review and rationale for use. *J Am Dent Assoc* 107: 623–630. 1983.

22. J. A. Buckley. Efficacy of epinephrine concentration in local anesthesia during periodontal surgery. *J Periodontal* 55: 653–657. 1984.

23. S. G. Ciancio. Clinical pharmacology for dental professionals. 3rd edition. Chicago, IL: Year Book Medical, pp. 146–148. 1989.

24. D. H. Roberts. Local analgesia in dentistry. 2nd edition. Bristol, UK: Wright, pp. 84–88. 1987.

25. S. Kim, G. Pecora, R. Rubinstein. Color atlas of microsurgery in endodontics. Philadelphia, PA: W.B. Saunders. 2001.

26. F. J. Vickers. Hemostatic efficacy and cardiovascular effects of agents used during endodontic surgery. *J Endod* 28(4): 322–323. 2003.

27. B. G. Jeansonne. Ferric sulfate hemostasis: effect on osseous wound healing. II. With curettage and irrigation. *J Endod* 19(4): 174–176. 1993.

28. J. L. Gutmann. Posterior endodontic surgery: anatomical considerations and clinical techniques. *Int Endod J* 18: 8–34. 1985.

29. L. B. Peters. Soft tissue management in endodontic surgery. *Dent Clin North Am* 41(30): 513–528. 1997.

30. J. W. Harrison. Wound healing in the tissue of the periodontium following periradicular surgery. I. The incisional wound. *J Endod* 17(9): 425–435. 1991.

31. D. E. Cutright. Microcirculation of the perioral regions in the Macaca rhesus: part 1. *Oral Surg* 29: 776. 1970.

32. N. P. Lang. The relationship between the width of keratinized gingiva and gingival health. *J Periodontal* 43: 623–627. 1972.

33. S. Kim. Hemostasis in endodontic microsurgery. *Dent Clin North Am* 41(3): 499–512. 1997.

34. J. V. Cambruzzi. Molar endodontic surgery. *J Canadian Dent Assoc* 49: 61–65. 1983.

35. G. B. Carr. Surgical endodontics. *Pathways of the Pulp*. 7th edition. St Louis, MO: Mosby-Year Book, pp. 608–656. 1998.

36. S. O. Dorn. Retrograde filling materials: a retrospective success-failure study of amalgam, EBA, and IRM. *J Endod* 16: 391–393. 1990.

37. A. L. Frank. Long-term evaluation of surgically placed amalgam fillings. *J Endod* 18: 391–398. 1992.

38. J. Oynick. A study for a new material for retrograde fillings. *J Endod* 4: 203–206. 1978.

39. R. P. O'Connor. Leakage of amalgam and super-EBA root-end fillings using two preparation techniques and surgical microscopy. *J Endod* 21: 74–78. 1995.

40. D. L. Bondra. Leakage in vitro with IRM, high copper amalgam, and EBA cement as retrofilling materials. *J Endod* 15: 157–160. 1989.

41. J. T. Briggs. Ten year in vitro assessment of the surface status of three retrofilling materials. *J Endod* 21: 521–525. 1995.

42. S. G. Forte. Microleakage of super-EBA with and without finishing as determined by the fluid filtration method. *J Endod* 24(12): 799. 1998.

43. M. Torabinejad. Physical and chemical properties of a new root-end filling material. *J Endod* 21: 349–353. 1995.

44. M. Torabinejad. Dye leakage of four root end filling materials: effects of blood contamination. *J Endod* 20: 159–163. 1994.

45. M. Torabinejad. Histologic assessment of mineral trioxide aggregate as a root-end filling in monkeys. *J Endod* 23: 225–228.1997.

46. E. S. Lee. A new mineral trioxide aggregate root-end filling technique. *J Enodod* 26(12): 764–765. 2000.

47. H. L. Levine. Repair following periodontal flap surgery with the retention of the gingival fibers. *J Periodontol* 43: 99–103. 1972.

48. G. E. Lilly. Reaction of oral tissues to suture materials: Part III. *Oral Surg* 28: 432–438. 1969.

49. G.E. Lilly. Reaction of oral tissues to suture materials: Part IV. *Oral Surg* 33: 152–157. 1972.

50. R. A. Rubinstein. Short-term observation of the results of endodontic surgery with the use of the surgical operating microscope and Super-EBA as root-end filling material. *J Endod* 25: 43–48. 1999.

51. R. A. Rubinstein. Long-term follow-up of cases considered healed one year after apical microsurgery. *J Endod* 28: 378–383. 2002.

52. M. L. Zuolo. Prognosis in periradicular surgery: a clinical prospective study. *Int Endod J* 33: 91–98. 2000.

53. D. E. Arens, M. Torabinejad, N. Chivian, R. Rubinstein. *Practical Lessons in Endodontic Surgery.* 1st edition. Chicago, IL: Quintessence. 1998.

I would like to express my deep appreciation for Dr. Alice P. Chen for her outstanding effort in editing and rewriting this chapter. I would also like to thank Dr. Syngcuk Kim for generously sharing some of his microsurgical slides. I am very grateful for the help I received from my assistants and staff in documenting and collecting clinical pictures and illustrations.

Chapter 7

The Evaluation and Treatment of Oral Lesions

Dr. Joseph D. Christensen and Dr. Karl R. Koerner

Introduction

When a general dentist discovers a lesion in the mouth of a patient, there are often several choices on how to proceed. This chapter will help the clinician properly evaluate, document, and manage a lesion within the oral cavity. It will outline and discuss the indications for biopsy, the materials and methods necessary to improve screening and early detection of lesions, and when to refer to someone with more knowledge and experience. Instructions on different types of biopsy and how to properly perform each will be described. Careful application of sound principles, good judgment, and clinical skill will help improve the dentist's ability to identify, evaluate, and treat—or refer—lesions found in the patients for whom we are responsible.

Patient Evaluation

In order to establish a diagnosis, the dentist should have a thorough history of the lesion, the patient's health history, and information from a clinical exam in order to put the questionable tissue into proper context. A patient's past health history, including medications, trauma, diet, previous surgeries, and habits all deserve thorough detective work on the part of the dentist. Answers to proper questions will often reveal the probable cause of the lesion and may help direct the clinician down an obvious path of treatment.

HEALTH HISTORY

The dentist should be in possession of a written health history that is both accurate and current. The patient's answers on the form should only be used as a starting point, however, and should provoke the dentist to probe further for a more complete picture of the patient's health. This history informs the clinician about situations that might cause or predispose a lesion. The history can also alert the clinician to various systemic conditions that could influence a decision regarding a proposed biopsy or other treatment. In these instances, it may be appropriate to investigate these issues further

201

through a physician consultation. Still other conditions may, at the very least, require special precautions such as with hypertension, brittle diabetes, heart defects, coagulapathies, and pregnancy.

The clinician must take into account that many oral lesions are manifestations of systemic conditions. Indeed, it is true that the oral cavity is a good barometer of overall health. Many diseases have an oral presentation as part of the disease process. Common examples of this include but certainly are not limited to Crohn's disease, HIV, Lupus, Sjogren's syndrome, diabetes, and many different viral, bacterial, and fungal infections. Being aware of the patient's systemic conditions and how they may present is part of the puzzle in helping the clinician determine a differential diagnosis.

Lesion History

In order to see an accurate picture, the dentist should retrieve as much information about the lesion as possible. Well-directed questioning of the patient will usually include the following:

1. **How long has the lesion been present?** Lesions that have been present for more than two weeks should be of the greatest concern. The patient should be asked whether they know the origin of the lesion and what may have led to its occurrence. The dentist should look for any source of trauma within the mouth (such as a denture irritation) and relieve it if necessary.
2. **Has the lesion changed in size, shape, or color?** The lesion may appear to the patient to be growing larger. Lesions that may have once been white in appearance but now are reddish or a speckled white-red should raise an immediate concern of seriousness, even possible malignancy, to the clinician. An ulcer may have recently been a vesicle or bulla. Has the tissue in question changed from one vesicle to

many vesicles or ulcers? If this is the case, the possibility of a viral process should be considered.

3. **Is the lesion causing pain?** If this is the case, then what stimulus brings on the pain? What makes the pain dissipate? Without any pain, the patient may not even be aware that the lesion is present. It should be noted that oral cancer, although assumed by many to be a painful disease, does not usually elicit any pain at all.
4. **Is there anesthesia or loss of sensation?** If no lesion were present, this symptom could be attributed to many things such as medication, diabetes, pernicious anemia, or even injury incurred due to dental treatment. However, the clinician should be aware that this is also a common symptom of malignancy.
5. **Is there any lymph node involvement?** Careful inspection and palpation of the lymph nodes may reveal tenderness and sensitivity. The patient may even complain that their lymph nodes seem swollen. This usually indicates an inflammatory response to an infection. Lymph nodes may also be affected by other conditions that could be present in the mouth, including oral cancer.
6. **Is there a history of trauma?** Trauma or oral habits are likely reasons that tissue may appear unusual. Denture trauma, a sharp tooth, cheek biting, use of tobacco products, burns associated with hot foods or liquid, cuts and abrasions from hard or sharp food, and chemical burns from aspirin or other medicines are just a few of the possible reasons why tissue may appear unusual.
7. **Are there any constitutional symptoms?** For example, is the patient febrile? Does the patient have dysphagia (difficulty swallowing), nausea, or general malaise? These are all signs that may have taken root from a general systemic condition, which may or may not be associated with the lesion, but that add information to an

overall picture. Fever and dysphagia particularly may suggest an inflammatory process requiring further investigation.

Examination

A proper examination and description of the lesion and the surrounding tissue should be accurately recorded in the patient's chart. Along with the written description, an illustration demonstrating the exact location and size of the lesion and affected lymph nodes (if any) should be included in the record as well. This information will be helpful if a lesion is to be followed over a short period of time for comparison, resolution, or change in appearance. If the dentist decides that referral to a specialist for further evaluation and more definitive treatment is warranted, a copy of all written information (see Figure 7.1), illustrations, radiographs, and a quality photograph (if possible) should be sent to

Diagnostic Laboratory

(LAB USE ONLY)
LAB # ________ - S - ________
DATE REC'D ________
PATHOLOGIST ________
Container: ____ Labeled ____ Unlabeled

REQUEST FOR MICROSCOPIC EXAMINATION

BIOPSY: ☐ Excisional ☐ Incisional ☐ Cytology ☐ X-rays # enclosed ____ ☐ Photos # enclosed ____

CONTRIBUTING DOCTOR OR OHSU STUDENT:	PATIENT: Surgery Date ___ / ___ / ___	BILLING:
Name ________	Name ________	___ BILL DOCTOR
Address ________	Address ________	
________	City ________	___ BILL PATIENT:
City ________	State ________ Zip ________ - ________	(completion of back page is required)
State ________ Zip ________ - ________	DOB ___ / ___ / ___ Age ________	
Phone ( ) ________	Sex ____ Race ____	
Fax ( ) ________	Pt Phone ( ) ________	
	Occupation	

PLEASE INDICATE LOCATION AND EXTENT OF LESION:

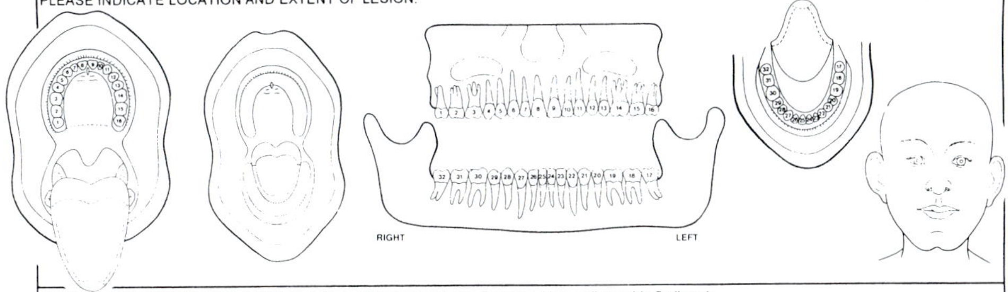

CLINICAL DESCRIPTION OF LESION: (Location, clinical appearance, firmness, size, radiographic findings.)
Please enclose radiographs/photographs when applicable.

HISTORY OF LESION: (Describe sequence of events & findings leading to the present state of the lesion -- duration, rapidity of growth, variation in appearance, pain or other symptoms, possible causes, pertinent lab tests.)

SIGNIFICANT PAST MEDICAL - DENTAL HISTORY:

PROVISIONAL CLINICAL DIAGNOSIS:

GROSS: (Dept. Use Only)

Figure 7-1. Biopsy diagnostic report form typical of those used by oral pathology laboratories and submitting clinicians.

the oral pathologist and/or the oral and maxillofacial surgeon.

During an examination, it is a common mistake to handle a lesion and the surrounding tissue before a written description can be made. This manipulation can cause characteristics of the lesion to change. For example, many lesions are friable and epithelium may tear, ulcerations may open and hemorrhage, and vesicles may rupture. A lesion may also change character, color, and size over time, so an accurate initial description, before manipulation, will help obtain the proper diagnosis and treatment and may serve as a comparison and reference in the future.[1]

There are a number of factors and questions that should be answered and recorded in order to place the lesion into proper perspective. Just as variability in the clinical presentation of a lesion is a factor, so too, can microscopic analysis be a challenge without the proper lesion history, medical history, and preoperative description.

When describing a lesion for the patient's clinical record, there is accepted medical terminology and descriptors that should be used to convey an accurate picture in a language common to all who will evaluate the tissue. This is especially true if a specimen is to be sent to an oral pathologist. This description should include many observed characteristics, such as location, size, shape, color, texture, consistency, overall character, single or multiple lesions, ulcerations, mobility or fixation to adjacent structures, fluctuance, inflammation, and associated lymphadenopathy. Table 7.1 gives definitions of proper terminology.

Clinical Judgment

After the collection and recording of information has been completed and a differential diagnosis made, the clinician must then make a professional judgment of how to proceed. It is important that a definitive diagnosis of all lesions be determined.[2] It is

Table 7-1. Clinical Descriptions

Bulla   Loculated fluid in or under the epithelium of skin or mucosa. A large blister, larger than 5mm.

Crusts   Dried or clotted serum protein on the surface of skin or mucosa.

Cyst   A pathologic epithelium-lined cavity often filled with liquid or semisolid contents.

Ecchymosis   A nonelevated area of hemorrhage. Larger than petechia.

Erosion   Superficial ulceration (excoriation).

Fissure   A narrow, slit-like ulceration or groove.

Granuloma   A focal area of chronic inflammation composed of vascularized granulation tissue.

Macule   Circumscribed area of color change without elevation.

Multilocular   A radiolucent lesion composed of multiple compartments.

Nodule   A large palpable mass elevated above the epithelial surface. Larger than 5mm in diameter.

Papillary   A tumor or growth exhibiting numerous surface projections.

Papule   A small palpable mass elevated above the epithelial surface. Less than 5mm in diameter.

Pedunculated   A tumor or growth whose base is narrower than the widest part of the lesion.

Petechia   A round, pinpoint area of hemorrhage.

Plaque   A flat elevated lesion. The confluence of papules.

Pustule   A cloudy or white vesicle—the color of which results from the presence of polymorphonuclear leukocytes (pus).

Scale   A macroscopic accumulation of keratin.

Sessile   A tumor or growth whose base is the widest part of the lesion.

Telangiectasia   A vascular lesion caused by dilatation of a small, superficial blood vessel.

Ulcer   Loss of epithelium

Unilocular   A radiolucent lesion having a single compartment.

Verrucous   A tumor or growth exhibiting a rough, warty surface.

Vesicle   A small loculation of fluid on or under the epithelium. A small blister under 5mm.

not consistent with the current standards of care to simply watch a lesion over an extended period of time. When local irritation is thought to be the reason for the problem, the area in question should be treated nonsurgically to allow the tissue to heal. Examples of nonsurgical treatment would include smoothing the sharp cusp of a tooth, acrylic relief or clasp adjustment on a denture, or just observing an area where it is suspected that sharp or hot food injured the tissue without the patient's knowledge or remembrance. In this situation, a watch-and-wait period of two weeks would be prudent. If in fact the lesion was trauma induced, the area should heal within this period of time. However, if after the waiting period the lesion still persists, then it must be assumed the causation is not traumatic in nature, and therefore biopsy would be indicated.

It should be noted that most oral cancers are asymptomatic in the early stages.[3] The consequence of this is that most cases are not detected and diagnosed until classic signs of malignancy appear late in disease progression. The classic signs of oral cancer include: erythroplakia, induration, ulceration, parasthesia, bleeding, and cervical adenopathy. Unfortunately, all of these signs may be associated with advanced disease and increased morbidity and mortality.[4] See Table 7.2.

The problem for the clinician lies in the difficulty of distinguishing precancerous and early-stage cancerous oral lesions from similarly appearing benign lesions.[5] Oral cancer in its early stages is insidious, difficult to identify, and does not always exhibit consistent characteristics. For example, Sandler found that 25 percent of 207 early stage oral cancer lesions did not demonstrate any classic signs of malignancy.[6] Unrealized to some practitioners, it does not always originate from the traditional predisposing risk factors either. Blot demonstrated this in their study that showed approximately 25 percent of oral cancers arise in patients who do not consume tobacco or heavy amounts of alcohol.[7]

Table 7-2. Possible Signs of Malignancy

Erythroplakia Although less common than leukoplakia, almost all true erythroplakias show malignant changes and have a much greater potential for dysplasia or invasive malignancy.

Leukoplakia Although not often malignant, this is by far the most common oral precancer, representing 85 percent of such lesions in tobacco smoking populations.

Ulceration Ulcerated areas that do not heal after 14 days must receive a prompt biopsy.

Parasthesia Oral cancer with deep invasion can cause loss of sensation when involved near or within nerves.

Loss of mobility Clinically this may present as fixation of the tongue or inability to fully open the mouth.

Induration This simply indicates firm or hard tissue, but in the case of malignancy, it is commonly seen with ulcerations, leukoplakia, and especially erythroplakia.

Persistence If after local trauma and irritation are removed, a lesion is highly suspicious—remaining longer than 2–3 weeks in duration.

Sciubba showed the difficulty with visual inspection and identification of oral cancer in a 1999 study.[8] That study surprisingly revealed that even specialists trained in oral and maxillofacial pathology, oral medicine, and oral and maxillofacial surgery had difficulty differentiating benign lesions from cancerous or precancerous ones. These experts identified and categorized 647 lesions out of 945 in the study as benign in appearance. Results from oral brush biopsy were returned on all 945 lesions. Of the 647 benign-appearing lesions, 29 of them returned with a result of atypical or positive by brush biopsy, and scalpel biopsy subsequently confirmed the presence of dysplasia or malignancy. In this multicenter study, the brush biopsy system revealed every precancerous and cancerous lesion among all patients within the trial.[9] This important study highlights the fact that visual inspection of the oral cavity alone is not a good predictor for determining whether a patient has early stage oral cancer.

The clinical lesion decision tree shown in Table 7.3 illustrates possible treatment scenarios upon discovering an oral abnormality. Oral cancer risk factors are listed in Table 7.4.

Biopsy

Biopsy, by definition, is the removal of tissue, cells, or fluids from the living body for diagnostic examination in order to confirm or establish the diagnosis of disease. The mere mention of the word biopsy traditionally has implied the eminent use of a sharp knife. Scalpel biopsy is still the gold standard

Table 7-3. Decision Tree for Treatment of Oral Lesions

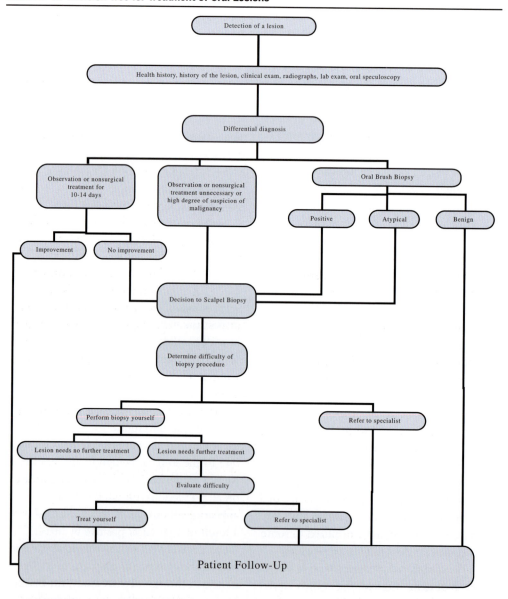

Adapted from L.J. Peterson, E. Ellis, J.R. Hupp, and M.R. Tucker. *Contemporary Oral and Maxillofacial Surgery*, 4th edition. St. Louis, MO: Mosby. 2003.

upon which all clinicians rely for a definitive diagnosis. In addition to this technique, the advent of the brush biopsy has allowed dentists the opportunity to perform a noninvasive biopsy on lesions they probably would have watched in the past. An obvious point to be made is that a clinician should not wait to biopsy or refer for biopsy any patient with tissue that raises the suspicion of malignancy. In fact, a highly suspicious lesion exhibiting any classic signs of cancer should, with tactful communication to the patient, be referred immediately to a specialist. If this situation arises, it is easier for the specialist to treat the patient if an initial biopsy **has not** been done. It is much easier for the specialist to evaluate the tissue in an undisturbed state rather than a manipulated and/or incised state.[2]

Five types of biopsy/diagnostic measures that help enhance and visualize suspect tissues will be discussed. These five procedures are 1) oral brush biopsy; 2) aspiration biopsy; 3) incisional biopsy; 4) excisional biopsy; and 5) oral speculoscopy. A description of each method and how to perform it is given in the following sections.

ORAL BRUSH BIOPSY

A computer-assisted method of analysis developed by Oral CDx (OralScan Laboratories, Suffern, NY) is an important adjunct in the clinical assessment of an oral lesion. As stated, the majority of oral cancer goes undiagnosed until obvious signs of malignancy are exhibited—usually late in the disease process.[10] Consequently, the five-year survival rate of oral cancer is low—approximately 52 percent[11] (see Table 7.5). The purpose of the oral brush biopsy is to identify lesions that otherwise may appear harmless but in fact histologically exhibit atypical cells, dysplasia, or frank carcinoma.

Brush biopsy is a convenient, inexpensive, and noninvasive alternative to watching a lesion for an indefinite amount of time. In the

Table 7-4. Risk Factors for Oral Malignancy

- Tobacco use responsible for 90 percent of oral cancer.
- Alcohol and tobacco used concurrently increases risk exponentially.
- Smokers and alcohol users older than age 40 at the highest risk.
- 25 percent of oral cancer patients have no risk factors.
- Sun exposure to the lip.
- Human Papilloma Virus (HPV16, HPV18, HPV31, and HPV33).
- Squamous cell carcinoma is multifactorial in its genesis.

past, many general dentists have been reluctant to perform a biopsy on a patient who has an innocuous-looking lesion, or even refer this patient for biopsy. They may have felt a scalpel biopsy was overkill for something that appeared so harmless. A watch-and-wait approach was most likely accepted by the patient and became an acceptable alternative to the knife. In contrast, the oral brush biopsy is a breakthrough advancement, bridging the gap between observation and surgery, bringing a reliable and perhaps lifesaving tool to the aid of our patients.[12] Just as important, this technique can confirm that a harmless-appearing lesion is in fact benign.

Another benefit of brush biopsy is patient

Table 7-5. Oral Cancer Statistics*

30,000	Americans diagnosed each year.
8,000	Die each year.
52%	Die within 5 yrs. of diagnosis.
70%	Diagnosed in late stage.
90%	Curable if caught early.
60%	Increase in tongue cancer with people under age 40 over the past three decades.

*Oral Health in America: A report of the Surgeon General. 2000 Reuters Health.

compliance. It is well documented that many patients referred to an oral surgeon for biopsy of a lesion delay, cancel, or avoid the appointment altogether.[13, 14] The simplicity of this noninvasive procedure allows the dentist to perform the biopsy at the same time the lesion is found, without the need for local anesthetic. Depending on lab results, it may also prevent the need for incisional or excisional biopsy in the future.

Procedure

A brush biopsy kit supplied from the manufacturer contains a brush biopsy instrument (round stiff nylon brush), a bar-coded glass slide, alcohol-based fixative, and a protective plastic case for mailing (see Figures 7.2A and 7.2B). Written instructions and a video are also available. The nylon brush is designed to collect cells from all three layers of epithelium: superficial, intermediate, and basal. This method of collection differentiates itself from the unreliable and traditional oral cytology, where only superficial epithelial cells were collected and evaluated. With oral brush biopsy, cells are taken from perhaps the most important and revealing portion of the lesion, the basal layer. Therefore, it is critical that the brush extract cells from this area of the lesion. This is accomplished by applying firm pressure on the lesion and rotating the brush 5–10 times. Pinpoint bleeding or exposure of pinkish-red mucosa usually signals that an adequate sample of cells has been taken.

After cell extraction, the nylon brush is rotated thoroughly and evenly across the glass slide in order to transfer as many cells as possible. The slide is then doused with the alcohol fixative included in the kit and allowed to dry before being transferred to the plastic container for mailing.

Because this test is designed to be effective on tissue exhibiting an **epithelial** abnormality, lesions with an intact, normal-looking epithelium or lesions originating in submu-

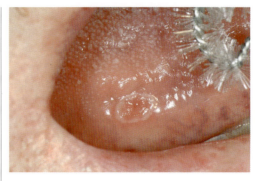

Figure 7-2A. Clinician approaching an oval lesion with a white border on the right lateral dorsum of the tongue.

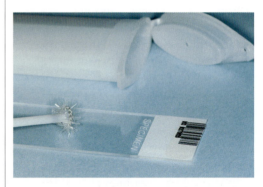

Figure 7-2B. Cells being smeared on a slide prior to adding the fixative. The Oral CDx lab reported that the cellular representation consisted of superficial, intermediate, and basal cells. The diagnosis was of benign epithelial cells, singly and in clusters—negative for premalignant or malignant epithelial change.

cosa, should not be tested by oral brush biopsy. This would then exclude fibromas, pigmented lesions, lipomas, salivary gland lesions (mucoceles), papillomas, and lesions found on the vermilion border of the lip.

Dentists new to this procedure may be concerned that their biopsy may have an insufficient number of cells and, therefore, risk a false-negative result. For this reason, safeguards have been put into place by OralScan Laboratories to ensure that only quality specimens are given an outcome. Each specimen is carefully examined to ensure that an adequate cellular representation of all epithelial layers is present. If this has not been achieved, it usually means the specimen is lacking sufficient cells from the basal layer and the dentist will be contacted in order to perform another biopsy. On the rare occasion that this occurs, the lab will replace the biopsy kit at no cost to the patient or dentist.

After the clinician submits the oral brush biopsy to the lab, it is analyzed by a sophisticated network of computers specifically designed for this type of pathological review. Each biopsy is photographed approximately 200 times and scanned by the computer for epithelial abnormalities associated with oral precancerous and cancerous cells.[15] After the computer analysis, an oral and maxillofacial pathologist then evaluates the biopsy. Results are subsequently given in one of three categories: negative, atypical, or positive.

A biopsy returned with a result of atypical or positive requires an incisional or excional biopsy to microscopically review the histologic architecture of the lesion for definitive diagnosis. A report or finding from the scalpel biopsy is returned to the referring dentist giving the results. If necessary, the lesion is then given a grading and staging specific to that tissue. Of course no matter what the finding, even a negative finding, all patients possessing lesions or abnormalities should be scrutinized and be provided with proper follow-up in the future. If during these visits the lesion persists or changes presentation, prudence would require an additional biopsy be performed.

ASPIRATION BIOPSY

Aspiration biopsy is removing contents of a lesion for the purpose of analysis or quick observation. This technique should not be confused with fine needle aspiration biopsy (FNA), which will be discussed later. Aspiration biopsy is typically used to rule out the possibility of a vascular lesion. This method of discovery is vastly preferable to

the unforgettable experience of finding a vascular lesion unexpectedly. Avoidance of succumbing to this misadventure requires the treating clinician be familiar with and be able to perform an aspiration biopsy on all suspected soft tissue vascular lesions and radiolucent osseous lesions before surgical exploration is undertaken. This may require referral to a specialist.

Not only is the aspiration biopsy helpful in ruling out vascular lesions, this technique is also helpful in identifying contents of various other lesions as well.

For example, if air is extracted into the syringe, a traumatic bone cavity has probably been accessed. If it is difficult to aspirate air or fluid at all from the tissue, the lesion is most likely solid, and a different type of biopsy may be indicated. If a purulent white fluid is obtained, then an infection may be present. If a yellow straw-like substance is present, then perhaps the fluid of a cyst was removed. The presence of blood on aspiration can indicate the most important lesion, which is the previously mentioned vascular lesion; however, it may also suggest the presence of other types of lesions. If blood is observed upon aspiration, the general dentist should need no further evidence in order to refer the patient to a specialist, where a more thorough exploration of the tissue can be accomplished in a controlled surgical setting.

Aspiration Biopsy Procedure

This technique requires the use of an 18-gauge needle and a 5–10 cc syringe. The patient should be anesthetized, after which the 18-gauge needle and syringe are inserted into the approximate area of the mass. The needle oftentimes may need successive repositioning in order to be correctly placed within the center of the lesion. Negative pressure (pulling back on the plunger) is then applied to the syringe in an attempt to achieve positive aspiration. If a bony lesion is to be accessed, the needle should be placed on the periosteum and twisted, and firm pressure applied. If the needle cannot be introduced through the cortex with the suggested technique, a flap should be reflected, after which a small dental bur can be used to penetrate the cortical plate, allowing for needle aspiration.

Once again, clinical judgment of the lesion, the patient, and the dentist's own knowledge, skill, and comfort level are essential in determining how to proceed and, more importantly, who should perform this treatment.

FINE NEEDLE ASPIRATION BIOPSY

Although not commonly performed by the general dentist, the FNA will be discussed in order that the practitioner may be aware of the technique, its application, and the difference between it and the similar aspiration biopsy.

This procedure is normally reserved for deep soft tissue lesions not easily obtained and incised by simple scalpel biopsy. It is normally performed by a pathologist on lesions of the oropharynx, lymph nodes in the neck and submandibular area, and suspected tumors of the salivary glands. Unlike the aspiration biopsy, which provides the practitioner with quick visual analysis of a lesion's nature, the FNA removes cells for histologic review and tentative diagnosis by a pathologist.

Procedure

The specialist utilizes a special fine needle that is directed to a deep part of the lesion. The mass is then pierced with the needle attached to a disposable 10cc syringe containing 2-3cc of air. FNA requires many quick passes within the mass while at the same time applying negative pressure. These jabbing passes should be taken in different areas of the tissue in order to capture cells representative of the entire lesion.[16] The air introduced into the syringe before aspiration helps dispel the specimen onto the glass slide once the biopsy is completed. Normal fixative procedures are then implemented and the biopsy is examined.

ORAL SPECULOSCOPY

This technique is a noninvasive adjunct to the normal full-mouth soft tissue examination. To be clear, this procedure is not a biopsy, but a diagnostic method. However, it may aid in the visualization and evaluation of an oral mucosal abnormality. Originally, this technique was adapted from OB-GYN's Visual Cervical Screening Test. Its application in dentistry has been appropriate because the epithelium located within the oral cavity is histologically the same as epithelium within the female reproductive tract. Not only is the tissue almost identical, oral cancer and cervical cancer are essentially the same disease process.

In a gynecological study, the traditional Papanicolaou (Pap) smear when used alone detected cervical neoplasia in 31 percent of the women studied. When the combination of acetic acid and chemiluminescent light (speculoscopy) was used in conjunction with the Pap smear, the number jumped to 83 percent.[17] Since oral cancer is the sixth most common type of cancer in the United States, ahead of cervical cancer, Hodgkin's disease, and malignant melanoma, there is a natural need to utilize this and other new methods made available to improve early detection.[18, 19] This procedure was introduced and made available to dental practitioners in 2002 by ViziLite (Zila Pharmaceuticals). Essentially, this product uses acetic acid to dehydrate the epithelium, making it easier to visualize abnormal tissue with short-wavelength light. Its recommended application is for patients who have risk factors for oral cancer and those patients who have a suspected lesion or questionable area of mucosa. See Figures 7.3 and 7.4.

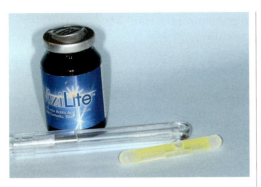

Figure 7-3. ViziLite vial of acetic acid, light stick, and light stick holder. This product helps the dentist visualize and evaluate possible oral abnormalities.

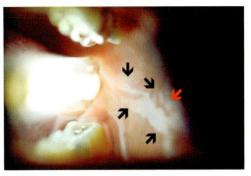

Figure 7-4B. The same tissue after application of acetic acid rinse for 30–60 seconds followed by visualization of tissue with chemiluminescent light.

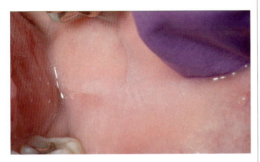

Figure 7-4A. White areas of tissue extending from the pterygomandibular raphe forward onto the buccal mucosa found during a routine dental exam.

According to a study by Huber and associates,[20] oral epithelium that is normal will absorb the chemiluminescent light used in oral speculoscopy, causing it to have a "blue-hue" appearance. In contrast, abnormal epithelium may reflect the light, making it appear acetowhite (see Figure 7.4B). It gives this appearance for either of these two reasons: 1) The tissue exhibits excessive keratinization, hyperparakeratinization, and/or significant inflammatory infiltrate; or 2) the cells have an altered nuclear-cytoplasmic density ratio. This altered nuclear-cytoplasmic ratio oftentimes means the cell has a large or enlarged nuclei, which is one of the characteristics of dysplastic or cancerous tissue.

This procedure should not only help reveal oral lesions but also impress upon the patient the need to reduce any risk factors they may have in their life. If test results are positive and determine that the patient requires a biopsy, this technique can help the patient go forward with the decision more confidently. Whether the biopsy is to be performed by the general dentist or specialist, the ViziLite application will help the clinician decide what specific area of the lesion should receive brush biopsy or scalpel biopsy.

Procedure

The provided examination kit contains instructions, a bottle of 1 percent acetic acid solution, a short-wave chemiluminescent light stick, and a two-piece retractor/holder for placement of the light stick (see Figure 7.4B). After the conventional oral examination is performed, the patient rinses with 1 percent acetic acid solution for 30–60 seconds. Following this, the light stick capsule is activated and placed into the holder, and the room lights are dimmed or turned off. The light stick is placed next to the oral mucosa in order to visualize any change in tissue appearance. If necessary, the process can be repeated. Be aware, however, that when repeating the procedure, the light stick will only stay activated for approximately 10 minutes. As with any procedure, there is a learning curve, and determining results from what is seen in the mouth can seem somewhat arbitrary. Because of this, the company provides good clinical color photographs for help in interpreting what is seen.[21]

Teaching prevention and early detection of oral cancer is the best way the dental professional can ward off this elusive threat. **Early detection** is most easily facilitated by revealing and uncovering the extent of lesions with the use of the acetic acid and chemiluminescent light. It helps not only with patients exhibiting obvious risk factors such as those who smoke and frequently consume alcohol but also with those with general questionable areas of tissue as well. The use of oral speculoscopy can provide additional information to the overall situation when a dentist is trying to determine if brush biopsy or scalpel biopsy should be recommended to a patient. If it is determined that the patient is in need of biopsy, this procedure may help the general dentist or specialist decide what portion of the lesion should be biopsied for histological exam. In addition, a full-mouth soft tissue exam used in combination with oral speculoscopy improves the finding and early detection of lesions within the oral cavity. Although this procedure could be useful with any patient, it is recommended for routine use on those patients exhibiting risk factors.

EXCISIONAL BIOPSY

This type of biopsy is described as the removal of an entire lesion including a representative portion of normal tissue surrounding the lesion. This is the preferred method of removal for small minor lesions that appear to be benign. This procedure is both diagnostic and definitive in nature in that the entire lesion is removed for examination and diagnosis. In most instances, these lesions will not need further surgical intervention.

In an ideal world, the excisional biopsy would be utilized almost exclusively. However, this procedure is not practical for every lesion and situation. It is best used by the general dentist on lesions that are 1 cm or less in diameter, are surgically accessible, and do not appear obviously malignant. Patients with more extensive or complicated situations should be referred.

INCISIONAL BIOPSY

Incisional biopsy is the removal of a representative portion of a lesion for microscopic examination. This type of biopsy is primarily used on large, diffuse, or malignant-appearing lesions. The intent of this procedure is to remove a portion of the tissue in question along with a sample of normal adjacent tissue for comparison.

The incisional biopsy, although not complicated, requires more forethought and planning for proper execution than the excisional biopsy. A pie-shaped wedge incision is usually made, starting 2–3 mm within normal tissue and extending into an adjacent portion of abnormal tissue. It is a common mistake for dentists to incise tissue too superficially in relation to the actual depth of the lesion. Cellular changes are most easily detected not in the superficial tissue that is often necrotic, but in the deeper cells located where the lesion originates. In this case, the old surgical adage applies, "It is better to incise tissue narrow and deep, than broad and shallow."

Surgical Principles for Soft Tissue Biopsy

The general practitioner should be familiar with and be able to perform a simple soft tissue biopsy. Every day, general dentists perform many complicated procedures including: extraction of bony impactions, molar root canal therapy, and surgical periodontal procedures. All of these procedures are more complicated, demand more knowledge and

THE EVALUATION AND TREATMENT OF ORAL LESIONS 213

skill, and require much more time to perform than a straightforward soft tissue biopsy. It is also true that not all scalpel biopsies are easily performed. Factors such as presentation of the lesion, surgical accessibility, and anatomic hazards may all contribute to referral of a difficult case. Nevertheless, the straightforward soft tissue biopsy can be one of the easiest dental procedures to accomplish. This section of the chapter will focus on describing the process of soft tissue biopsy and instructing the general dentist how this is to be performed.

As stated earlier, before any biopsy can be considered, the patient's health history must be evaluated for any contraindications or relative contraindications. If a scalpel biopsy (incisional or excisional) is to be performed, local anatomy within and around the area to be incised should be considered. Care should be taken to plan incisions that, wherever possible, will run parallel with and not across significant anatomical structures. For example, are the palatal vessels nearby? Are there any salivary ducts close to the proposed incision? Are the mental or lingual nerves within the proposed surgical site? Familiarity with and identification of the local anatomy is essential before any surgical procedure is planned and undertaken.[22] See Table 7.6.

ANESTHESIA

Regional block anesthesia is the most desired method of anesthesia when performing a biopsy. Although block anesthesia ensures that histologic integrity of the lesion remains intact, practicality may require local infiltration with a vasoconstrictor such as epinephrine in order to control bleeding. The possibility of changing the microscopic architecture of a lesion or causing an artifact to be present is heightened when infiltrating anesthetic within or very close to a lesion; therefore, caution must used in its application. If infiltration is needed to assist in anesthetizing the tissue or to reduce hemorrhage

Table 7-6. Instrumentation/Supply List for Biopsy

Scalpel handle #3
Scalpel blade #15
Minnesota retractor
Small hemostat (2)
Dean scissors
Curved tenotomy scissors
Needle holder
3-0 silk suture for traction
Additional closing sutures
Adson tissue forceps
Gauze sponges
Specimen bottle with 10 percent formalin

by way of vasoconstrictor, it should be deposited no closer than 1 cm from the lesion.[1] This general rule of thumb will help preserve an area of undisturbed tissue for the oral pathologist to evaluate.

INCISION

Whether an incisional or excisional biopsy is being made, the same elliptical pie-shaped wedge should be taken where possible. Although the shape of the wedge is usually the same for both types of scalpel biopsy, the small lesion requiring an excisional biopsy should include at least 2 mm of normal tissue around the entire periphery of the lesion (see Figure 7.5A). However, the incisional biopsy, depending upon the size and character of the tissue, is usually taken from the area of the lesion that shows the most clinical change and may extend partly across or fully across the lesion. Regardless of where in the mouth the tissue is removed from, it is very important that the dentist include a band of normal tissue underneath and adjacent to the lesion for comparison. If the tissue looks suspiciously malignant or fast growing or is diffuse, vascular, or pigmented, it is best to include 5 mm of normal tissue

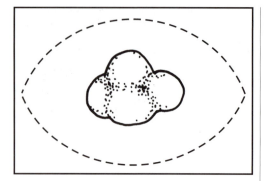

Figure 7-5A. Elliptical incision lines for an excisional biopsy that show leaving a margin of normal tissue adjacent to the lesion.

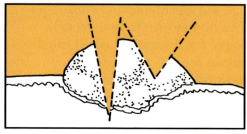

Figure 7-6. The incisional biopsy on the left side of the lesion shows the ideal removal of cells below the basement layer of the lesion. Less ideally, the wedge on the right demonstrates an incision that does not capture the entire height of the lesion. It is better to incise narrow and deep, than wide and shallow.

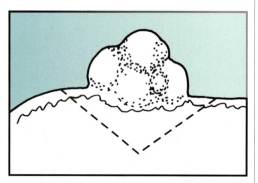

Figure 7-5B. Elliptical incisions (as shown in Figure 7-5A) that meet underneath the lesion. Traction is placed on the lesion with tissue pickups or suture to facilitate tissue control and get cleanly beneath the lesion.

surrounding the specimen. Ideally, in a longitudinal view, the incision would create a "V" that captures normal tissue below the basement layer of cells adjacent to the lesion (see Figure 7.5B).

If the lesion is located within unattached tissue (buccal mucosa, tongue, floor of mouth, and soft palate), then the length of the incision should equal about three times the width of the lesion. After removal of the tissue, the wound should be undermined (if necessary) with blunt dissecting scissors (tenotomy scissors) to relieve any tension from the submucosa layer.[2] These techniques assist the tissue to heal by primary intention and help reduce stress being placed on the suture line, thereby minimizing scar formation. See Figure 7.6.

If the lesion is located within attached mucosa, such as the palate and the attached gingiva, it is not necessary to incise longer and wider than what is required for the histological examination. The main reason for this is because the tissue usually cannot be brought together for primary closure. Although sometimes quite painful, the biopsy site located within attached mucosa is left to heal by granulation and secondary intention. The patient with a biopsy in this area can have a periodontal dressing placed to help alleviate pain postoperatively. If the incision was made on the palate, an acrylic stent can be fabricated to hold a dressing in place on the underside of the prosthesis.

It should be kept in mind that a biopsy is taken in order to determine histologic identity or change in a given area. Therefore, if the lesion is large, is not uniform in its appearance, or has multiple areas of presentation, more than one biopsy may be necessary in order to properly characterize the tissue. Regardless of whether a single site has been biopsied or multiple sites have been excised, the dentist must be able to identify and illustrate to the pathologist exactly where the lesion or lesions were taken from and document this on the tissue submission form.

Suture material, used for purposes of identification, can be helpful to the pathologist in two different ways. If there is suspicion of malignancy, a suture may be placed in a designated area of the lesion, such as the superior margin. That suture position is then written both in the patient's record and the tissue submission form, which is then forwarded to the pathologist. This orientation of the lesion, or **tagging**, then helps the dentist communicate to the oral pathologist an accurate characterization of the tissue and gives the precise location of something of particular interest. Identifying the orientation of a lesion and each of its margins also facilitates the planning of future surgical intervention if it is needed.

When incising tissue in a small enclosed area like the mouth, management of the tissue, especially the tongue, is essential. Retraction is critical in management of the oral tissues during biopsy and helps the clinician and assistant visualize the task they are performing. There are many methods of retraction, and the dentist must use what specific method feels comfortable to him or her. Different techniques include the following: finger stabilization by an assistant with gauze, chalazion forceps for lesions of the lip and buccal mucosa, placement of traction sutures, tongue retractor/probe for use on the floor of the mouth, and an atraumatic towel clip for manipulation of the tongue itself. The chalazion forcep, in particular, is useful in obtaining hemostasis because it acts like a tourniquet as well as a forcep, providing a bloodless field in which to operate (see Figures 7.7A and 7.7B).

If the lesion is small, tissue may be incised more easily if an anchoring suture is placed within the specimen itself. This not only helps with traction of the lesion, it also minimizes tissue damage easily made with tissue forceps that tend to crush when not used in a gentle manner. For larger lesions in the un-

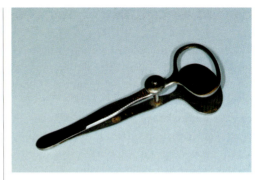

Figure 7-7A. The Chalazion forcep is commonly used to stabilize tissue for the removal of lesions in alveolar mucosa, such as mucocels and fibromas.

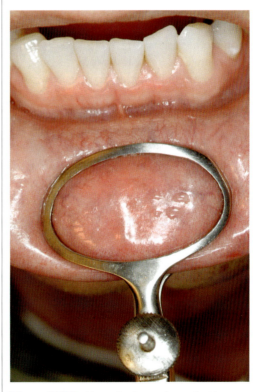

Figure 7-7B. Here, the forcep is applied to a mucosal area, allowing a fluid-filled mucocel within the soft tissue to be more easily excised.

attached areas of the oral cavity such as the tongue, buccal mucosa, soft palate, and floor of the mouth, traction sutures may be placed adjacent to the biopsy site and held by hand or hemostats for better manipulation.

Hemorrhage control

A natural consequence of incising tissue is hemorrhage. Use of dental suction to control bleeding, especially with high-volume evacuators, should be avoided if possible. This is especially true if a small lesion is to be excised. Generally a specimen is not best visualized microscopically after being fished out of a filthy, debris-ridden suction trap. Most oral pathologists, if polled, would probably agree. However, if a suction device must be used, a low-volume evacuator with overlying gauze can be implemented. Gauze compresses and applied pressure to the donor site will usually control most bleeding situations.

In recent years, many dentists have found electrosurgical cautery units to be of great use in controlling bleeding, especially when performing prosthodontic procedures. Soft tissue biopsy might initially be seen to some as another appropriate place to utilize the unique hemorrhage control that this device affords. However, just as direct infiltration of anesthetic solution and rough handling with instrumentation can distort tissue, so too can electrocautery alter and cause destruction of the specimen. These electrosurgical units may appropriately be used, however, for hemorrhage control of the donor site after the lesion has been removed. See Figures 7.8A–E.

Tissue Management

When performing a biopsy, extreme care must be taken in order to preserve the structural integrity of the lesion and associated normal tissue that will be evaluated microscopically. Avoiding unnecessary damage to the specimen is something more easily talked about than accomplished. By its very nature, biopsy is an invasive traumatic procedure where tissue is cut and removed from the human body. Although damage to the inflicted area is the immediate result, the long-

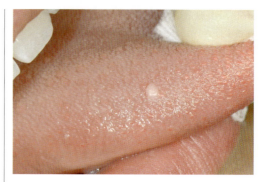

Figure 7-8A. Small lesion on the dorsum of the tongue.

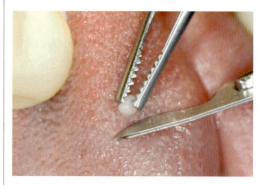

Figure 7-8B. With traction on the lesion, a scalpel is ready to make the first elliptical incision on one side.

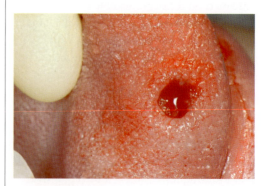

Figure 7-8C. After a cut on both sides of the lesion; cuts that meet underneath while traction is applied; the lesion is removed. The defect is ready to suture.

term prospect, if done correctly, is diagnostic and healing in nature. Fortunately, use of modern surgical principles and instrumentation can help the clinician remove the lesion

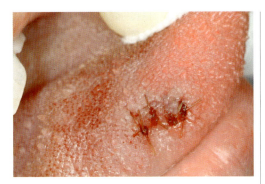

Figure 7-8D. The defect is sutured with four 4-0 chromic sutures.

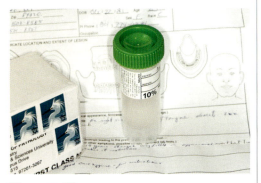

Figure 7-8E. The lesion has been placed in a specimen jar, the report form has been filled out, and it is ready to be mailed to the oral pathology laboratory. The lesion was diagnosed at a dental school pathology laboratory as a squamous papilloma.

as atraumatically as possible, while still maintaining the architecture of the tissue.

A common mistake made by practitioners when performing this procedure is delivering excess pressure with tissue forceps, and consequently damaging the lesion. These forceps should ideally only be used to handle normal tissue adjacent to the lesion. If not used in the correct place and in a careful gentle manner, these pick-ups will crush and distort the tissue, thereby altering the natural structure of the specimen. A hemostat or needle-holder should not be used to grasp the lesion.

After the tissue is carefully removed from the operative site, it should be placed immediately in a jar of 10% neutral buffered formalin to avoid tissue autolysis. The clinician should acquire this jar complete with fixative and an identification sticker, a tissue submission form, and written mailing instructions, prior to performing the biopsy. It is important that when the lesion is placed within the container, it does not adhere to the wall of the jar, but is fully immersed, free floating within the solution. It should be noted that if multiple biopsies are obtained, each specimen should be placed in a separate container of fixative and labeled appropriately. The volume of the formalin should equal or exceed 10 times the volume of the tissue. This is important because, with the exception of academic clinicians, most dentists do not practice within a short distance of an oral pathologist and will have to mail their specimens for evaluation. The volume of formalin and other specific packaging requirements by the lab ensure that there will be no chance of the tissue absorbing all of the solution and becoming dehydrated or necrotic while in transit.

TISSUE SUBMISSION FORM

It is important that the oral pathologist receive as much information as possible in order to identify and correctly characterize the submitted lesion. Therefore, a copy of all necessary information should be included to help solve an often difficult puzzle. The patient's obvious demographics should be enclosed along with the medical history, lesion history, differential diagnosis, patient habits, and an illustration of the biopsy site and associated lymph nodes (if involved). If the lesion is within bone or is located near hard tissue, radiographs should also be included. If the dentist has possession of a high-quality camera capable of taking excellent intraoral photographs, a picture could prove useful to the pathologist as well (see Figure 7.1).

On the form there is an area where the referring clinician describes the appearance of the lesion and any additional comments that may prove pertinent in helping to find a definitive diagnosis. This description may include size, shape, color, location, texture, consistency, induration, and so on. If the lesion was suspicious in nature, orientations of tissue margins were hopefully identified with suture. The location of tissue margins and the corresponding suture should be given to the oral pathologist in written word and drawn illustration for clear communication.

Conclusion

It is vital that general dentists grasp the importance of their role in oral cancer detection. In the patient's oral exam and also the head and neck exam, an opportunity is presented to identify lesions and follow-up until they are diagnosed and, if necessary, treated. These could present as suspicious lesions in the mouth, on the lips, on the face, or on the neck. The generalist can make note of the abnormality, make the patient aware, and treat with diagnostic testing, biopsy, or referral—depending on the knowledge and comfort level of the dentist and the nature of the problem. Referral of a patient to another clinician for consultation and/or treatment is rarely a poor decision.

In this chapter, principles of oral lesion management and soft tissue biopsy are emphasized in simple terms from a general dentist's perspective. An acute awareness of the importance of these principles, combined with continual practice, can help make many of these techniques and procedures part of the general dentist's routine dental treatment.

References

1. L. J. Peterson, E. Ellis, J. R. Hupp, M. R. Tucker. *Contemporary Oral and Maxillofacial Surgery,* 3rd ed. p. 460. Mosby-Year Book. 2002.
2. D. P. Golden, J. R. Hooley. Oral mucosal biopsy procedures. *Dental Clinics of North America* 38(2): 279–300. 1994.
3. D. C. Shugars, L. L. Patton. Detecting, diagnosing, and preventing oral cancer. *Nurse Practitioner* 22: 105, 109–110. 1997.
4. A. Mashberg, L. J. Feldman. Clinical criteria for identifying early oral and oropharyngeal carcinoma: erythroplasia revisited. *Am J Surg* 156: 273–75. 1988.
5. S. Silverman. Oral cancer. *Semin Dermatol* 13: 132–137. 1994.
6. H. Sandler. Cytological screening for early mouth cancer. *Cancer* 15: 1119–24. 1962.
7. W. J. Blot, J. K. McLaughlin, D. M. Winn, et al. Smoking and drinking correlation to oral and pharyngeal cancer. *Cancer Res* 48: 3282–87. 1988.
8. J. J. Sciubba. Improving detection of precancerous and cancerous oral lesions: computer-assisted analysis of the oral brush biopsy—U.S. Collaborative OralCDX Study Group. *J Am Dent Assoc* 130: 1445–57. 1999.
9. D. Eisen. The oral brush biopsy: a new reason to screen every patient for oral cancer. *General Dentistry* 48: 97. 2000.
10. A. Mashberg, F. Merletti, P. Boffetta, et al. Appearance, site of occurrence, and physical and clinical characteristics of oral carcinoma in Torino, Italy. *Cancer* 63: 2522–7. 1989.
11. P. A. Wingo, L. A. Ries, H. M. Rosenberg, D. S. Miller, B. K. Edwards. Cancer incidence and mortality, 1973–1995: a report card for the U.S. *Cancer* 82: 1197–1207. 1998.
12. S. L. Zunt. Transepithelial brush biopsy: an adjunctive diagnostic procedure. *J Indiana Dent Assoc* 80: 6–8. 2001
13. M. N. Prout, J. N. Sidari, R. A. Witzburg, G. A. Grillone, and C. W. Vaughan. Head and neck cancer screening among 4611 tobacco users older than forty years. *Otolaryngol Head Neck Surg* 116: 201–8. 1997.
14. G. L. Frenandez, R. Sankaranarayanan, J. J. Lence Anta, S. A. Rodriguez, P. D. Maxwell. An evaluation of the oral cancer control program in Cuba. *Epidemiology* 6: 428–31. 1995.
15. J. P. Handlers. Diagnosis and management of oral soft-tissue lesions: the use of biopsy, toluidine blue staining, and brush biopsy. *CDA J* 29(8): 602–06. 2001.
16. H. Dym, O. E. Ogle. *Atlas of Minor Oral Surgery.* p. 180. Philadelphia, PA: W.B. Saunders. 2001.
17. W. Mann, N. Lonky, S. Massad, R. Scotti, J. Blanco, S. Vasilev. *Int J Gynecol Obstet* 43: 289–96. 1993

18. R. T. Greenlee, M. B. Hill-Harmon, T. Murray, M. Thun. Cancer statistics, 2001. *CA Cancer J Clin* 51(1): 15–36. 2001.

19. N. Johnson. Oral cancer: a worldwide problem. *FDI World* 6(3): 19–21. 1997.

20. M. A. Huber, S. A. Bsoul, G. T. Terezhalmy. Acetic acid wash and chemiluminescent illumination as an adjunct to conventional oral soft tissue examination for the detection of dysplasia: a pilot study. *Quintessence International* 35(5): 378–84. 2004

21. Christensen Research Associates. Intraoral precancerous and cancerous lesion screening. *CRA Found Newsl* January: 3. 2005.

22. R. A. Convissar. Soft tissue biopsy techniques for the General Practitioner, Part 2. *Dentistry Today* 19: 46–49. 2000.

Chapter 8

Anxiolysis for Oral Surgery and Other Dental Procedures

Dr. Fred Quarnstrom

Introduction

This chapter discusses the need for sedation, the risks of various modalities of sedation, techniques to minimize the risks, and two safe techniques to control fear and apprehension in the dental office. The biggest risk of sedation is respiratory depression. Mechanisms of respiratory control will be reviewed, and various forms of monitoring will be discussed along with respiratory conditions that complicate sedations. Nitrous oxide/oxygen sedation are covered, as are oral sedatives—with emphasis on benzodiazepines and specifically the use of triazolam (Halcion) for conscious sedation to control fear and apprehensive.

Oral surgery is somewhat traumatic for all patients. Because of this, many oral surgeons will suggest deep intravenous (IV) sedation/general anesthesia for even simple surgery procedures. Most of the in-office surgery procedures can be done with local anesthesia; however, many patients prefer some form of sedation for their surgery. The surgery is easier and faster for the surgeon if the patient is comfortable. The use of nitrous oxide/oxygen

sedation with and without oral triazolam are discussed. With these two drugs, almost all surgery procedures can be completed on even quite fearful patients without the need for the more hazardous general anesthesia.

A second issue is the dental patient who is a dental phobic. A *USA Today* article quoted American Dental Association (ADA) figures detailing that 12 million Americans are dental phobics. Another source estimated that 12 to 24 million suffer dental anxiety.[1] Coping with the difficult-to-manage fearful patient has long plagued the profession, and one of the major challenges of dentistry is apprehension control. Fear and pain control are closely related. Fear of future treatment is often the result of lack of pain control in past appointments. Pain control is most often achieved with local anesthesia. According to Weinstein,[2] patients report the incidence of failure of the local anesthetic injection to be as high as 26.4 percent. It is suggested that fear has a high correlation with those who have anesthetic-related problems.[3]

About half the U.S. population avoids yearly dental care. Between 6 and 14 percent of patients avoid **any** treatment whatsoever because of fear. This phenomenon is not unique to the United States. Others have shown similar problems in Sweden and Japan.[4–6]

Government regulations that dictate who can and cannot be hospitalized (Medicare, Medicaid) and the threat of litigation have caused many dentists to avoid providing dental treatment on all but the most cooperative and easily managed patients. Some dentists refuse to see those patients unable to receive dental care in the usual manner.[7]

In the late 1990s and early 2000s the greatest barrier to using sedation has become dental politics. The target is primarily oral sedation and those practitioners who provide this service. The American Dental Association's committee H proposed guidelines that were passed by the ADA House of Delegates in 2004, severely limiting the use of oral sedatives. Many states' licensing bodies have started adopting these guidelines. The American Association of Oral and Maxillofacial Surgeons has encouraged state licensing boards to limit the use of oral sedation. In one letter sent to state boards, they suggested that the use of oral sedation should have the same certification required of IV sedation.

In this chapter, considerable space is spent referring to the patient who is unconscious, asleep, dozing, and napping—and explaining why I am not comfortable with such a patient. On the other hand, the patient who is orally sedated but awake and will respond to verbal directions is a safe patient. So long as this patient remains conscious, the operator can relax and enjoy performing dentistry. With a proper preoperative evaluation, careful use of the right drug and calculation of its dose, a dentist should never have a patient lose consciousness; that is, "go to sleep." Should this occur, all else should cease until the patient is again verbally responsive or awake. Some states have regulations dictating dentist training and equipment for treating patients receiving general anesthesia, and rightfully so. It is a little late to start buying equipment and getting training when a patient is unconscious. General dentists administering oral conscious sedation need training and special equipment.

As we discuss triazolam, it will become obvious that the chance of problems arising with this drug, when it is used properly, is very slight. But even if complications should occur, with the availability of a selective reversal agent, flumazenil (Romazicon), we reverse the effect that is going beyond the levels we wanted. As you will see later, flumazenil is reported to rapidly reverse the sedation of benzodiazepine drugs, much as naloxone (Narcan) does the opiate drugs.

Various forms of oral sedation have been used by dentists to help apprehensive patients. Patient comfort can be achieved by the practitioner who uses oral sedation, and/or nitrous oxide to allay patient's anxiety and apprehension. Anxiolysis (a relief of anxiety) also decreases the likelihood of stress-induced medical emergencies. The difficulty of using oral agents is the time it takes to get an effect. Since these drugs must be swallowed and absorbed via the small intestine it often takes over an hour to get the drugs into the circulation and see the maximum effect.

What Are the Levels of Sedation?

Sedation needs to be matched to the level of apprehension along with the physical and mental stimulation the patient will have to endure while their dentistry is being provided. Apprehension control is a continuum of the levels of sedation—from no sedation through general anesthesia. A patient with minimal apprehension and a short simple procedure will need less help than a severely phobic patient who will be undergoing a painful, lengthy, noisy, stressful procedure. The levels have been named anxiolysis, moderate sedation/analgesia, deep sedation, and general anesthesia.

ANXIOLYSIS FOR ORAL SURGERY AND OTHER DENTAL PROCEDURES

Anxiolysis is a drug-induced state during which the patient responds normally to verbal commands. Their cognitive functions and coordination may be impaired, but ventilatory and cardiovascular functions are normal. This level could be compared to a glass or two of wine. These patients are exposed to little, if any, risk. Anxiolysis may be protective for patients with mild to moderate medical conditions that can worsen due to the stress of dentistry. This level of sedation is achieved with light oral sedation and/or nitrous oxide/oxygen sedation.

Moderate sedation/analgesia is a bit deeper; the patient will respond to verbal commands, but you might have to add light tactile stimulation to get a response. They are able to maintain their airway, and spontaneous ventilation is adequate. Their cardiovascular system is normal. This level of sedation is most often achieved with an oral sedative, but light IV sedation could also achieve these levels.

Deep sedation/analgesia takes a patient to a level where they respond only after repeated or painful stimulation. They may not be able to maintain their airway and may need an assist to maintain adequate ventilation. This level requires advanced training for the practitioner, as protective reflexes are now obtunded or absent. Cardiovascular function is maintained.

General anesthesia is a complete loss of consciousness. Often patients will need help to maintain their airway, and their respiratory function may need assistance. They will have lost the protective swallowing, gag, and laryngeal reflexes. General anesthesia can be achieved by the inhalation of potent anesthetics, with IV drugs, with oral drugs if high enough doses are given, or a combination of these. It is imperative if this level is achieved that the practitioner is capable of monitoring the patient's vital signs, maintaining the airway, assisting respiration if necessary, and handling all the various life-threatening emergencies that can occur. Children are much more difficult because they are less forgiving of alterations from normal. Their respiratory physiology has a narrower margin of safety (see Figure 8.1).

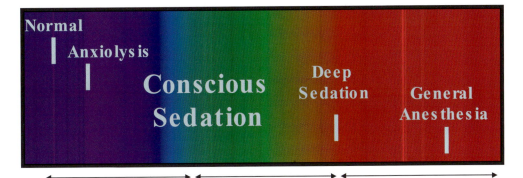

Figure 8-1. This chapter will discuss only area 1 of the spectrum of anesthesia. Areas 2 and 3 require advanced training and come with greater risk to the patient.

How Safe Is Sedation?

Dentists with proper training can perform oral sedation safely and effectively. Most dental therapy can be accomplished on phobic patients using local anesthesia and sedation. Therefore, adequate use of local anesthesia must be considered as the first step of not only pain control but also anxiety control. Many central nervous system (CNS) depressants can alter the level of consciousness. Most of these can produce a hypnotic state if given in higher doses, but only a select few can actually produce a complete state of general anesthesia.

The potential for complications is not limited to the general anesthetic state. It may accompany any degree of drug-induced CNS depression. Respiratory and cardiovascular depression are the most feared complications. Respiratory depression represents the principal negative variable introduced with conscious sedation and, left unrecognized and untreated, is the cause of most serious complications.

Further complicating the question, "To Sedate or Not To Sedate?" is the fact that nearly all dentistry is elective. It is very rare to face the situation in which a life will be lost if treatment is not initiated. A nerve may die; a tooth may be lost; all the teeth may be lost; but the patient will still be alive and reasonably healthy. It is very difficult to accept a dental procedure where there is even a slight risk of death. This is not to say that there is not a very slight risk with even the most simple procedures. Even administration of local anesthesia has resulted in death. But, whatever we do, safety protocol is of the utmost importance (see Figure 8.2).

Sedation and deep sedation/general anesthesia has a remarkable safety record; however, there have been studies showing that the deeper the sedation, particularly when administered to medically compromised patients such as the very young and the elderly, the greater the risk. Dionne reported that overall mortality in the United States associated with general anesthesia, based on self-

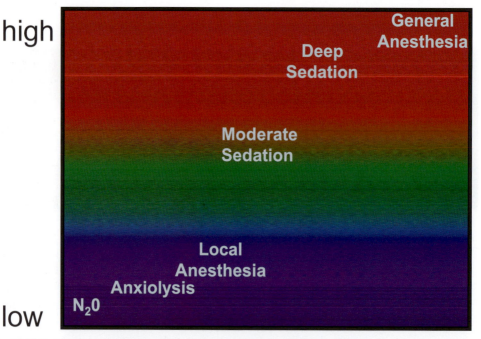

Figure 8-2. The relative risks of various forms of sedation anesthesia. Because of the high levels of oxygen, nitrous oxide is protective for almost all patients. Anxiolysis with oral sedation of a benzodiazepine drug is nearly as safe. With help from Dr. Mark Donaldson B.Sc., Pharm.D.

report of oral surgeons, has ranged from 1:740,000 to 1:349,000; however, self-reporting is usually given little credence because not all cases are acknowledged. A more credible study came out of records from the United Kingdom, where the overall mortality risk was 1:248,000 for general anesthesia and 1:1,000,000 for conscious sedation. Only very low risk could be determined for local anesthesia.[8]

The risk of sedation and anesthesia can be dramatically decreased with modern monitoring devices and the use of persons trained in monitoring and administrating anesthesia. It has been shown that the risk of anesthesia is dramatically reduced when a separate practitioner trained in general anesthesia administers and controls the sedation/anesthesia. In the case of two-operator administered anesthesia, the risk went from 1:248,000 to 1:598,000.[9] This is particularly true when treating patients with underlying medical problems.

Patient Ambulation

A problem that was unique to dentistry but is now affecting our medical colleagues who use day surgery is the need for rapid ambulation. We need to get our patients back to a state that allows them to leave the office in a timely manner. Their reflexes need to be such that they can walk unassisted after a short period of time, even though this author insists that another adult take their arm for additional support. It may be wise to use a wheelchair to transport the patient from the dental chair to their auto. They should not drive, undertake any task that might be hazardous, be placed in a position of responsibility (for example, taking care of children), or make important decisions. Even climbing stairs should be avoided. They need to be accompanied and supervised by a responsible adult for the rest of the day, during which time their activities should be very limited. Operating the remote control of a television

is about as complex a cognitive activity as they should attempt. It should be stressed to the patient that although they might feel normal, their reflexes could still be depressed. They need to take the remainder of the day off.

It should be mentioned that some of the benzodiazepine drugs are initially bound to plasma proteins. This binding tends to reverse about six hours after administration. This phenomenon is known as a "second peak effect."[10] When using most benzodiazepines, it is necessary to inform our patients that they will experience an increase in sedation about 5–8 hours after leaving the office. Interestingly, even after this time, blood concentrations of active drug have been reported to be close to 50 percent of what they were during sedation. For this reason, it is imperative that they not undertake any activity requiring cognitive or coordination skills the rest of the day. Because of the long half-life of diazepam (Valium), some practitioners have felt there was reason for some concern even the next day.

Drug Selection

Our choice of drugs is guided by consideration of elimination half-lives and side effects. When we examine sedative systems, we find a continuum of effects from slightly noticeable changes through more profound sedation to general anesthesia, eventually leading to death, if enough drug is administered. "General anesthesia is less safe than conscious sedation, which is less safe than local anesthesia."[11]

It is our goal to choose a sedation system with a very wide difference between desired effect and death in a very broad range of patients. It is ideal if the effects of the drugs can be reversed at will if our system seems to be getting out of control.

It is also our goal to create a state of tranquility that will allow the patient to comfortably undergo the needed procedure. If we can alleviate apprehension without changing any of the patient's other parameters, we have achieved success. In fact, we always cause some change in our patients' physiology; however, with modern drugs these changes are much less hazardous than what was accepted a few years ago.

Routes of Drug Administration

In attempting to create a state of tranquility, we must get a certain concentration of agent to the appropriate location in the central nervous system. When considering routes, we should consider patient comfort, time to achieve effect, control of the effect, ease of administration, the skill needed for administration of the drug, necessary equipment for administration, and monitoring of the patient. Unfortunately, we must also consider medical-legal questions of insurance and regulation by governmental organizations.

In general, the faster the drug reaches the CNS and has an effect, the better the control we have over the sedation. By titrating for effect, we can give just that amount of drug that is necessary to control apprehension. Both intravenous and inhalation agents can be readily controlled in this manner. Other routes of administration require administering an appropriate dose and waiting up to an hour to see the desired effect. These routes require very specific dosages, usually associated with body size. They require conservative dosages, as hypersensitivity to a medication will not be obvious until it is much too late to adjust the dosage. It is imperative that a drug with a very wide range of safety be used when these slower routes of uptake are utilized. Ideally, we will have reversal agents that can deactivate the drug in the case of overdose when using these routes.

We, in dentistry, have used and continue to use a variety of agents and combinations of agents. Multiple agents often complicate the treatment, as each has side effects that can be additive. They all are CNS depressants and some have unwanted depressing effects on respiratory and the cardiovascular systems. The combination of all these effects can lead to problems that are hard to predict and even more difficult to control and treat. However, if only one agent is used, the side effects are often more predictable and more treatable.

It is easier and safer to use a single agent, as we then only have one set of side effects. This assumes a single agent will provide the needed result at a concentration where few side effects are present. When Dionne looked at drug mixtures used by 264 dentists, he found 82 distinct combinations.[12] He said, "The scientific basis for the use of such a diverse group of agents and combinations is unclear."[13]

INHALATION SEDATION

The inhalation route of administration offers a major advantage when we consider an overdose. By removing the source of the drug (having the patient breathe room air or 100 percent oxygen), the patient will excrete most inhalation agents via the lungs, thus reversing the overdose.

ORAL SEDATION

Several factors come to light when we consider oral sedatives. The time from ingestion to sedation becomes very important. For any effect to take place, the drug must be absorbed into the bloodstream and delivered to the site of action, usually thought to be in the central nervous system, in sufficient quantities to be effective. Some drugs can be absorbed sublingually; others must be swallowed and absorbed from the small intestine. Depending on the time necessary for absorption, it might be necessary to have the patient take the drug at home before coming to the office. This author prefers to administer the drug in the office because then you know how much was taken, when it was taken, and by whom it was taken. You don't have to worry about the patient trying to drive to the appointment as the drug starts to take effect, and should there be a reaction to the drug, the patient is in the office where aid can be administered.

One downside is that because it will take 45 minutes to one hour to get the desired sedation, it is time-consuming to titrate or alter the dose if a patient is not adequately sedated.

INTRAVENOUS SEDATION

With the regulations that are now in place in many states, it is nearly impossible for the average general dentist to use intravenous sedation. Many states require a 60-hour course with 20 patient sedations in addition to any training that was received in dental school. Intravenous sedation has several advantages, however. When giving a drug IV, one slowly titrates the amount to the level of sedation desired. For most drugs, these effects began to diminish in a short period of time—first, due to redistribution to other tissues in the body (primarily fat stores), and then more slowly as the drug is metabolized into inactive forms or eliminated in the urine or feces.

Although this should be the safest route of administration, it is possible to go from conscious to deep general anesthesia in a matter of seconds. Although this should be a very safe technique, this is where we are seeing deaths.

Drug Options

Historically, many drugs and routes of administration have been used to control apprehension in dental offices. As stated earlier, insurance companies, state regulatory bodies, and other entities have all but eliminated intravenous sedation from the armamentarium of general dentists. If we look into other methods of sedation, however, we will see that all is not lost for the phobic patient.

NITROUS OXIDE

Nitrous oxide is possibly the safest of all sedatives. It is estimated that close to 40 percent of dentists are equipped to administer nitrous oxide. It has been used in dentistry for more than 150 years. Trace nitrous oxide released into the air of the dental office, and its effect on the dental staff, however, must be considered. It is recommended that there be postoperative oxygenation for not only nitrous oxide but also other sedatives. If one is looking for a very safe anxiolytic drug from which the patient recovers quickly and with which the patient is able to drive to and from the office, nitrous oxide is the only choice.

ALCOHOL

Alcohol has been used by some patients for years to help with their dental treatments. It is not unusual for a patient to self-medicate with a bit of liquid reinforcement before coming to an appointment. **It is important when considering the use of sedatives for apprehension control that patients be warned against using any other substance that is a central nervous system depressant**. The combination of benzodiazepines and alcohol has lead to very serious respiratory depression and death.

CHLORAL HYDRATE

This drug has been a favorite, particularly for children. Evidence is emerging, however, that indicates it may not be as safe as we believed. Chloral hydrate's sedative action comes from its metabolite, trichloroethanol. The peak activity occurs in the plasma within 20 to 60 minutes after oral administration. Its half-life is 4–12 hours. It acts primarily on the CNS and has little effect on the respiratory and cardiovascular systems of healthy patients.

In higher doses, chloral hydrate becomes a cardiac irritant. There have been several reported cases of overdose leading to hypotension. In one report of two patients, when this hypotension was treated with catecholamines or agents that released catecholamines, both patients experienced cardiac arrest; one survived, the other did not. Any other CNS depressant will enhance the sedation-depression of chloral hydrate, including nitrous oxide and narcotics.[14] Deaths have occurred in combination with local anesthetics when used with small children. It is thought that often this is due to using a toxic dose of local anesthesia: four cartridges—one for each quadrant to be treated. Even two cartridges of local anesthesia can be a toxic dose for small children.

BARBITURATES

Barbiturates were the standard antianxiety agent for both medical and dental patients for many years. Barbiturates make a patient drowsy, and sleepy patients tend to be less apprehensive. In larger doses, barbiturates have the potential to render patients asleep. It is in this way that the short- and ultra-short-acting barbiturates were used as induction agents for general anesthesia and for very brief general anesthetics.

The ratio of the dose necessary for sleep and the dose that will end in death—the **therapeutic index**—is usually stated to be a factor of two, as compared to diazepam, with a ratio of 20.[15] Unfortunately, barbiturate drugs in higher doses tend to be potent cardiac and respiratory depressants. Because of their addictive nature, they are not administered for long-term anxiety control.[16]

BENZODIAZEPINES

Benzodiazepine (BZD) drugs come in many varieties. They differ in the rapidity that they take effect, the time it takes for them to wear off, time to peak blood levels, and half-lives.

While the names are different they are more similar than different in their effect (beyond uptake and deactivation times). Dentistry has several BZDs that are ideal for use with apprehensive patients, and the effect can be tailored to the time necessary to perform the procedures being contemplated. One, triazolam, is well suited to dentistry. Triazolam came to market as a sleep aid and has become very popular and controversial. Triazolam will be discussed in detail.

THE TWO MOST USEFUL SEDATIVE DRUGS FOR THE GENERAL DENTIST

Nitrous oxide has an interesting history. Originally it was used as an attraction at public science shows. It was at such a program that a dentist, Horris Wells, saw a participant in a nitrous frolic receive a serious injury causing a dramatic wound . . . with no pain. He took this knowledge to his office and began offering painless dentistry using nitrous oxide as a general anesthetic.

Its history as a general anesthetic has brought dentistry some criticism. Nitrous oxide is a weak anesthetic agent. At one atmosphere of pressure, 80 percent nitrous oxide is usually considered to be the minimum concentration that will achieve general anesthesia. Even at this concentration, it is not possible to render some patients unconscious. If we go to a higher concentration, we begin to encroach on the 21 percent oxygen found in the atmosphere and expose our patients to hypoxia.

The standard of the past was to watch the patient's color. When they began to show a blue tinge of cyanosis, the procedure was started. (I like to state, tongue in cheek, that dentists hoped the pain of the extraction would restart the heart.) Anesthetics were very short. One tooth in the forceps, one in the air and one hitting the bucket, simultaneously, was the goal. Actually, many general anesthetics were done by this technique with an amazing safety record, which may be more testimony to a patient's desire to live than to the safety of the procedure. Today, this hypoxic anesthesia technique would be severely criticized, as it should be.

Because nitrous oxide is absorbed and removed from the blood stream via the lungs essentially unchanged, nitrous oxide is a very safe sedative. But its major disadvantage—its relative weakness—is also its major advantage. Although sedation with nitrous oxide is not adequate for our severely phobic patients because it is such a weak anesthetic agent, there is little risk of sedation rendering the patient unconscious—that is, in a state of general anesthesia. However, it is not impossible. I have had two patients in 40 years who were under general anesthesia with very modest concentrations (less than 40 percent) nitrous oxide. Neither had taken any other drugs. If the patient is not responding even at low concentrations this might be the problem. The mask should be removed and the patient allowed to breathe room air or just oxygen.

Our primary concern in anesthesia is the loss of swallowing and laryngeal reflexes that can lead to regurgitation of stomach contents and aspiration of the low-pH stomach contents into the lungs. So long as a 50 percent concentration of nitrous oxide is not exceeded, there is little chance of general anesthesia or other complications.

The complications that may arise are not serious ones. Occasional vomiting may be seen, but since our patients are always conscious, this is not serious, as protective laryngeal reflexes are present. The patient is definitely uncomfortable, and vomiting certainly can be messy, but it is usually not life-threatening.

Patients will occasionally hallucinate with nitrous. Again, this can be uncomfortable for them. Treatment consists of removing the source of nitrous oxide and reassuring the patient, typically by telling them they are all right and will return to normal in a few minutes. It is helpful to repeatedly assure the patient until the hallucination is over. Use their first name and remind them they are in the dental office—that they should relax and will be back to normal in a few minutes.

Another potential problem deserves mention—that of sexual aberrations. A certain number of female patients will experience sexual feelings while on nitrous oxide.[17] This can happen at relatively low concentrations. Some patients describe the sensation of a sexual orgasm. It is not all that easy to identify when this is taking place. However, if it looks like a duck, walks like a duck, and quacks like a duck, the chances are we are observing a duck. This may, in fact, be the ultimate distraction to dental treatment. Fortunately, it is very rare. For this reason it is important that a male dentist, hygienist, or assistant always be accompanied by a female dental assistant when treating female patients with nitrous oxide. This phenomenon has never been documented in male patients.

A potentially more serious problem can arise if we treat chronic obstructive pulmonary disease (COPD) patients with nitrous oxide. Should a patient be overdosed with nitrous oxide, it is a simple matter to remove the source of the gas, and provided the patient is breathing, they will eliminate the excessive concentration of nitrous oxide. If they are not breathing, we should be ready and able to assist their respiration. This would be a very unusual complication and probably would suggest the patient had other sedatives or was given excessive nitrous oxide (greater than 80 percent). It should be stressed that nitrous oxide is a very safe sedative for almost all patients, provided equipment has been properly installed and maintained.

Nitrous Usage

It is estimated that about 50 percent of dentists have the equipment to administer this mix and that more than 424,000 dental personnel are exposed to the trace amounts of gas as a result of its administration.[18]

Many dental and dental hygiene schools now take a very cautious attitude toward the use of nitrous oxide. This has come about because of the publication of a number of papers concerned with the effect of waste gases on office personnel, particularly those who are pregnant.

The first indication that anesthetic gases might be a problem for humans was a report in 1967 by Vaisman, who studied Russian female anesthesiologists and reported that 18 of 31 pregnancies ended in spontaneous abortion.[19] Studies have shown similar problems in U.S. operating rooms.[20] It was clear the operating room had the potential to be a hazardous place to work, but it was not clear which chemicals were the causative agents.

Animal Studies

Potent anesthetic agents have been shown to have teratogenic effects in animal studies. Because nitrous oxide was part of many anesthetic administrations, it needed to be evaluated. Many studies showed problems for animals exposed to high levels of nitrous oxide.[21–31] It was shown that nitrous oxide decreases vitamin B_{12}, which can impair DNA synthesis.[32] These studies hint that if the levels are kept low enough the problems can be lessened.

Retroactive Human Studies

The dental office was an ideal study site as there were two types of offices, those that used nitrous oxide and those that did not. Cowen did two such studies in conjunction with the American Dental Association. These studies suggested there is a problem with higher levels of exposure for pregnant staff.[33, 34] Although there may be some problems with these retrospective studies,[35] they did point to a concern for females who were pregnant and working in dental offices where nitrous oxide was used. The studies did not suggest at which level exposure became a problem.

Occupational Hygiene Agencies

There are three governmental bodies associated with setting appropriate levels of exposure to chemicals: OSHA, NIOSH, and ACGIH.[36] The NIOSH publication, *Alert*, suggests the recommended exposure limit (REL) of 25 parts per million (ppm) on a time-weighted average (TWA) of 25-ppm. These levels were recommended after reviewing two studies by Bruce.[37, 38]

The Problem Studies

The TWA level of 25-ppm came from two studies done by Bruce, Bach, and Arbit. In the first study, a difference was shown when subjects were exposed to 50-ppm nitrous oxide with 1-ppm halothane but not to 500-ppm nitrous oxide, except for a digit span test.[39] The second study showed a slight effect to subjects exposed to 500-ppm nitrous oxide for four hours.[40] Note that Bruce recanted this study as flawed in two letters— one in 1983 the other in 1991. He stated,

> "Several years later, we learned that most of the subjects we studied were a unique population that used no mood altering substances and as such, might have been abnormally sensitive to depressant drugs such as nitrous oxide and halothane. There is no longer any need to refer to our conclusions as 'controversial.' They were wrong, derived from data subject to inadvertent sampling bias and not applicable to the general population. The NIOSH standards should be revised".[41,42]

Many papers have been published in the dental literature that mention the motor skill effect, which was not shown for just nitrous oxide in either study. These two studies and the publications of NIOSH that arose from these studies have been referenced in so many dental journals they have become fact, ignoring the two retraction letters. After a paper is published, it is very nearly impossible to retract the paper.

What Is a Safe Level of Exposure?

What studies have been done with humans that suggest appropriate exposure levels? Ahlborg showed Swedish midwives exposed to nitrous oxide and shift work had no difficulty getting pregnant unless they used nitrous oxide 30 or more times a month to assist with deliveries.[43] In another study of midwives, he showed no increase in spontaneous abortions with exposure to nitrous oxide, but he saw an increase with night shifts, high work loads, and no nitrous.[44] Sweeney performed a study on 20 practicing dentists. The exposures ranged from 50 ppm to more than 5,000 ppm on a time-weighted average. The only depression seen was in three dentists with exposure of more than 1,800 ppm. To set levels that would ensure safety, Sweeney suggested we should not exceed 450 ppm on an 8-hour.[45, 46]

Rowland looked at the ability of female dental assistants to become pregnant (fecundability). He showed no problems if scavenging was used.[47] These two studies strongly suggest that if we use scavenging and keep levels below 450 ppm, the dental office staff is at no risk.

What Levels of Exposure Can Be Achieved?

Early studies showed that the Brown mask, a mask within a mask with suction, could achieve levels of 50 ppm under ideal settings. OSHA reviewed these data and suggested that since this was achievable, it should be our goal. Donaldson has shown that many scavenging devices being used in practicing dental offices can achieve levels in the 40 to 60 ppm range.[48]

How Can Levels Be Controlled?

It is clear that offices should have one of the available scavenging systems on each nitrous oxide/oxygen unit. Today's scavenging systems are predominantly systems with suction placed on the mask over the pop-off valve. Some systems attempt to suck up additional air that is around the mask, and they may remove traces of nitrous oxide that the patient exhaled through their mouth or that leaked from around the mask.

Every nitrous machine must have a scavenging system with adequate suction. There should be a reasonable exchange of air in our dental offices. Outside air should be brought into the office by our heating and cooling systems. It is suggested that the minimum air exchange is five changes per hour, although is it recognized that 15 to 20 changes per hour is better. Hoses and connectors should be checked for leaks. Masks should be selected that fit the patient, and the patient should be discouraged from speaking while receiving nitrous oxide sedation. If all these suggestions are followed, it is possible to stay in the 50-ppm range[49]—well below the 450-ppm exposure level suggested by several authors.

OXYGENATION AFTER NITROUS OXIDE OXYGEN

Oxygen is the one drug that should be available in all dental offices. Oxygen can be used with little regard for side effects or other problems and should be available in every office as part of the emergency protocol. There are exceptions to this generality and times when it should not be used. For example, oxygen should be used cautiously for COPD patients (severe emphysema). If a COPD patient's disease has progressed to its final stages, his or her breathing may be on an oxygen drive—not the primary carbon dioxide drive. Giving high levels of oxygen to one of these patients could cause him or her to go into respiratory arrest. These patients are normally quite easy to identify because of their obvious respiratory difficulty.

Oxygen is routinely administered after general anesthesia when nitrous oxide was used in order to avoid diffusion hypoxia. This phenomenon was first described by Fink to explain a transient hypoxia after anesthesia in conjunction with nitrous oxide.[50] Nitrous oxide would diffuse out of the blood and fill the alveoli of the lungs and the rest of the respiratory tree. Nitrous oxide crosses from the blood to the alveoli of the lung much more quickly than either oxygen or nitrogen, and thus, nitrous oxide would tend to fill the dead space in the lungs. On the first inspiration of room air, the patient would have a mixture of nitrous oxide from the dead space (150cc of 100 percent nitrous oxide) and 350cc of room air. In theory, this would result in hypoxia that could be a problem for a sick patient, a patient with a compromised respiratory system, or a patient with respiratory depression due to the anesthesia drugs. In the case of general anesthesia, this could be a serious issue.

What is the harm in using some oxygen? Nothing, unless the two gas lines have been switched. In such a case, although the machine reads 100 percent oxygen, it is in reality delivering 100 percent nitrous oxide. There are many ways this can happen. One case occurred in a surgery practice using general anesthesia and resulted in the death of a young, healthy, adult patient.

You can use a pulse oximeter to investigate the need for oxygen after nitrous oxide/oxygen administration. One study failed to show any drop in oxygen saturation if the mask was simply removed at the end of the appointment where nitrous oxide had been used.[51] The study has now been repeated by others with the same results.[52, 53]

An overriding reason for leaving a patient on oxygen, however, is to scavenge the gas the patient is exhaling. With our present knowledge of the risks of trace contaminants of nitrous oxide, we believe we should leave our patients on 100-percent oxygen for five minutes to ensure that the nitrous oxygen they exhale is removed from the atmosphere we breathe. However, if a patient ever becomes unresponsive while on 100-percent oxygen, remove the mask. It may be that the gases have been switched.

Respiratory Effects of Drugs Used for Sedation

Sedation can be performed safely and effectively by dentists with proper training. Respiratory depression is the principal concern when sedation is administered. If we are going to get into trouble, the most likely cause will be due to respiratory depression or respiratory inadequacy due to airway obstruction.

In all cases of dental sedation, patients should remain awake. If the patient tends to fall asleep, they should be awakened. General anesthesia has been described as great amounts of boredom occasionally dispersed with moments of stark terror. Unless you are well equipped, well trained, and certified, you do not want patients to be unconscious. It is not possible to tell napping, dozing, or sleep from general anesthesia without trying to wake the person. If the patient awakes, keep them awake. If they do not awaken, you are not doing conscious sedation. The patient is under general anesthesia. If the patient is not awake, you need to reverse the sedation.

With some drugs, our concern may be that we have depressed the respiration to the point that an adequate exchange of gas is not taking place. The presence of an open airway should be established, evaluation of the level of respiration assessed, and vital signs should be taken. It should be noted that several studies have shown that watching the chest and/or reservoir bag move is not adequate to ensure an adequate minute volume. Skin color has been relied on in the past as a way of ensuring adequate tissue profusion. The arterial oxygen level can be dangerously low, however, before we see the blue tinge of cyanosis. Cyanosis is no longer considered to be an adequate monitor of arterial oxygen levels. A pulse oximeter and/or capnograph are invaluable in assessing the adequacy of ventilation (see Figures 8.3 and 8.4).

Physiologic Basis of Ventilation

To properly appreciate the importance of monitoring respiration along with reviewing the respiratory advantages of benzodiazepine drugs, we need to review a topic we all studied in dental school but most likely have not thought about since then—respiratory physiology. This is not intended to be a complete discussion. Yet, it will review a minimal level of knowledge that we should have when using sedative drugs.

Our breathing is controlled by several mechanisms. When we consciously take a breath, we have conscious control. Normally, though, our breathing rate and depth are stimulated by carbon dioxide (CO_2), a by-product of our metabolism. CO_2 alters the hydrogen ion concentration, or the pH of our blood. This pH change is the primary stimulus to breathing (see Figure 8.5). Breathing is also stimulated, to a lesser extent, by low concentrations of oxygen. Many drugs affect the CO_2 drive, but nitrous oxide depresses the secondary drive because of a lower oxygen level (see Figure 8.6).

The solution to the aforementioned problems lies in several areas. We should use drugs that minimally depress respiration. Avoid combinations of different drugs that affect several things at once. Monitor the

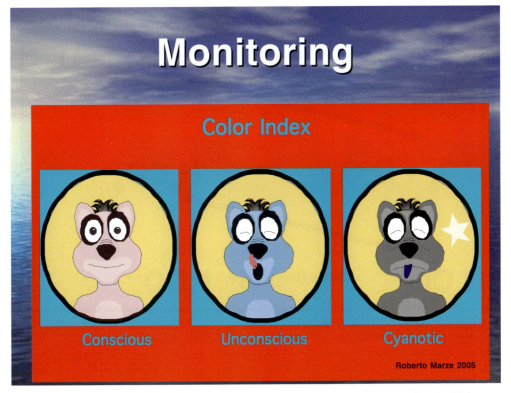

Figure 8-3. Early dental anesthesia with nitrous oxide was monitored by the patient's color. Pink was awake. Slight cyanosis was time to do the extractions. Deep cyanosis was time to give oxygen.

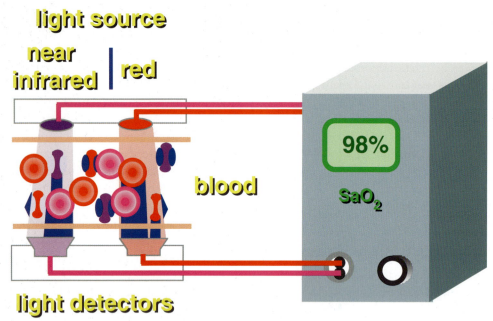

Figure 8-4. A pulse oximeter shines light through tissue, usually a finger. Receptors read the levels of each light. This information is analyzed, and the percentage of oxygen saturation is displayed on the monitor.

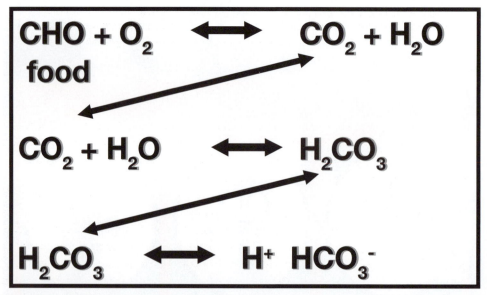

Figure 8-5. Food is oxidized in our bodies and becomes CO_2 and water. The CO_2 is absorbed in the water of the plasma to become carbonic acid. Carbonic acid disassociates into hydrogen ions and bicarbonate ions. The negative log of the hydrogen ion concentration is known as pH. The hydrogen ion is the prime stimulus to respiration. In the COPD patient, bicarbonate ions are absorbed by the kidneys, forcing the hydrogen ions back to carbonic acid. In this way, the stimulation of the hydrogen ion is blunted, forcing them to breathe on oxygen drive. The oxygen drive is depressed by nitrous oxide. High levels of O_2 can do the same.

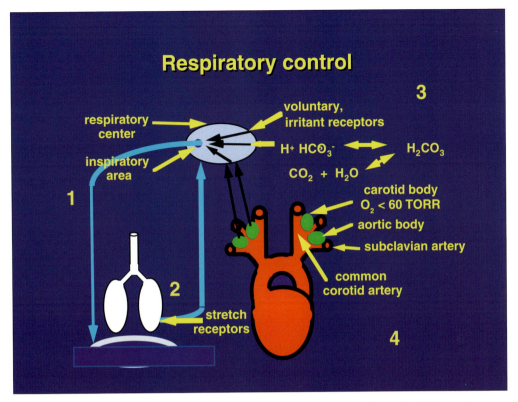

Figure 8-6. Stimulus to the inspiratory area of the respiratory center stimulates the diaphram to contract. This increases the volume of the chest cavity, drawing air into the lungs as they expand. Stretch receptors send an inhibitory signal to the respiratory center. The diaphragm relaxes, and the elastic fibers of the lungs cause them to collapse, forcing the air out. The mechanism can be stimulated by high hydrogen ion concentrations, low pH, high CO_2 concentrations, or low O_2 levels.

patient to ensure that adequate arterial oxygen levels are maintained and that CO_2 levels do not increase. Hypoventilation is characterized by a reduction in arterial oxygen tension and an elevation of CO_2 tension. With the advent of pulse oximetry, it is now possible to easily monitor oxygen saturation of hemoglobin.

Pulse oximetry shows the oxygen saturation of hemoglobin. In addition, most machines also display pulse rate. Knowing the saturation of hemoglobin, one can approximate the arterial oxygen tension, assuming a normal pH of the blood. Although 90 percent saturation provides reasonable assurance of adequate arterial oxygen tension, 95 percent is preferred. Although oximetry is not equivalent to capnography, it is valuable in alerting the dentist that ventilation is depressed.[54]

The importance of monitoring a patient's respiration cannot be overemphasized. If a patient is awake and responding to verbal commands, we can assume the patient is safe. If the patient is unconscious (asleep?), we must have more concern. Several studies of medical and dental anesthesia have shown inadequate ventilation to be the most common cause of death or brain damage. As practitioners, we must be prepared to monitor and assist respiration should it become necessary.

The Reservoir Bag

In the 1960s, watching the reservoir bag was used on several popular television programs as a means of determining when it was time to discontinue surgery and give condolences to the next of kin. We have now all been taught via television to read electrocardiographs (ECGs) and to recognize flat line. Some feel the movement of the bag can be used to monitor respiration. There have been several studies that show one should not depend on movement of the bag as an accurate indication of the adequacy of respiratory exchange. It will indicate respiratory rate.

Pulse Oximeter

The advent of an affordable pulse oximeter has made our lives much easier and patients' lives more secure. By passing two different frequencies of light through various tissues, reading the absorption of the two frequencies, and evaluating these differences, a pulse oximeter can determine the percentage of oxygen saturation of the arterial blood with great accuracy. In addition to O_2 saturation, most equipment also shows pulse rate, and some shows a pletysmograph of the pulse wave. The use of such monitoring has made general anesthesia much safer and, consequently, has decreased the frequency of tragic outcomes.

However, there is at least one possible caveat to their use: If a patient is given supplemental oxygen, his or her hemoglobin saturation will approach 100 percent. In patients with severe respiratory complications, oxygen saturation could be normal even though exchange rates were inadequate to cleanse the blood of CO_2. This could lead to high CO_2 levels and result in low pH of the blood. This potential problem can be circumvented by limiting sedation to patients with no significant respiratory problems.

Capnography

Capnography is very sensitive to respiratory depression or apnea. This equipment measures the CO_2 of a patient's expired gas. It then gives a reading of the concentration of CO_2 in these gases. This information can be invaluable when monitoring patients with respiratory problems or those undergoing general anesthesia, but it is not necessary for the sedated patient.

Benzodiazepines

It was established that barbiturates, meprobamate, and alcohol all affect the chlorine channel in brain neurons. They hyperpolarize the neuron, increasing its threshold for depolarization. Benzodiazepines act at a different but closely related site. Alcohol, barbiturates, and meprobamate all act at the same site, and all put animals to sleep with only modestly higher doses than are required for sedation.

It was shown that all these drugs interact with the neurotransmitter gamma amino butyric acid (GABA). When GABA binds with a receptor site on the neurons, it slows the neuron's rate of firing. It serves to modulate the nervous system.

Specific benzodiazepine receptors exist in the brain. If either GABA or a benzodiazepine is present, the other's binding ability is enhanced. Thus, the effects of the benzodiazepines are explained by the increased activity of GABA.[55][56]

The receptor sites are concentrated in parts of the brain that regulate emotional behavior. The advantage to benzodiazepines is their ability to relieve anxiety. They produce some drowsiness and, unfortunately, are somewhat addicting. Tolerance develops with continued use, and withdrawal occurs when the drug is stopped. However, the extent of tolerance and withdrawal are less than what is seen with barbiturates.

Historically, we have used barbiturates

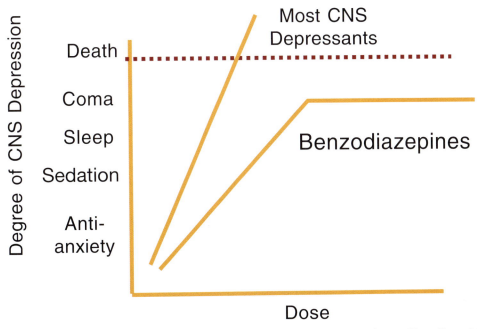

Figure 8-7. Most central nervous system (CNS) drugs if given in large enough quantities will result in death, usually from respiratory depression. When given as a single agent, benzodiazepines can be given in very large doses without causing death. They have a wide margin of safety.

and narcotics, both of which have significant effects on respiration and circulation. The most clear-cut advantage of the single-agent, benzodiazepine sedation is the fact that overdoses are rarely lethal. In the case of barbiturates, the lethal dose is only a few times greater than the dose necessary to cause sleep (see Figure 8.7).

To deactivate most oral sedatives, we must wait for the drug to be excreted or metabolized. In the case of diazepam it is metabolized in liver to another sedative, oxazepam (Serax), which is available as a long-term sedative on its own. Triazolam, along with midazolam (Versed), have the shortest half-life of the benzodiazepine drugs; both are in the one- to two-hour range. Midazolam is normally considered to be an intravenous drug, although it is being used orally and as a nasal spray. It is available in Europe as a tablet. Unfortunately, it has been shown to have a noticeable respiratory depressant effect in higher doses.

THE ADVANTAGES OF ORAL TRIAZOLAM SEDATION

Oral sedation with triazolam is simple to administer, and because of the nature of the drug, it is convenient and safe to use. Triazolam is readily available from any pharmacy. Reports of adverse drug reactions are rare and tend to be relatively mild. A major plus for all oral sedatives is that it is not necessary to administer an injection or start an intravenous line. (The last thing most phobic patients need is a needle puncture before they are sedated.) Getting an IV started in a phobic patient can be the most difficult part of a dental appointment. Patients readily accept oral sedation.

Triazolam is a drug that has been around

for some time but has been used primarily as a sleep aid. In this context, it has received bad press because of side effects that have shown up in patients who used it over an extended period of time. In the early 1990s, it is the most commonly prescribed sleeping pill used in the United States; 7.2 million prescriptions were written annually.[57] It should be emphasized that triazolam is not approved by the FDA as a sedative for dental purposes.[58–60] This is an "off-label" use.

Triazolam comes close to being an ideal drug for dental sedation.[61] It has the advantage of being absorbed rapidly, achieving peak blood levels in 1.3 hours. Its half-life is two to three hours. In addition, it may be up to eight times more effective as a hypnotic than diazepam. Yet, triazolam has very little effect on the circulatory or respiratory systems. Several studies have shown no changes in blood pressure, pulse, or percentage of oxygen saturation, and only a slight change in respiratory rate. The high incidence of anterograde amnesia on conscious patients further endears it to the dental practitioner. Patients do not have to be asleep for their dental treatments if they can be relaxed enough for us to do the required procedures and not have any memory of the procedure.[62–65]

Triazolam's relative lack of respiratory and cardiovascular sedation is important for safety. Safety is dependant on the ratio of the L/D 50 dose (that dose usually fatal to 50 percent of study animals) to the E/D 50 dose (concentration that provides sedation to 50 percent of study animals).

It would be ideal if this ratio were constant for humans. If this ratio held for humans, it would take a tablet about the size of a bowling ball to have fatal consequences. Unfortunately, this is not true. The greater the difference between the E/D 50 and L/D 50, the safer the drug. Several patients have committed suicide with triazolam. From postmortem blood samples, it was estimated that one person ingested 26 0.25-mg tablets.

Another individual was found dead in a hot tub. It was estimated she had taken 10 tablets. So it is possible to overdose and die, but the amounts necessary are well beyond what is necessary for dental sedation.[66]

Ambien (zolpidem) has been used by some dentists to replace triazolam. Ambien is an agonist of the GABA-benzodiazepine omega-1 receptor site. It has a similar half-life to triazolam, but is a nonbenzodiazepine hypnotic of the imidazopyridine class. Some claim it has a little faster absorption than triazolam; however, the manufacturer reports maximum blood levels occurred at 59 and 121 minutes for 5- and 10-mg doses. It has a half-life of 1.4–4.5 hours

Yagiela suggested lorazepam (Ativan) would be an alternative to multiple doses of triazolam.[67] Lorazepam has a 10–20-hour half-life and a slower uptake. He suggested it should be taken two hours prior to starting treatment. Five hours later, less than half of the drug has been deactivated. Ten to 20 hours later half the effect is still present. Be concerned about the patient driving the day after treatment. It makes more sense to use a drug with a shorter half-life and give a supplemental dose after one to two half-lives have passed. In this way, recovery should be faster. Lorazepam makes sense if you will give only one dose of a sedative drug, and you need sedation for four or more hours.

Pharmacology of Triazolam

The unique properties of triazolam are attributed to its chemical configuration. The nitrogen atom prevents it from being water-soluble. Midazolam has a carbon in this position and, thus, is water soluble and suitable for IV administration.

One chlorine atom is responsible for potency. Without this chlorine, the drug is one-fifth as potent. Larger alkyl substitutions also decrease potency. The second chlorine is necessary for benzodiazepine action. Bromo and nitro substitution are only weakly anxiolytic. The nitro version is also anticonvulsant, as illustrated by clonazepam. The triazolo ring and attached methyl group are responsible for the rapid oxidation by the liver enzymes, resulting in a short elimination half-life and conversion to metabolites that are rapidly excreted. The methyl group also makes a drug more potent.[68, 69]

ABSORPTION

Triazolam reaches a rapid peak within 1.3 hours.[70] It works faster in the elderly and in young women.[71] It also works more rapidly in daytime than at night, due to a longer predose fasting period. It is as much as two times quicker after a 12-hour fast.[72] One study reported that 85 percent of the drug is absorbed into the bloodstream. The study also found that it is absorbed 28 percent more quickly if given sublingually, where some of it is absorbed but most of it is swallowed.[73]

DISTRIBUTION

The distribution of triazolam shows no difference in obese and normal patients. It is 89 percent bound to plasma and 49 percent bound to serum proteins and crosses readily into the central nervous system because of high lipid solubility. It also crosses the placental barrier and has been found in milk of rats.

METABOLISM AND ELIMINATION

Triazolam is oxidized in the first pass through the liver and the lining of the gut by the cytochrome P450-mono-oxygenase system. The P450 system is made up of many enzymes. Triazolam is metabolized by the 3A4 enzyme. Tagamet, cimetidine, erythromycin, isoniazid, possibly some oral contraceptives, some anti-HIV drugs, delavirdine (DLV), efavirenz (EFV), and grapefruit depress the cytochrome P450-mediated oxidative system, thus reducing the first-pass liver clearance by decreased metabolism and reduction in hepatic blood flow.[74] The absence of an enzyme in some people can be idiosyncratic or associated with certain patient subsets. Southeast Asians may have less 3A4 enzyme (see Figure 8.8).

Triazolam has no active metabolites. As mentioned, its half-life is approximately two to three hours but is slower at night. The half-life is longer in the elderly because of lower liver oxidizing capacity. There is no change with kidney dialysis, but the half-life is slower with cirrhosis. Ninety-one percent is eliminated in urine and 9 percent in feces within 72 hours.[75 76]

CENTRAL NERVOUS SYSTEM EFFECT

All the benzodiazepines have clinically useful antianxiety, sedative-hypnotic, anticonvulsant, and skeletal muscle relaxant properties. They all depress the CNS to some degree, tending to be more antianxiety oriented as compared with barbiturates and other sedative-hypnotics. They depress the limbic system and areas of the brain associated with emotion and behavior, particularly the hippocampus and the amygdaloid nucleus. The major effects are attributed to an interaction with the GABA receptor complex.

CARDIOVASCULAR SYSTEM EFFECT

In normal therapeutic doses, the benzodiazepines cause few alterations in cardiac output or blood pressure when administered intravenously to healthy persons. Slightly greater than normal doses cause slight decreases in blood pressure, cardiac output, and stroke volume in normal subjects and patients with cardiac disease, but these changes are not usually clinically significant. Triazolam did not affect cardiovascular dynamics in doses four to eight times greater than normal.[77]

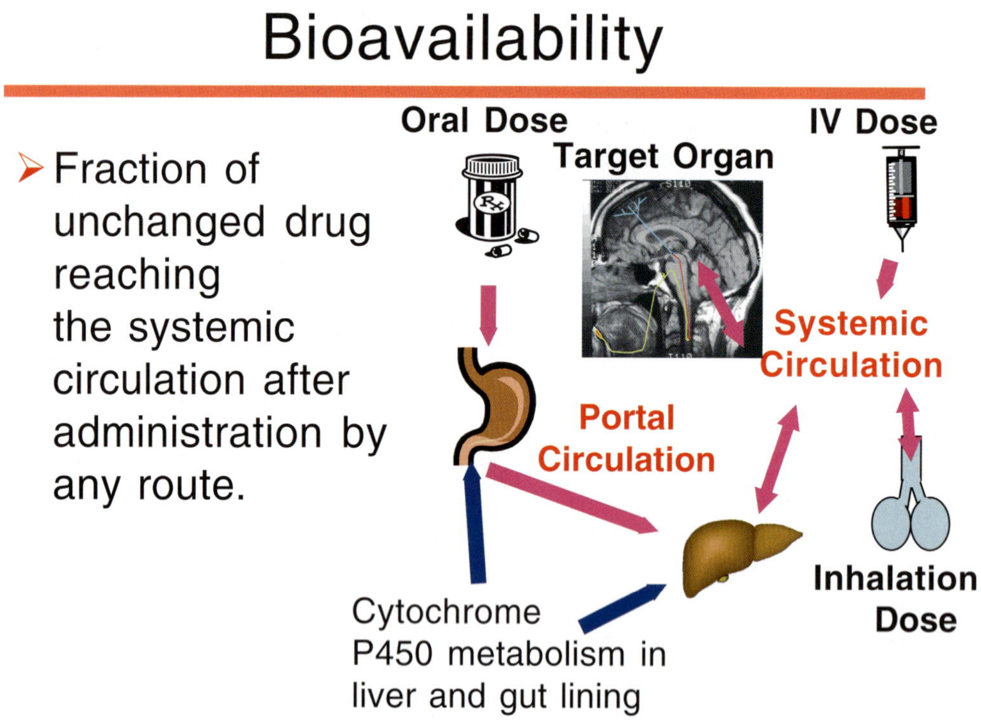

Bioavailability

> ➤ Fraction of unchanged drug reaching the systemic circulation after administration by any route.

Oral Dose

Target Organ

IV Dose

Systemic Circulation

Portal Circulation

Inhalation Dose

Cytochrome P450 metabolism in liver and gut lining

Figure 8-8. Benzodiazepine drugs are absorbed through the intestinal wall, where metabolic breakdown is initiated by the cytochrome P450 metabolic enzymes. They travel to the liver via the portal circulation. When in the liver, further metabolism occurs prior to entering the systemic circulation. When in the systemic circulation the drugs can affect the target organ, the brain.

RESPIRATORY SYSTEM EFFECT

Most benzodiazepines are mild respiratory depressants. Given alone to a healthy patient they have little effect; however, they can potentate other CNS depressants. Midazolam is one that can cause respiratory depression and apnea. Triazolam did not depress respiratory response to CO_2 in doses four to eight times normal.

REPRODUCTION

In rats, slightly reduced fertility occurred, but the drug did not affect their postnatal development.

RECOVERY

One method of measuring recovery, a visual coordination study (following a randomly moving dot with their finger), had patients back to normal in five hours after ingesting 0.25mg and in 11.5 hours after ingesting 0.5mg benzodiazepins. Reported side effects include 8 percent sleepiness; 4 percent headache; and dizziness, neuritis, and dry mouth.

TRIAZOLAM PHARMACOLOGY

Before practitioners use any medication, they should be knowledgeable of its pharmacology. Likewise, every practitioner, but particularly those using sedatives, should be able to initiate resuscitation (including cardiopulmonary resuscitation) and ventilation. The equipment necessary to provide these emergency treatments must, of course, be available.

There are a few absolute contraindications to the use of triazolam. Patients who are known to be hypersensitive to triazolam or other benzodiazepine drugs should avoid its use. Myasthenia gravis patients should not be treated, as triazolam has a muscle relaxation effect. Glaucoma patients should avoid all benzodiazepines, as these drugs raise intraocular pressure by increasing the outflow resistance to aqueous humor.[78] (This can often be reversed by pilocarpine.) All the benzodiazepine drugs are teratogenic and should not be given to pregnant women. As triazolam has been shown to pass through the mammary glands of mice into the milk, it should not be given to lactating mothers. As it is a CNS depressant, it should be given cautiously to anyone on other CNS depressants or drugs that suppress the P450 metabolic system.[79]

Relative Contraindications

There are no detailed studies of triazolam's use as a sedative with pediatric and geriatric populations, and practitioners should be cautious when giving triazolam to these groups. Some clinicians teach not to use it with patients under 18 or over 65 years of age. There have been reports of suicide attempts by psychiatric patients. Suicidal tendencies were unmasked, creating this paradoxical behavior.[80] Several European countries have outlawed triazolam. One report showed an incidence of psychotic episodes after triazolam. However, the study was done in a psychiatric hospital, where many patients have psychotic tendencies. The final relative contraindication is the fact that triazolam has not been approved by the FDA for dental sedation or the sedation of children.

Adverse Effects

Adverse effects have been reported in less than 4 percent of patients. Most adverse effects were with doses greater than 0.5mg or when combined with other CNS depressants. As with all sedatives, patients cannot drive, operate machinery, or undertake any activity that could be hazardous. This includes such activities as walking unaided, climbing stairs, and so on. They should not undertake positions of responsibility or care of children and should not make important decisions (legal, monetary, and so on) for the rest of the day. They should not have alcohol or other sedatives for 24 hours.[81]

The office should have an effective, efficient emergency protocol. This should include a person to be continuously in the room with the patient from the time of administration of the drug until the patient is judged able to leave the office. The patient should not be allowed to sleep at any time. Oxygen saturation should be continuously monitored and recorded starting before administration of the drug. Vital signs should be taken at regular intervals such as every 15 minutes or even more often if there is any indication of over-sedation.

Management of adverse reactions should be planned before the drug is used and should be reviewed on a periodic basis. It should be noted that most adverse effects would be prevented by complete history taking, physical examination, and appropriate adjustment of drug dosage. Recognition of an emergency situation must be followed by initiation of a stabilization routine. This essentially entails the A-airway, B-breathing, and C-circulation of basic cardiac life support. Opening and maintaining a patient's airway is of paramount importance, as is monitoring vital signs. Calling the Emergency Medical Service by dialing 911 should follow if any doubt exists as to how to proceed.

Use in the General Dental Office

Over 15 years, this author has used triazolam more than 400 times. The patients come to the office one hour before we want to start their dental procedure. They are monitored by recording blood pressure, pulse rate, and pulse oximetry. The drug dose is determined by the patient's weight and purposely kept conservative—less than might be necessary. We usually administer a supplemental dose sublingually if at the 30-minute mark we see no signs of sedation.

My patient population has ranged from 7 to 83 years of age and from 60 to 320 lbs.[103] All patients were ASA 1 or 2 with no history of recent illness. All adult patients were dental phobics who requested IV sedation or general anesthesia for their procedures. The children had previous attempts at treatment with conventional methods, including nitrous oxide, which were unsuccessful.

Cardiovascular and respiratory parameters measured and recorded included blood pressure (systolic and diastolic), heart rate, and oxygen saturation. With uncooperative children, only heart rate and oxygen saturation could be measured. Cardiovascular parameters were recorded every 15 minutes. During the procedure, oxygen saturation was continuously monitored with a pulse oximeter.

After recording initial baseline data, oral triazolam was dispensed. Many authors have reported on the appropriate dosage for sleep enhancement. Suggested dosages range from 0.125mg to 0.5mg.[82, 83, 84, 85, 86, 87]

After a discussion and completion of an informed consent document and recording of preoperative vital signs, a dose of triazolam is administered. An assistant stays in the operatory with the patient for the next hour, taking vital signs, blood pressure, pulse, and respiration every 15 minutes with instructions to alert me if there is any change. The assistant is instructed to talk with the patient to ensure that they remain awake. I check to see whether there is any sign of sedation at 30 minutes. If there is no sedation evident, we will administer one-half the original dose. If even slight sedation is noted at that time, we normally will have adequate sedation for the procedure. (Many patients will be disappointed at the end of the 40 minutes by the relative lack of sedation. They are assured that this is normal, and they will be adequately sedated by the time we start.)

As mentioned, we decide to administer one-half the initial dose after 30 minutes if there is no evidence of sedation. Supplemental dosages were necessary for about 10 percent of patients. We used the following protocol to determine the dosages. Dose in mg = 0.25 mg + 0.125 mg for every 70-pound weight increment over 40 pounds.[88]

Patients reported a decrease in apprehension that was greatest the first 30 minutes, with the second largest drop between 30 and 60 minutes. About 50 percent had moderate to complete forgetfulness of the appointment, and most did not remember the ride home. There were no significant changes in blood pressure, pulse rate, or oxygen saturation.

It should be emphasized that no patients slept, snoozed, snored, or napped. All were awake and responded to verbal commands without painful stimulation. We have had no adverse effects on any of my patients. We did have three who were not sedated adequately to treat.

Protocol in Our Office

It should be stressed, and I will repeat again, that we do not want a patient who is asleep. If a patient sleeps, they are oversedated and should be kept awake by verbal commands, or if this does not work, the drug should be reversed. We do not worry whether the patient is disappointed by their level of sedation because the amnesia that is common to this technique will allow them to forget most, if not all, of the appointment. It should be emphasized with children that they might still cry during the appointment. If they are controlled enough to allow dentistry to be safely done, they are adequately relaxed. Crying, although distracting to the practitioner, is an indication of adequate ventilation. I would suggest not using any form of sedation on children under 7 years of age, unless you are trained in pediatric

ANXIOLYSIS FOR ORAL SURGERY AND OTHER DENTAL PROCEDURES 243

anesthesiology and are equipped and trained to handle general anesthesia and all the complications of anesthesia.

The Procedure

At a pre-appointment interview, the medical history is reviewed to determine that there are no contraindications to triazolam, the procedures, or from possible risks. Benefits and options are discussed with the patient or, in the case of children, with their parents.

Patient Selection

1. The patient is over 7 years of age and 70 lbs of weight.
2. The patient is ASA 1 or 2. I suggest not treating any person who has any medical problem, however slight.
3. Have a signed consent form.
4. Start with a dose of triazolam appropriate for the patient's size.
   a. 70 to 110 lbs gets 0.25 mg
   b. 110 to 180 lbs gets 0.375 mg
   c. 180 to 240 lbs get 0.5 mg
   d. 240 plus get 0.625 mg (see Figures 8.9 and 8.10)

5. If after 30 minutes you see absolutely no effect and if the patient tells you they do not feel any different, give half the original dose sublingually. If they show even a very slight effect, no second dose is necessary (see Figure 8.11).
6. Two hours later you can give half the total dose if you have another hour to go and the patient is much less sedated than they were at 60 minutes. You are giving a dose equal to the amount that has been metabolized.
7. If you need a little more sedation toward the end of a case, augment with nitrous oxide.
8. Only use one oral drug, triazolam. Have the reversal agent and be prepared to inject it into the floor of the mouth if the patient does not respond to verbal command without any tactical stimulation. A pinch will arouse the patient until you can inject the reversal agent. Reverse the sedation as they are starting to get deeper, not after they are under general anesthesia.
9. We are not talking SLEEP, DOZE, SNORE, or NAP. We are talking awake with anxiolysis.

$$\text{Dose (mg)} = 0.25\text{mg} + 0.125\text{mg (for every 70lb weight increase} > 40\text{lbs)}$$

$$\text{Therefore mean dose} = 0.005\text{mg/lb or } 0.5\text{mg for 180-pound man}$$

➤ Triazolam (Halcion) oral sedation can be used effectively over traditional intravenous or inhalation sedation.
  ➤ 70 lb to 110 lb = 0.25 mg
  ➤ 110 lb to 180 lb = 0.375 mg
  ➤ 180 lb to 250 lb = 0.5 mg
  ➤ 250 lb and greater 0.625 mg
➤ Dosing is simple (based on the "Q-factor").
  ➤ Give half the original dose if no effect at 30min.
  ➤ Give half the original dose every 2 hr. if sedation lightens.
➤ Good body of evidence reporting its successful use.

Figure 8-9. Dosage calculation: Dose in mg = 0.25mg + 0.125mg for every 70 lb weight increase over 40 lbs. This equals 0.5 mg for a 180-pound man. If no sedation is observed at 30 minutes, a second dose is administered that is half the original dose. For long cases additional doses may be necessary as the drug is metabolized.

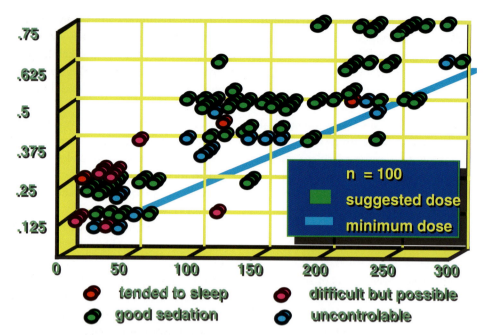

Figure 8-10. Weight vs. dose of triazolam. This was an early graph of our use of triazolam in 110 patients. It was from these data that I developed a dosing scheme relating to the patient's weight.

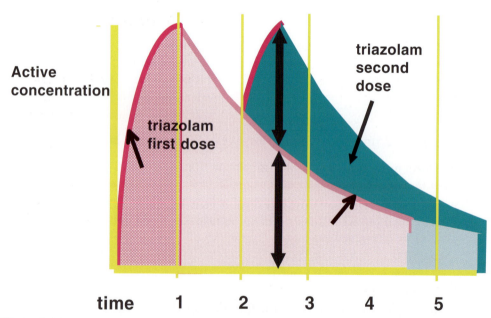

Figure 8-11. Titration of triazolam: Long cases may require a second dose that equals the amount of drug that has been metabolized. Based on information from the following two references: (1) Friedman, H. et al. 1886. Population study of triazolam pharmacokinetics. *Br J Clin Pharm.* 22(6):639–42. (2) Derry, C.L. et al. 1995. Pharmacokinetics and pharmacodynamics of triazolam after two intermittent doses in obese and normal-weight men. *J Clin Psychopharmacol.* 15(3):197–205.

10. Never leave the patient alone in the room.
11. Never leave a male dentist, hygienist, or assistant alone with a female patient.
12. Monitor BP, pulse, and oxygen saturation continuously after you give the initial dose.
13. If the patient needs to use the restroom, they must be accompanied by a same-sex staff person.
14. The patient must be with a responsible adult the rest of the day.
    a. They are to have no alcohol or other sedatives for 24 hours before the appointment.
    b. There should be no chance that they are pregnant.
    c. They should have none of the other contraindications.
    d. They cannot drive, operate machinery, or undertake any activity that could be hazardous. This includes such things as walking unaided, climbing stairs, and so on.
    e. They should not undertake positions of responsibility, such as care of children, and should not make important decisions—legal, monetary, and so on, for the rest of the day.[89, 90, 91]

It is stressed that we are not attempting nor is it our intent to have the patient sleep, although they might experience amnesia for some or all of the appointment. I have found that about 75 percent of patients have amnesia from the time we start the procedure (60 minutes after administering triazolam). The amnesia lasts for 2–3 hours. All patients have had some amnesia or forgetfulness of the appointment.

When the appointment is complete, we keep the patient in the dental chair until they are able to walk out with someone holding their arm. The dentist is the one to determine whether they are able to safely leave the office. You are looking for a noticeable decrease in sedation. Postoperative in-

structions, the same as were given to the patient in the pre-appointment, are reviewed with the adult who is going to take the patient home and watch over them the rest of the day. I assess and record the patient's level of sedation prior to his or her leaving the office. In addition, my home phone is given to this accompanying adult, who is encouraged to call if they have any questions or problems. Finally, an assistant accompanies the patient out to the car, supporting the patient so there is no chance of a fall. The patient is seated in the passenger seat, and the seat belt is buckled.

It should be noted that a second appointment will normally be easier than the first. It has never been necessary to use a higher dose at the second appointment if the dose on the first appointment was adequate. Also, as this is a class IV drug, it is necessary to keep careful accounting records of its use.

Status of Triazolam

UPJOHN

The Upjohn company distributes triazolam in the United States. They make no claims of its usefulness as a dental sedative, nor has it been tested for use with children. The Upjohn company made it very clear to me in a letter that the use of this drug for dental sedation and with children is investigational in nature and not supported or encouraged by the company. The patent has run out for triazolam. Consequently, there is little chance that it will ever be certified for dental sedation.

FDA

The FDA does not recognize triazolam's use for either dental or pediatric sedation. A practitioner must recognize that should there be a problem, the lack of FDA approval would create problems from a medical-legal standpoint. Lack of FDA approval does not,

246 CHAPTER 8

however, prevent our using the drug for sedation.

RECORDKEEPING REQUIREMENTS

The Drug Enforcement Administration, a division of the U.S. Department of Justice, has a booklet that is available from any DEA office, entitled, *Physician's Manual, An Informational Outline of the Controlled Substances Act of 1970.* This manual spells out the requirements of recordkeeping, storage, inventory, security, and so on required for prescribing and dispensing a controlled substance. Triazolam is a schedule IV substance.

To administer, prescribe, or dispense any controlled substance, a physician (dentist) must be registered with the DEA. The DEA requires that "The registration must be renewed every three years and the certificate of registration must be maintained at the registered location."

"It is necessary for dentists to keep records of drugs purchased, distributed and dispensed. Having this closed system, a controlled substance can be traced from the time it is manufactured, to the time it is dispensed to the ultimate user."

"All controlled substance records must be filed in a readily retrievable location from all other business documents, retained for two years, and made available for inspection by the DEA. Controlled substance records maintained as part of the patient file will require that this file be made available for inspection by the DEA."

"A physician (dentist) who dispenses controlled substances is required to keep a record of each transaction."

Inventory requirements

"A physician (dentist) who dispenses or regularly engages in administering controlled substances is required to keep records and must take an inventory every two years of all stocks of the substances on hand."

Security

"A physician (dentist) must keep these drugs in a securely locked, substantially constructed cabinet or safe."

In my office, the triazolam is kept locked in a keyed locker, which is permanently attached to an office wall. Inventory sheets are kept in a book with patient record forms. This sheet shows date and patient name, age, and weight and has space for comments. The inventory total is changed with each drug administration so as to provide a running total of the drug inventory. When restocking the drug supply, a copy of the prescription is attached to the inventory sheet.

PATIENT RECORDS

Patient records are kept for all treatments. These records would be the same for any sedative agent except when nitrous oxide is used with no other sedative drugs. These records include the consent form, post-sedation evaluation, and a sedation record that includes blood pressure records, pulse rates, and pulse oximeter readings. These values are taken and recorded preoperatively and at 15-minute increments from the drug administration until the case is completed. The patient's medical status (ASA rating) is recorded along with age, sex, weight, amounts of drug administered, name, date, and whether this is the first administration of this sedative.

Sedation records are necessary for several reasons. First, they establish a baseline and would be one of the first indicators of a potential problem. If any of the measured parameters start to change, we should immediately be alerted and start corrective action. Second, the stress of an emergency makes time sequencing difficult for the practitioner. It becomes all but impossible to recall vital signs and the times they were recorded. Complete records can provide clues about the case and possible solutions to our problem as it progresses. (At what point did we lose verbal contact? How long has the patient been at this level? Did the change come on rapidly or have vital signs been slowly changing for some time?) Lastly, in the event of legal action, complete and accurate records are a must for one's defense.

Flumazenil (Romazicon) Reversal Agent

It would be a great advantage to have a medication that would reverse the effects of any drug we use. This is particularly true of any drug that requires excretion or metabolism to be deactivated. When using drugs intravenously, small test doses can be given and augmented as necessary to achieve the desired effect. These test doses go directly to the CNS and show their effect. They are then redistributed to the rest of the tissues of the body, effectively diluting the effect in the case of an overdose or sensitivity to an agent. Titration with oral drugs is very slow. It takes considerable time before it is obvious that we have a problem. Redistribution and saturation into the body have already taken place and are of little aid. In the case of overdose, there is little we can do except treat the symptoms of the overdose and support respiration and circulation. For this reason, a reversal agent for oral drugs is very desirable. The reversal agent for benzodiazepines is flumazenil.

HISTORY

In 1974, Haefely hypothesized and showed that benzodiazepines act by increasing the effectiveness of the most important inhibitory neurotransmitter, GABA. Later, several compounds were produced that had a greater affinity for this site than diazepam. One of these, flumazenil, was selected as an antagonist for clinical trials.[92]

PHARMACOLOGY

Flumazenil was shown to prevent benzodiazepine sedation if given before the benzodiazepine and to reverse the effect if given during or after the sedative drug. To reverse sedation or general anesthesia of benzodiazepine drugs, flumazenil is administered intravenously in titrated doses from 0.2-to-1.0 mg doses. In the case of overdose, 2.0 to 3.0 mg may be necessary.[93]

TOXICITY AND SAFETY

"Flumazenil has a high therapeutic index and a wide margin of safety." It showed minimal effect on patients with ischemic heart disease. No withdrawal symptoms were seen when it was given to patients who had been on diazepam or triazolam for up to 14 days. Some symptoms were seen in patients who had been on lorazepam. It should not be given to patients with severe head injuries and unstable intracranial pressures.[94] When given to patients with panic disorder, 2mg of flumazenil intravenously precipitated panic attacks. It had no effect on healthy patients.[95]

Use with Children

Jones administered flumazenil to 40 healthy children aged 3–12 years of age after they had received midazolam for the induction of anesthesia. The drug was given along with a placebo, and the efficacy of antagonism was assessed. Those receiving the active drug awoke approximately four times faster. There were no cases of resedation and minimal changes in the cardio-respiratory variables.[96]

Use with Adults

The half-life of flumazenil at 54 minutes (.7 to 1.3 hr) is less than triazolam, midazolam, and diazepam, so you may see some rebound of effect (see "Resedation" section later in this chapter). Sedation was gone within 2 to 5 minutes. I have seen the reversal drug used sublingually in the floor of the mouth. The pain of this injection noticeably aroused the patient. Their sedation was obviously lessened within two minutes; however, maximum reversal took 10 minutes for IV administration and 20 minutes for sublingual. In both cases, most of the effect occurred in the first five minutes.

Contraindications

Flumazenil is contraindicated in patients with a known hypersensitivity to flumazenil or to benzodiazepines, in patients who have been given a benzodiazepine for control of a potentially life-threatening condition (for example, control of intracranial pressure or status epilepticus), and in patients who are showing signs of serious cyclic antidepressant overdose.[97]

RESEDATION

Because of the relatively short half-life of flumazenil, 54 minutes, it is possible that its reversal effect could disappear before the sedative effect of triazolam, with its half-life of one to two hours (see Figure 8.12). Midazolam has a similar half-life (one to two hours), and several studies have failed to show significant resedation if appropriate doses of midazolam had been used.[98–100] Resedation has been shown with diazepam,[101] which has a much longer half-life (20–50 hours), and with larger doses of midazolam.[102] Until studies have been reported showing no resedation with triazolam, a patient who requires flumazenil should be ob-

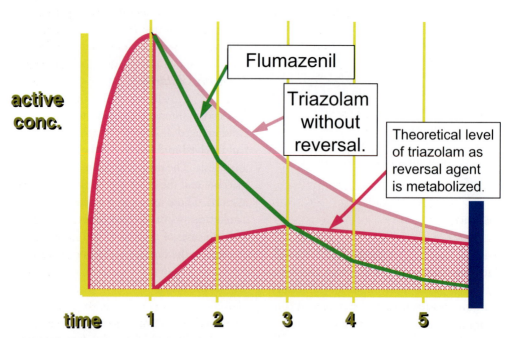

Figure 8-12. The figure shows the reversal with Flumazenil. At time 1 the triazolam is completely reversed. At time 2 one hour later, half the Flumazenil has been metabolized, and part of the effect of the triazolam has rebounded. This effect increases through hour 3.

served for several hours after reversal to be positive resedation does not occur. There is a risk that with reversal the patients may feel normal and attempt activities they are not capable of safely performing.

With the introduction of this reversal agent, we are able to use triazolam with the comfort of knowing that we can reverse its sedation should we achieve an overdose. Of course, this in no way should cause us to use excessive doses of triazolam, nor does it relieve us of the responsibility of monitoring a patient's physical status and responding accordingly in the case of cardiovascular or respiratory depression.

Politics of Sedation

Oral conscious sedation has become a controversial subject for dentistry. The American Dental Association, specialty groups, and some state boards have attempted to severely limit the use of this very necessary and important technique.

In general, benzodiazepine drugs, and specifically triazolam, are very safe when used conservatively. Triazolam has become a drug of choice in dentistry because of its rapid uptake, short half-life, and amnesia. Oral sedation has come a long way toward addressing the unmet needs of phobic patients.

The ADA's guidelines state that titration or "giving a second dose of an oral sedative" is unpredictable and can lead to deeper levels of sedation. These guidelines limit the dose of an oral sedative to the maximum recommended dose (MRD). MRD is a FDA term. In the case of triazolam, it refers to the dose used as a sleep-aid for a patient who may be home alone and has nothing to do with dental sedation. The MRD for triazolam is 0.50 mg.

When you face a sedation/anesthesia emergency, you need all the skill and training you have acquired, previous experience handling such emergencies, and a little luck. This is an area where dental patients can and

do die. Conservative dosing of triazolam for oral conscious sedation will never expose the practitioner to these moments of terror or the patient to theses risks. Always remember DO NO HARM! Death is forever.

Case Reports

It can be helpful to clinicians to have examples of situations in which a medication was actually used with a patient. Following are two care reports using triazolam in clinical settings.

PATIENT NO. 1

A seven-year-old was sedated for dental treatment by a pediatric dentist. The patient left the office able to walk holding the hand of her mother. She went home and tended to sleep if left alone. The dentist's home phone line was out of order that evening. After trying to reach the dentist, her mother became concerned and called a local emergency room, who told her to watch the patient and that triazolam was not approved for use with children. The mother then called poison control and was again told that triazolam should not be used with children. The dentist relieved the mother's concerns when she reached him in the office the next day.

PATIENT NO. 2

A 40-year-old black male about 6′1″ tall and 230 pounds had an uneventful sedation. At the close of the case, when he was judged to be ready to leave, his wife, a rather petite woman of 5′6″, was brought in and given postoperative instructions. At this time she mentioned they would be taking public transportation, a bus, home. Because I was concerned about her being able to help the patient on and off the bus, we kept him an extra hour to ensure that his wife would not have any problem getting him home. We did not insist that the patient be transported by auto. The patient arrived home safely.

Bibliography

1. C. Bennett, C. Richard. Dissociative-sedation. *Compend. Contin. Educ. Dentl*, Vol XI, No.1 Jan., p. 34–38. 1990
2. P. Weinstein, P. Milgrom, E. Kaufman, L. Fiset, D. Ramsay. Patient perceptionsof failure to achieve optimal local anesthesia. *General Dentistry*, May–June, p. 218–220. 1985.
3. P. Milgrom, P. Weinstein, R. Kleinknecht, T. Getz. *Treating fearful dental patients*. Reston, VA: Reston Publishing Co., Inc.. 1985.
4. P. Domoto, P. Weinstein, S. Melnick, M. Ohmura, H. Uchida, K. Ohmachi, M. Hori, Y. Okazaki, T. Shimamoto, S. Matsurma, T. Shimono. Results of a dental fear survey in Japan: implications for dental public health in Asia. *Community Dental Oral Epidemiol* 16: 199–201. 1988.
5. E. Friedaon, J. Feldman. The public looks at dental care. *JADA*, 57: 325–335. 1953.
6. R. Kleinknecht, F. McGlynn, R. Thordnike, J. Harkavy. Factor analysis of the Dental Fear Survey with cross validation. *JADA*, 108: 59–61. 1984.
7. N. Trieger. Current Status of Education in Anesthesia and Sedation; Predoctoral Education in the USA. *Anes Prog*, vol. 36, no. 4/5, p. 217, July-October. 1989.
8. R. A. Dionne. Pharmacologic considerations in the training of dentists in anesthesia and sedation, *Anes Prog* 36: 113–116. 1989.
9. M. P. Coplans, R. A. Green. A Mortality and morbity studies. In M. P. Coplans and R. A. Green (eds.), *Anesthesia and Sedation in Dentistry*. Amsterdam: Elsevier, 131–147. 1983.
10. J. W. Dundee. Advantages and problems with benzodiazepine sedation. 6th International Dental Congress on Modern Pain Control—proceedings Washington, D.C., May, p. 75. 1991.
11. R. A. Dionne. Pharmacologic considerations in the training of dentists in anesthesia and sedation. *Anes Prog* 36: 113–116. 1989.
12. R. A. Dionne, H. C. Gift. Drugs used for parental sedation in dental practice. *Anes. Prog* 35: 199–205. 1988.
13. R. A. Dionne. Pharmacologic considerations in the training of dentists in anesthesia and sedation. *Anes Prog* 36: 113–116. 1989.
14. J. A. Yagiela, E. A. Neidle. *Pharmacology and thearapeutics for dentistry.* St. Louis: CV Mosby, p. 198, 201. 1989.
15. J. A. Yagiela, E. A. Neidle. *Pharmacology and thearapeutics for dentistry.* St. Louis: CV Mosby, p. 190. 1989.
16. S. H. Snyder, Solomon. *Drugs and the Brain*. New York, NY: Scientific American Library Books, Inc. , p. 156. 1986.
17. J. T. Jastak, S. F. Malamed. Nitrous oxide sedation and sexual phenomena. *Dent J Am Dent Assoc.* Jul;101(1): 38–40. 1980.
18. NIOSH Alert: Request for assistance in Controlling Exposures to Nitrous Oxide During Anesthetic Administration, National Institute of Occupational Safety and Health, US Department of Health and Human Service. 1994.
19. A. I. Vaisman,. Working conditions in surgery and their effect on the health of anesthesiologists. *Anesthesiology*, 29: 565. 1968.
20. H. A. C. Lassen, et al. Treatment of tetanus: Severe bone marrow depression after prolonged nitrous oxide anesthesia. *Lancet* 1: 527–530.
21. E. L. Eger. Fetal Injury and Abortion Associated with Occupational Exposure to Inhaled Anesthetics. *AANA Journal*, vol. 59, No. 4 p. 309–312. 1991.
22. H. S. Abdul-Kareem, R. P. Sharma, D. B. Drown. Effects of Repeated Intermittent Exposures to Nitrous Oxide on Central Neurotransmitters and Hepatic Methionine Synthetase Activity in CD-1 Mice. *Toxicology and Industrial Health*, Vol. 7, no. 1/2 p. 97–108. 1991.
23. C. E. Healy, D. B. Drown, R. P. Sharma. Short Term Toxicity of Nitrous Oxide an the Immune, Hemopoetic, and Endocrine System in CD-1 Mice. *Toxicology and Industrial Health*, Vol. 6, No. 1, p. 57–70. 1990.
24. M. Fujinaga, J. M. Baden, T. H. Shepard, R. I. Mazz. Nitrous oxide Alters Body Laterality in Rats. *Teratology*, Vol. 41, No. 2, p. 131–135. 1990.
25. E. Viera, P. Kleaton-Jones, J. C. Austin, D. G. Moyes, R. Shaw. Effects of Low Concentrations of Nitrous Oxide on Rat Fetuses. *Anesth. Analgesia*. Vol. 59, p. 175–177. 1980.

26. B. J. Kripke, A. D. Kelman, N. K. Shah, K. Balogh, A. H. Handler. Testicular Reaction to Prolonged Exposure to Nitrous Oxide. *Anesthesiology*, Vol. 44 p. 104. 1976.

27. P. Cleanton-Jones et al. Effect of Intermittent Exposure to a Low Concentration of Nitrous Oxide on Hematopoesis in Rats. *Anesthesiology* 49: 233. 1977.

28. W. B. Coate, B. M. Ulland, T. R. Lewis. Chronic Exposure to Low Concentrations of Halothane-Nitrous Oxide: Lack of Carcinogenic Effect in the Rat. *Anesthesiology* 50: 306. 1979.

29. J. M. Baden et al. Carcinogen Bioassay of Nitrous Oxide in Mice. *Anesthesiology* 50: 306. 1979.

30. E. Vieira et al. Effects of Low Concentrations of Nitrous Oxides on Fetuses. *Anesth. Anal.* 59: 175. 1980.

31. R. D. Hardin et al. Testing of Selected Workplace Chemical for Teratogenic Potential. *Scand. J. Work. Environ. Health* 7(4): 66. 1981.

32. N. M. Sharer et al. Effects of Chronic Exposure to Nitrous Oxide on Methionine Synthetase Activity. *Br. J. Anesth.* 55: 693. 1983.

33. E. N. Cohen, B. W. Brown, M. L. Wu, C. E. Whitcher, J. B. Brodsky, H. C. Gift, W. Greenfield, T. W. Jones, E. J. Driscoll. Occupational disease in dentistry and chronic exposure to trace anesthetic gases. *JADA*, 101: 21–31. 1980.

34. J. B. Brodsky, E. N. Cohen, B. W. Brown, Jr., M. L. Wu, C. E. Whitcher. Exposure to nitrous oxide and neurologic disease among dental professionals. *Anesth Analg*60: 297–301. 1981.

35. J. A. Yagiela. Health Hazards and Nitrous Oxide: A Time for Reappraisal. *Anesth Prog* 38: 1–11, Jan. 1991.

36. ADA News. ADA seeks data on nitrous exposure. American Dental Association, November 23, vol. 23. 1992.

37. D. L. Bruce, M. J. Bach. Effects of trace anesthetic gases on behavioral performance of volunteers. *British J Anesth* 48: 871–876. 1976.

38. D. L. Bruce, M. J. Bach, J. Arbit. Trace Anesthetic Effects on Perceptual, Cognitive and Motor Skills. *Anesthesiology*, v 40, 5 May, 1974.

39. D. L. Bruce, M. J. Bach. Effects of trace anesthetic gases on behavioral performance of volunteers. *British J Anesth* 48: 871–876. 1976.

40. D. L. Bruce, M. J. Bach, J. Arbit. Trace Anesthetic Effects on Perceptual, Cognitive and Motor Skills. *Anesthesiology*, v 40, 5. May, 1974.

41. D. L. Bruce. Recantation Revisited. *Anesthesiology*, Vol.,74, No. 6, p. 1160–61. June, 1991.

42. D. L. Bruce, T. H. Stanley. Research replication may be subject specific. *Anesth. Analg.* No 62, p. 617–21. 1983.

43. G. Ahlborg, G. Axelsson, L. Bodin. Shift work, nitrous oxide exposure and subfertility among Swedish midwives. *International Journal of Epidemiology*, Aug., vol.25, NO. 4, p. 783–790. 1996.

44. G. Ahlborg, G. Axelsson, L. Bodin. Shift work, nitrous oxide exposure and spontaneous abortion among Swedish midwives. *Occupational and Environmental Medicine*, Vol. 53, No. 6, p. 374–378. 1996.

45. J. F. Nunn et al. Serum methionine and hepatic enzyme activity in anesthetists exposed to nitrous oxide. *Br. J. Anesth.* 55: 593. 1982.

46. Sweeney et al. *British Medical Journal.* 1985.

47. A. S. Rowland, D. D. Baird, C. R. Wienberg, D. L. Shore, C. M. Shy, A. J. Wilcox. Reduced fertility among women employed as dental assistants exposed to high levels of nitrous oxide. *New England Journal of Medicine*, Vol. 327, No. 14, p. 993–997.

48. D. Donaldson, J. Orr. A comparison of the effectiveness of nitrous oxide scavenging devices. *Journal Canadian Dental Association.* Vol 55, No. 7, p. 535–537. July, 1989.

49. D. Donaldson, J. Orr. A comparison of the effectiveness of nitrous oxide scavenging devices. *Journal Canadian Dental Association.* Vol 55, No. 7, p. 535–537. July, 1989.

50. B. R. Fink. Diffusion anoxia. *Anes.* Jul; 16(4): 511–9. 1955

51. F. C. Quarnstrom, P. Milgrom, M. J. Bishop, T. A. DeRouen. Diffusion Hypoxia Clinical Study of Diffusion Hypoxia after Nitrous Oxide Analgesia. *Anesthesia Progress.* vol. 38, no. 1, p. 21–23. 1991.

52. J. B. Brodsky, R. E. McKlveen, J. Zelcer, J. J. Margary. Diffusion hypoxia: a reappraisal using pulse oximetry. *J Clin Monit.* Oct; 4(4):244–6. 1988.

53. M. B. Papageorge, L. W. Noonan, M. Rosenberg. Diffusion hypoxia: another view. *Anesth Pain Control Dent.* Summer; 2(3): 143–9. 1993

54. D. E. Becker. The respiratory effects of drugs used for conscious sedation and general anesthesia. *JADA*, vol. 119, p. 153–156. July, 1989.

55. S. H. Snyder. *Drugs and the Brain.* New York, NY: Scientific American Library, Scientific American Books Inc., p. 151–177. 1986.

56. D. L. Gottlieb. GABAergic Neurons. *Scientific America*n, no. 2, p. 82–89. February, 1988.

57. G. Cowley, K. Springen, D. Iarovici, M. Hager. Sweet dreams or nightmare? *Newsweek.* August 19, p. 48. 1991.

58. R. P. Juhl, V. M. Daugherty, P. D. Kroboth. Incidence of next-day anterograde amnesia caused by flurazepam hydrochloride and Triazolam. *Clin Pharm* (Nov–Dec) 3(6): 622—5. 1984

59. R. H. Meyboom. The triazolam affair in 1979, a false alarm? *Ned Tijdschr Geneeskd.* Nov 4; 133(44): 2185–90. 1989.

60. L. Lasagna. The triazolam story: trial by media. *Lancet* (Apr 12) 1(8172): 815–6. 1980.

61. R. Riefkoh, R. Kosanin. Experience with triazolam as a preoperative sedative for outpatient surgery under local anesthesia. *Aesthetic Plast Surg.* 8(3): 155–7. 1984.

62. E. D. Burgess, K. R. Burgess, T. R. Reroah, W. A. Whitelaw. Respiratory drive in patients with end-stage renal disease at rest and after administration of meperidine and triazolam. *Clin Res,*35: 173a. 1987.

63. R. T. Longbottor, B. J. Pleuvry. Respiratory and sedative effects of triazolam in volunteers. *Br J Anaesth,* 56: 179–185. 1984.

64. R. B. Knapp, E. L. Boyd, B. Linsenmeyer, O. I. Linet. A comparison of the cardiopulmonary safety and effects of triazolam, flurazepam and placebo in pre-surgical patients. *Excerpta Med Int Cong Ser.* 542: 246. 1979.

65. R. B. Knapp, E. L. Boyd, B. Linsenmeyer, O. I. Linet. An evaluation of the cardiopulmonary safety and efficacy of triazolam, flurazepam and placebo as oral hypnotic agents. *Clin Pharmacol Ther,* 21: 107–108. 1977.

66. B. Joynt. *Journal of Analytical Toxicology.* vol.17 p. 171–177. May/June, 1993.

67. J. Yagiela. Recent Developments in Local Anesthesia and Oral Sedation. Compendium. Sept. vol.25, no 9, p. 697–707. 2004.

68. Anonymous. New benzodiazepine sedatives assessed at recent symposium. *Pharm Pract News,* 14(5): 25–27. 1987.

69. P. D. Garzone, P. D. Kroboth. *Pharmacokinetics of the newer benzodiazepines.* Auckland, New Zealand: Adis Press p. 347. 1989.

70. G. E. Pakes, R. N. Brogden, R. C. Heel, T. M. Speight, G. S. Avery. *Triazolam: A Review of its Pharmacological Properties and Therapeutic Efficacy in Patients with Insomnia.* Auckland, New Zealand: Adis Press. p. 91. 1981.

71. P. D. Garzone, P. D. Kroboth. *Pharmacokinetics of the newer benzodiazepines.* Auckland, New Zealand: Adis Press. p. 346. 1989.

72. P. D. Garzone, P. D. Kroboth. *Pharmacokinetics of the newer benzodiazepines.* Auckland, New Zealand: Adis Press. p. 347. 1989.

73. P. D. Garzone, P. D. Kroboth. *Pharmacokinetics of the newer benzodiazepines.* Auckland, New Zealand: Adis Press. p. 348. 1989.

74. P. D. Garzone, P. D. Kroboth. *Pharmacokinetics of the newer benzodiazepines.* Auckland, New Zealand: Adis Press. p. 347. 1989.

75. P. D. Garzone, P. D. Kroboth. *Pharmacokinetics of the newer benzodiazepines.* Auckland, New Zealand: Adis Press. p. 348–976. 1989.

76. G. E. Pakes, R. N. Brogden, R. C. Heel, T. M. Speight, G. S. Avery. *triazolam: A review of its pharmacological properties and therapeutic efficacy in patients with insomnia.* Auckland, New Zealand: Adis Press. p. 93. 1981.

77. G. E. Pakes, R. N. Brogden, R. C. Heel, T. M. Speight, G. S. Avery. *triazolam: A review of its pharmacological properties and therapeutic efficacy in patients with insomnia.* Auckland, New Zealand: Adis Press. p. 91. 1981.

78. J. A. Yagiela, E. A. Meidle. *Pharmacology and therapeutics for dentistry.* St Louis, MO: CV Mosby, p. 132. 1989.

79. W. A. Parker, R. A. MacLachlan. Prolonged hypnotic response to triazolam-cimetidine combination in an elderly patient. *Drug Intell Clin Pharm* (Dec) 18(12): 980–1. 1984.

80. J. B. Weilburg, G. Sachs, W. E. Falk. Triazolam-induced brief episodes of secondary mania in a depressed patient. *J Clin Psychiatry* (Dec) 48(12): 492–3. 1987.

81. Young, R. Earle, Mason, Douglas. Triazolam and oral sedative for the dental practitioner. *J Canad Dent Assoc,* vol. 54, no.7. July, 1988.

82. H. Heinzl, C. Axhausen, U. Bahler, H. Gehrer. Comparison of the effectiveness of triazolam (Halcion) and flunitrazepam (Rohypnol) in the preoperative period. A double-blind crossover study*, Schweiz Med Wochenschr* (Nov 15) 110(46): 1745–8. 1980.

83. A. A. Borbely, M. Loepfe, P. Mattmann, I. Tobler. Midazolam and triazolam: hypnotic action and residual effects after a single bedtime dose. *Arzneimittelforschung* 33(10): 1500–2. 1983.

84. P. D. Kroboth, R. P. Juhl. New drug evaluations. Triazolam. *Drug Intell Clin Pharm* (Jul–Aug) 17(7–8): 495–500. 1983.

85. T. Roth, T. A. Roehrs, F. J. Zorick. Pharmacology and hypnotic efficacy of triazolam. *Pharmacotherapy* (May–Jun) 3(3): 137–48. 1983.

86. K. Morgan, K. Adam, I. Oswald. Effect of loprazolam and of triazolam on psychological functions. *Psychopharmacology* (Berlin) 82(4): 386–8. 1984.

87. L. F. Fabre, Jr., W. T. Smith. Multi-clinic crossover comparison of triazolam (Triazolam) and placebo in the treatment of co-existing insomnia and anxiety in anxious out-patients. *Dis Nerv Syst.* (Jun) 38(6): 487–91. 1977.

88. F. Quarnstrom, M. Donaldson. Triazolam use in the dental setting: A report of 270 uses over 15 years. *General Dentistry.* Nov/Dec p 434–9. 2004.

89. D. E. Boatwright. Triazolam, handwriting, and amnestic states: two cases. *J Forensic Sci.* (Jul) 32(4): 1118–24. 1987.

90. H. H. Morris, 3d, M. L. Estes. Traveler's amnesia. Transient global amnesia secondary to Triazolam. *JAMA* (Aug 21) 258(7): 945–6. 1987.

91. M. Leibowitz, A. Sunshine. Long-term hypnotic efficacy and safety of Triazolam and flurazepam. *J Clin Pharmacol.* (May–Jun) 18(5–6): 302–9. 1978.

92. H. Heinzl, C. Axhausen, U. Bahler, H. Gehrer. Comparison of the effectiveness of triazolam (Triazolam) and flunitrazepam (Rohypnol) in the preoperative period. A double blind crossover study. *Schweiz Med Wochenschr.* (Nov 15) 110(46): 1745–8. 1980.

93. B. K. Philip. *Flumazenil a review of the literature. Excerpta Medica*, Prinction. p. 8. 1992.

94. B. K. Philip. *Flumazenil a review of the literature. Excerpta Medica*, Prinction. p. 9–10. 1992.

95. R. N. Brogden, K. L. Goa. Flumazenil: A reappraisal of its pharmacological properties and therapeutic efficacy as a benzodiazepine antagonist. Auckland, New Zealand: Adis International Ltd. p. 1063.

96. R. D. M. Jones, A. D. Lawson, L. J. Andrew, W. N. S. Gunawardene, J. Bacon-Shone. Antagonism of the hypnotic effect of Midazolam in children: A randomized, double-blind study of placebo and flumazenil administered after Midazolam induced anesthesia. *British Journal of Anesthesia.* 66: 660–666. 1991.

97. *Mazicon, drug insert.* Nutley, NJ: Roach Laboratories. Dec., 1991.

98. A. A. Dunk, A. C. Norton, M. Hudson. *Aliment Pharmacol Ther.* 4: 35–42. 1990.

99. A. W. Harrop-Griffiths, N. A. Watson, D. A. Jewkes. *Br J Anaesth.* 64: 586–589. 1990.

100. J. G. Whitwam. *Acta Anaesthesio Scand.* 34(suppl 92): 70–74. 1990.

101. A. M. Holloway, D. A. Logan. The use of flumazenil to reverse diazepam sedation after endoscopy. *Eur J Anaesthesiol.* suppl 2: 191–194. 1988.

102. R. N. Brogden, K. L. Goa. Flumazenil: A reappraisal of its pharmacological properties and therapeutic efficacy as a benzodiazepine antagonist. Auckland, New Zealand: Adis International Ltd. p. 1074.

Chapter 9

Infections and Antibiotic Administration

Dr. R. Thane Hales

Introduction

Infections of the oral cavity and the surrounding structures of the head and neck can be some of the most complex and serious to manage. Minor infections, however, are usually easily treated when the correct antibiotic and debridement regimen is used. This regimen must include a comprehensive understanding of the infectious organism and the action of the antibiotic used, along with its corresponding dosage.

Oral infections are frequently mild or low-grade localized infections. However, these may spread to become moderate, and if left unattended, grow into a more severe complex condition. Appropriate treatment in the early stages will usually prevent the need for more serious fascial space infections that can be life threatening. Infections can rapidly become severe, especially in a medically compromised patient.

In this chapter, the most common oral infections and their causative pathogens will be discussed—along with current therapies. As we know, the science of oral microbiology is evolving and requires constant updating and study in order to stay proficient at treating patients. The material in this chapter is current at the time of writing, but change is ongoing, and the serious clinician must update frequently for the benefit of the patient.

Bacterial Characteristics

Bacteria differ from viruses in that they are single-celled organisms. Viruses are far simpler, consisting of one type of biochemical (a nucleic acid, such as DNA or RNA) wrapped in another (a protein). Most biologists do not consider viruses to be living things but, instead, infectious particles. Antibiotic drugs attack bacteria, **not** viruses. In the drawing shown in Figure 9.1, we would need to draw the virus four times smaller to make it correct in size relative to the size of the bacteria.[1]

Perhaps the most relevant problem we face today is that we are rapidly reaching a critical point in the use of effective antibiotics to destroy microorganisms. One of the most significant reasons is the lack of understanding and clinical skill of the clinician.

255

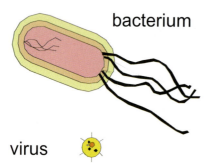

Figure 9-1. Bacterium and a virus particle. The virus would actually be several times smaller than illustrated here. Adapted from Ricki Lewis; FDA Consumer, Vol. 29, Sept. 1995.

Many providers prescribe antimicrobial drugs to treat viral infections when they are absolutely contraindicated. Another reason is that clinicians are not giving the right antibiotics in the appropriate dosages.

When microbes began resisting penicillin shortly after its discovery in the 1940s, medical researchers fought back with chemical cousins, such as methicillin and oxacillin. By 1953, the antibiotic armamentarium included chloramphenicol, neomycin, terramycin, tetracycline, and cephalosporins. But today, researchers fear that we may be nearing an end to the seemingly endless flow of antibiotic drugs.

The drug of last resort has long been Vancomycin. This is a derivative of Lincomycin, which was derived from soil bacteria near Lincoln Nebraska. Vancomycin, once our last line of defense, is now reported to be ineffective against certain hospital strains of enterococcus and strains of staphylococcus.

MICROORGANISMS PRODUCE ANTIBIOTICS

Penicillium and Cephalosporium produce the beta-lactam antibiotics penicillin and cephalosporin. Actinomycetes, mainly the *Streptomyces* species, produce tetracyclines, aminoglycosides (streptomycin and its relatives), macrolides (erythromycin and its relatives), chloramphenicol, and most clinically useful antibiotics that are not beta-lactams.

Bacillus species, such as *B. polymyxa* and *B. subtilis,* produce polypeptide antibiotics (that is, polymyxin and bacitracin), and *B. cereus* produces zwittermicin. These organisms live in a soil habitat forming a spore or resting structure. Antibiotics are secondary metabolites of these microorganisms. They are produced at the same time the cells begin sporulation (division) processes. Because of their complexity, it may require 30 separate steps to synthesize them. Some of the major antibiotics and the organisms they are produced from are listed in Table 9.1.[2]

ANATOMY OF BACTERIA

The review of the anatomy of single-cell bacteria is necessary to understand the discussion that follows. The components of bacteria are basically the cell wall, cytoplasm, DNA nucleus, plasmids, ribosomes, and other external structures shown in Figure 9.2.

Table 9-1. Antibiotic Origins and Actions

Antibiotic	Produced From	Activity	Site of Action
Penicillin	*Penicillium chrysogenum*	Gram pos/neg	Cell wall
Cephalosporin	*Cephalosporium acremonium*	Broad spectrum	Cell wall
Erythromycin	*Streptomyces erythres*	Gram pos	Protein synthesis
Tetracycline	*Streptomyces nimnosus*	Broad spectrum	Protein Synthesis
Metronidazol	Synthetic antiprotozoal	Gram neg	DNA replication
Clavulanic acid	*Streptomyces clavuligerus*	Gram neg	Blocks β-lactamases
Amoxicillin	*Penicillium notatum*	Gram pos/neg	Cell wall

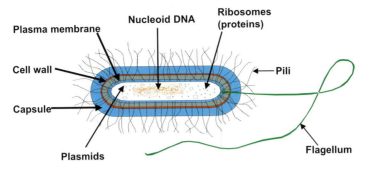

Figure 9-2. Anatomy of a single cell bacterium.

BACTERIAL RESISTANCE

There are at least three known ways bacterial resistance can occur.

1. Spontaneous mutation of the DNA.

    In spontaneous DNA mutation, bacterial DNA (genetic material) may mutate (change) spontaneously. This can occur with low levels of antibiotic therapy or noncompliance on the patient's part to "take as directed." Patients must take the medications for two days after symptoms disappear (see Figure 9.3).

2. Microbial sex transformation.

    The passage of genes from cell to cell by direct contact through a sex pilus or bridge is termed **conjugation.** This is an important way bacteria can change or adapt. It happens when one bacterium takes up DNA during replication or transformation from another bacterium that is already resistant (see Figure 9.4).

3. Plasmid transfer resistance.

    One of the more serious changes of bacteria is resistance acquired from a small circle of DNA called a plasmid. A plasmid can transfer from one type of bacterium to another. A single plasmid can provide several resistances. In 1968, 12,500 people in Guatemala died in an epidemic of Shigella diarrhea. The microbe harbored a plasmid carrying resistances to four antibiotics![1] See Figure 9.5.

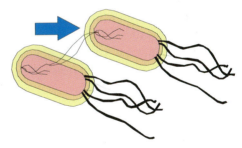

Figure 9-4. Microbial sex transformation. Adapted from Ricki Lewis, FDA Consumer, Vol. 29, Sept. 1995.

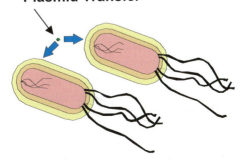

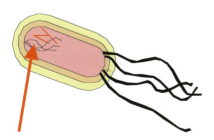

Figure 9-3. Spontaneous DNA mutation. Adapted from Ricki Lewis, FDA Consumer, Vol. 29, Sept. 1995.

Figure 9-5. Plasmid transfer. Adapted from Ricki Lewis, FDA Consumer, Vol. 29, Sept. 1995.

Indiscriminate Prescribing

We have taken antibiotics for granted. It seems that every time we get a cough, the sniffles, or a slight earache, the plastic bottle of magic medicine is the answer. Even sinus headache is treated unwarrantedly with antibiotics. Most sinusitis problems are viral, and the useless administration of antibiotics is helping the bacterial resistance to escalate. The use of antibiotics in the treatment of a well-localized and easily drained dentoalveolar abscess is usually unnecessary because drainage and dental therapy usually resolve the infection. On the other hand, when there are systemic signs and symptoms such as trismus, elevated temperature, poorly localized or diffuse cellulitis, diabetes, or immunocompromized diseases, antibiotic therapy is required.

The careful use of antibiotics is essential if we are to do our part in preserving the antibiotics that we have. Most odontogenic infections are caused by a few predictable groups of bacteria with which we must become familiar. A little time and effort in studying these microbes will make a practitioner's ability to diagnose and treat infections more predictable.

Bacteria Associated with Odontogenic Infections

Many different strains of bacteria exist in the oral cavity. Oral bacteria in certain infections may number from 350 to 500[3] different species. However, if we know the predominant ones, we will have a greater advantage over infectious disease.

The most common oral infections are those arising from pulpal necrosis and the subsequent overflow into the surrounding tissue, or periodontal infections that result from the invasion of bacteria into bone or soft tissue. This could be in the third molar region, where pericoronitis allows the bacteria into the underlying and surrounding tissues. Pericoronitis is not to be taken lightly as it can be a precursor to more serious infections even after the third molar is extracted. The extraction site must be irrigated thoroughly with copious amounts of sterile water and the patient placed on an antibiotic.

The abscessed tooth is the most common of all infections that dentists treat, and the second most common is periodontal infection. There are infections that arise due to the condition of the host, where defense mechanisms are compromised by illness or by drug therapy. This creates an imbalance that lets certain flora flourish. Currently, laboratory culture tests are able to cultivate only five or six of the major pathogens in an odontogenic infection,[4] but these few culturable bacteria are usually the major cause of the infection. Cultures and sensitivity tests then are very useful in choosing the right antibiotic regimen.

Aerobic and Anaerobic Bacteria

Infectious bacteria in the mouth are either aerobic or anaerobic. They either need oxygen or they do not. The bacteria that cause infections in the mouth are indigenous to the host. They all are prevalent in a balanced environment. This balanced environment is designed to keep each pathogen in check, maintaining function while living in a mutual coexistence. The effect of one bacterium upon another was first witnessed when streptococcus bacteria were noticed affecting diphtheria (*Corynebacterium diphtheriae*) before the advent of immunization. Sprays of streptococcus viridians were applied to the throat of victims of the disease in an effort to control the infection.

Most odontogenic infections that typically invade the host patient are a mix of aerobic or anaerobic bacteria. About 60 percent of all oral infections are a mix of these two types of flora. Infections that are aerobic only amount to about 5 percent of oral infections. Those that are anerobic only are the cause of roughly 35 percent.[3]

GRAM STAINING

Gram stain (an empirical staining procedure devised by Gram) is a process in which microorganisms are stained with crystal violet treated with a 1:15 dilution of Lugol's iodine, decolorized with ethanol or ethanol-acetone, and counterstained with a contrasting dye—usually safranin. Microorganisms that retain the crystal violet stain are said to be gram-positive, and those that lose the crystal violet stain by decolorization but stain with the counter stain are said to be gram-negative.

Bacteria that retain the stain have a thicker wall of peptidogylcan layers and, consequently, retain the stain (see Figure 9.5). This layer is very thin and beneath a cell wall in gram-negative bacteria, so the stain is decolorized. The ability to retain the stain or resist decolorization by alcohol in Gram's method of staining is a primary characteristic of gram-positive bacteria.

Gram-negative bacteria lose the stain and are decolorized by alcohol in Gram's method of staining. This is a primary characteristic of gram-negative bacteria—having a cell wall composed of a thin layer of peptidoglycan covered by an outer membrane of lipoprotein and lipopolysaccharide (see Figure 9.6).

The cell walls of bacteria are essential for their normal growth and development. Peptidoglycan is a heteropolymeric component of the cell wall that provides rigid mechanical stability by virtue of its highly cross-linked latticework structure. In gram-positive microorganisms, the cell wall is 50 to 100 molecules thick, but in gram-negative bacteria, it is only one or two molecules thick. Peptidoglycan is composed of glycan chains, which are linear strands of two alternating amino sugars (N-acetylglucosamine and N-acetylmuramic acid) cross-linked by peptide chains.

PRODUCTION OF BETA LACTAMASE

The most recognized cause of bacterial resistance is the production, by certain gram-negative anaerobes, of the enzyme beta lactamase. This enzyme attaches to the penicillin molecule at the beta lactum ring. If the β-lactam ring is enzymatically cleaved by bacterial β-lactamases, the resulting product, penicilloic acid, lacks antibacterial activity. The same scenario holds true for cephlosporins as their structure is similar. See Figure 9.7.

KILLING BACTERIA THAT CAUSE INFECTION

Antibiotics generally work in one of five ways:

1. Inhibition of nucleic acid synthesis (for example, Rifampicin)
2. Inhibition of protein synthesis (for example, tetracyclines, erythromycins)
3. Action on cell membrane (for example, polyenes; Polymyxin)
4. Interference with enzyme system (for example, Sulphamethoxazole)
5. Action on cell wall (for example, penicillins; cephlosporins, Vancomycin)

Penicillin works by blocking the formation of peptide bonds in the bacterial cell wall and, thereby, weakening it, leaving the bacterium susceptible to osmotic lysis. Although there appears to be a wide assortment of antibiotics and mechanisms of action, there are a very limited number of targets through which bacteria are susceptible to antibacterial activity. Researchers are constantly looking for new ways to combat bacteria.

The causative organisms can be treated either empirically or by isolating the bacteria by culture. The culture is treated with different antibiotic chips to see which one is the most effective in destroying the organism.

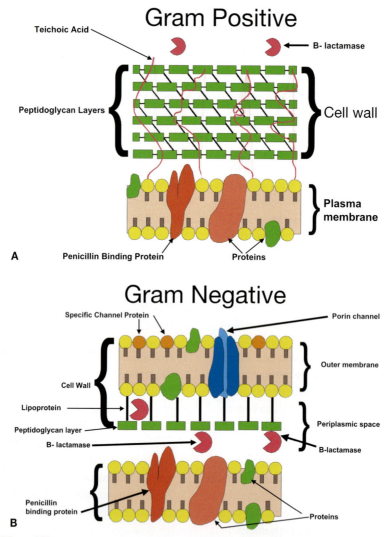

Figure 9-6A and B. Structure of the cell wall. Comparison of the structure and composition of gram-positive and gram-negative cell walls. (Adapted from Tortora et al., 1989.)

This is a sophisticated methodology using pus aspirates placed on a medium inducing their growth. The results of these tests can provide enough information to give a close picture of what is happening at different intervals during the infection. These intervals are usually related to the invasiveness of the organism. The more invasive an infection is, especially in the early stages of a cellulitis, the more an empirical decision can be made that this undefined borderless infection is due to aerobic bacteria. When aerobic bacteria reduce the oxygen potential and an infection becomes more localized, it takes the form of an abscess with more defined boarders. At this point, even without cultures, we can assume that the anaerobes have joined the process and we have a mixed microbial infection. It is postulated that anaerobic bacteria become opportunistic and feed on the essential nutrients and by-products of the aerobic bacteria as well as thriving in the oxygen-depleted environment.

In the last few years, science has been able to improve the aseptic collection of cultures. Also, through DNA mapping, they have

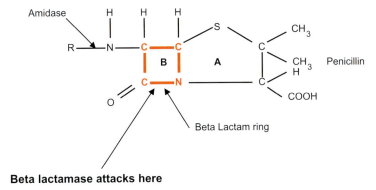

Figure 9-7. Penicillin.

more clearly defined what microbes we are trying to eliminate. Even though the treatment of infectious disease of the oral environment without culture is not absolute, we can be sure that in most cases a large majority of them follow patterns that are predictable. Every dental infection cannot be subjected to the cost of these modern tests. We can, however, order these tests when we are involved in treating severe infections to give us a clear picture of the usual causative bacteria.

Common oral flora contain the following gram-positive bacteria: *Streptococcus viridans* spp. *S. viridans* has many different species. See Table 9.2. These oral bacteria are alpha-hemolytic. The definition of alpha-hemolytic is alpha hemolysis; a greenish discoloration and partial hemolysis of the red blood cells immediately surrounding colonies of some streptococci on blood agar plates. Compare that to beta-hemolytic. Beta hemolysis: A sharply defined clear colorless zone of hemolysis surrounding colonies of certain streptococci on blood agar plates. So the properties of each of these two types of oral flora react differently when metabolizing blood and sugars.

Streptococcus viridans

About 85 percent of all oral infections contain bacteria of the aerobic strep viridans

Table 9-2. *Streptococcus viridans* Group

S. milleri
S. sanguis
S. salivaris
S. mutans
S. pyogenes

group. The viridans group is the group of bacteria we are treating in the prophylactic prevention of subacute bacterial endocarditis. They are sticky and have the ability to attach to epithelium, especially damaged epitheium. All of the alpha hemolytic strep are sensitive to penicillin and other antibiotics with a similar spectrum to penicillin. Other bacteria seen occasionally are *Streptococcus Pyogenes* and Staphylococci, but they do not play a significant role in oral infections.

Anaerobic Bacteria

Anaerobic bacteria far outnumber the aerobic bacteria in oral infections. They consist of two groups, gram-positive cocci and gram-negative rods. The gram-positive cocci are the anaerobic streptococcus and peptostreptococcus. These bacteria are found in about 33 percent of oral infections. They, like their cousins of the aerobic strep, are sensitive to penicillin and other antibiotics with a similar spectrum.

Table 9-3. Bacteriodes

Prevotella	Porphyromonas
P. melanogenica	P. asaccharolyticus
P. buccae	P. gingivalis
P. intermedia	P. endodontalis
P. oralis	
P. loeschii	

ANAEROBIC GRAM-NEGATIVE RODS

Anaerobic gram-negative rods are accountable for about 50 percent of the bacteria in oral infections.[5] The two most prevalent genre are fusobacterium and bacteriodes. The bacteriodes of the oral cavity were thought to be related to or the same as the gut flora bacteriodes. Gut bacteriodes are of the fragilis group and differ from the oral bacteriodes group. The two reclassified bacteriodes are prevotella and porphyromonas. Each of these genera has different species. For the sake of simplicity, we will address them as their genera only. Table 9.3 is provided to show some of their specific species that are currently identified.

The most common gram-negative rod isolated from infections is prevotella. Prevotella have a natural resistance to penicillin, with 40 percent to 80 percent being resistant.[3]

Porphyromonas are rarely found in oral infections with the exception of *P. gingivalis*, which is found to be one of the most common causes of periodontitis.

Another group of gram-negative rods are the fusobacterium genus. They are very pathogenic and destroy tissue like prevotella. This is done by the production of proteolytic enzymes and endotoxins. They are sensitive to penicillin, but 50 percent are not responsive to erythromycin. Fusobacteria are often associated with the most severe infections and often these include the viridians type aerobic *Streptococcus milleri*. This combination of virulence is common in severe infections that invade the lateral and retropharyngeal spaces. These can eventually progress downward into the mediastinum. Mediastinal and retropharyngeal infections are among the most serious infections and are very difficult to manage. They can lead to death of the patient.

BACTERICIDAL AND BACTERIOSTATIC ANTIBIOTICS

In discussing how best to treat the various infections, it is imperative that the doctor understand each of the antibiotics and the type of infection they are treating. This is an ever-changing science with the development of more and more resistant bacteria and hopefully new antibiotics.

One of the ways antibiotics are classified is the manner in which they destroy the pathogens. A **bactericidal** drug like penicillin actually destroys the bacteria by attacking the cell wall of the invading microorganism. The action of breaking down the cell wall is accomplished by interfering with a specific step in cell wall synthesis. Penicillin actually binds to a specific protein in the cell wall.

Bacteriostatic antibiotics merely retard the growth of the bacteria by attaching to the ribosomes and DNA inside the cell. They also interfere with cellular metabolism. These actions do not allow the bacteria to replicate certain essential proteins. Erythromycins are all primarily bacteriostatic and bind to the 50S subunit of the ribosome. This inhibits bacterial protein synthesis. It then allows the body's defense mechanism to work synergistically to eventually overcome the bacteria.[5] See Table 9.4.

Periodontal Infection

Of all oral infections, periodontal infection is probably the least understood in general practice. The changing world of infection and reclassification of certain organisms is

INFECTIONS AND ANTIBIOTIC ADMINISTRATION 263

Table 9-4. Bactericidal and Bacteriostatic Drugs

Bactericidal Antibiotics	Bacteriostatic Antibiotics
Penicillins	Erythromycin
Cephalosporins	Tetracycline
Aminoglycosides	Clarithromycin
Vancomycin	Clindamycin at 150mg
Metronidazole	Arithromycin
Imipenem	Sulfa
Fluoroquinalones	
Clindamycin at 300mg	

partially to blame. Prior to 1970, most investigators focused their attention on supragingival plaque rather than subgingival plaque. The subgingival flora is composed mainly of anaerobes, most of which could not be cultured. When grown, they could not be assigned to known species. Consequently, microbial specificity in periodontal disease was difficult to demonstrate. More recently, anaerobic culturing by the use of quantitative procedures has led to the isolation of several new species associated with various clinical entities. However, mere association is not evidence of causation, and the etiologic role of some of these species remains to be proven.

The most current information on periodontal infections tells us that the causative bacteria are mostly gram-negative anaerobes such as *Treponema denticola, Porphyromonas gingivalis, Bacteroides forsythus,* and *Actinobacillus actinomycetemcomitans*. They are all treatable with antibiotics that are effective against gram-negative pathogens.

Treponema denticola

The first of the four most common organisms in subingival plaque to be discussed is *Treponema denticola*. This spirochete is classified under the genus but precise identification of species is difficult. This flora is so named because of its surface-to-volume ratio, which facilitates nutrient uptake. Spirochetes are recognized by a helical shape

and vigorous motility when observed using a dark-field or phase-contrast microscope. *Trepenoma* are extremely difficult to grow, and they produce an array of proteolytic enzymes that invade the tissue. They comprise almost one-half of the flora in subgingival plaque. *Treponema vincentii* and other spirochetes are one of the primary causes of acute necrotizing ulcerative gingivitis (ANUG), along with *Fusobacterium* spp. *Prevotella intermedia* and other gram-negative rods that are also present.[6]

Bacteriodes (Prevotella, Porophyromonas)

Other bacteria cultured from subgingival plaque were thought to be of the bacteria melanogenisis family, a genus commonly found in the gut. However, recent more sophisticated DNA studies have shown that these black-pigmented bacteria are in reality nine or more species and are distinctly different from intestinal Bacteroides. Two new genera have therefore been proposed. The new genera are divided into two types: Asaccharolytic (non-carbohydrate-fermenting) organisms were assigned to the genus *Porphyromonas,* and those species capable of fermenting both carbohydrates and peptides were assigned to the genus *Prevotella.*

Porphyromonas gingivalis

Porphyromonas gingivalis is a virulent organism found in periodontitis. It is extremely aggressive and produces collagenase and other proteolytic enzymes. It is found in patients who do not respond to debridement therapy. It survives and thrives on a variety of molecules found in inflammation. The added dimension of collagenase production by macrophages stimulated by bacterial endotoxin coupled with bone resorption stimulated by-products of activated mononuclear cells indirectly enhances the process of tissue destruction.

Tannerella forsythensis

The other bacteroides that has been isolated is *Tannerella forsythensis* (formally *B. forsythes*).[4] It is an anaerobic, gram-negative, pleomorphic, nonmotile, long thin rod. Since it is extremely difficult to grow in the lab, detailed study of this organism, and more specifically its virulent mechanisms, has been disouraged. It may not even be a true member of the bacteroides family. Yet it is present in all periodontal infections and, in fact, is the most prevalent bacteria in this type of infection.[7]

Actinobacillus actinomycetemcomitans

A. actinomycetemcomitans is a small, gram-negative, microaerophilic coccobacillus. There is substantial evidence that it is the bacterial agent responsible for localized juvenile periodontitis (LJP). This coccobacillus is found in young people that have been exposed to other members of the family that have a history of LJP.[8] *A. actinomycetemcomitans* produces a leukotoxin that inhibits neutrophils in vitro, so in theory, it could locally disarm neutrophils in the pocket. The host's main protective barrier would thereby be removed, allowing the organism to penetrate into the connective tissue. This would result in destruction of the periodontal attachment.

Other organisms found in periodontal infections include *Fusobacterium nucleatum*, *Prevotella intermedia, Eubacterium,* and *Treponema*. Again there are several hundred bacterial species found in plaque and pockets,[9] but just a few are responsible for inflammatory periodontal disease. See Table 9.5.

Treatment of Periodontal infections

Most early periodontal infections can easily be treated with simple prophylaxis or debridement. This allows the majority of the invasive flora to be mechanically removed so the host can stabilize its own flora without the aid of chemical intervention. However, in severe or chronic periodontitis or abscesses, antibiotic therapy should be initiated. Scaling to interrupt biofilm and facilitate the efficacy of the antibiotic should be accomplished.

We must consider all that is happening in a periodontitis infection. There are direct and indirect mechanisms that exist as a result of the bacteria and their by-products. Direct mechanisms are those in which bacterial substances directly injure and destroy tissue. These are substances like collagenase (a histologic enzyme) and lukotoxin produced by the bacteria *A. actinomycetemcomitans*. Indirect influence gives the added dimension of collagenase production by macrophages stimulated by bacterial endotoxins. Products of activated mononuclear cells like interleukin and prostaglandin E-2 are examples that indirectly stimulate bone resorption.

Table 9-5. Pathogens Common in Periodontal Disease Listed by Prevalence in Periodontitis

Very Prevalent	Prevalent	Moderately Prevalent
A. actinomycetemcomitans	P. intermedia	Streptococcus intermedius
P. gingivalis	C. rectus	Peptostreptococcus micros
T. forsythenis*	E. notatum	F. neucleatum
Spirochetes of ANUG	Treponema sp.	E. corrodens
	Eubacterium	

Source: Modified from G. Greenstein. Changing Periodontal Concepts Compend. Dent. Ed. 26(2):81–89, 2005. The list is not all inclusive. Previously *Bacteroides forsythus*.

*Previously Bacteroides forsythus: Treatment Considerations.

INFECTIONS AND ANTIBIOTIC ADMINISTRATION

Recent studies reveal a complex interplay between the bacteria and host responses that cause a destructive process in the bone.[7]

Which Antibiotics to Use in Periodontitis?

The drugs that have the most effect on the gram-negative anaerobes are metronidazol and tetracycline (in the forms of Flagyl Doxycycline). Penicillin may be used in combination with other bactericidal drugs like metronidazol for any of the aerobic strains because of its effect on at least half of the bacteriodes. Affecting aerobic bacteria also stops their exudates by eliminating their source. In theory, some of the anaerobic bacteria flourish on the exudates of streptococcus viridans group. However, in recent studies, the penicillins have shown little effect on the pathogens of periodontitis.[10]

The advancement of the infection can happen over time or rapidly, and it is almost always treated with antibiotic therapy. The use of antibiotics will not manage the infection alone. Treatment must include incision, drainage, and debridement to prevent recurrence. In many cases the architecture of the tissues and bone must be remodeled to a more physiologic state to prevent recurrence. When choosing chemical means to facilitate the cure, a thorough debridement is also recommended.

Culturing and sensitivity testing are not feasible for treatment of a periodontal abscess because obtaining a sample that is not going to violate the oxygen-sensitive anaerobes is difficult and not within the ability of normal dental office. The use of empirical knowledge is used for immediate treatment. Penicillin, even though it is commonly used, is not a recommended regimen by itself because of the many gram-negative organisms that are not affected by it. Therefore, the use of a more specific antibiotic like Doxycycline, which has shown its ability to destroy many gram-negative anaerobes and collect in gingival crevicular fluid, is advocated. One tablet of Doxycycline 100 mg can be given daily for 7–10 days. The infection is then reevaluated, and the antibiotic continued if necessary. Tetracycline can also be used, but the compliance is compromised since the patient needs to take this drug one hour before and two hours after eating. It is given as 250 mg qid. Metronidazol is a very good treatment of choice in severe periodontal abscesses because of its effect on gram-negative anaerobes. It is given as 250 mg qid for 7–10 days. Clindamycin can be given, but there is the potential of a negative influence on the flora of the gut due to its spectrum. It is usually given 300 mg tid for eight days.

Do not mix penicillin (bactericidal) and any tetracycline (bacteriostatic) for treatment, as they render each other less effective. Giving both a bactericidal and a bacteriostatic drug together is contraindicated.

The effect of antibiotic therapy in periodontal infections is determined by several factors including the total bacterial load in relation to the maximum achievable antibiotic concentration. You must take into consideration the health of the patient and whether there are compromising systemic diseases, like diabetes. Smoking further complicates the process and affects the host defenses. Pregnancy also limits the use of antibiotics as shown in Table 9.5. Use antibiotics only in the more serious infections and coordinate with the attending physician. The FDA classifies only penicillin, clindamycin, and metronidazol as pregnancy category B.[11] This indicates they are probably safe after the first trimester, but if the disease can be handled without chemical intervention, this would be preferred.

ORAL RINSES

Mouth rinses are used in many infectious diseases. Chlorhexidine, which was first introduced in Europe around 1970 and the United States in 1986, is quite effective against supragingival plaque. It is used after a variety of surgical procedures and except for staining of the teeth doesn't seem to have any serious side effects when used long term. Some patients with physical disabilities can use chlorhexidine effectively. It is used in many postsurgical situations to lower the level of bacteria. There have been reports of taste disturbance while it is being used.[12]

It should be noted that the delivery of oral rinses and systemic antibiotic therapy alone is not without problems. First, it is difficult to achieve effective drug levels in the fluids of the pocket. Only a very small amount of an antibiotic enters the gingival tissue, and eventually the pocket. Irrigating pockets after surgery or after scaling with chlorhexidine or other rinses does not place enough medication into the pocket to be effective. Irrigation after scaling and root planning does have positive effects, probably by flushing out colonies of subgingival bacteria. Second, it exposes nontarget tissue to the drug.

LOCAL DELIVERY

Controlled delivery of chemotherapeutic agents (such as Arestin and Atridox) within periodontal pockets can alter the pathogenic flora and improve clinical signs of periodontitis. The benefit of local antibiotic delivery is that the drug can be delivered to the site of disease activity in high bactericidal concentrations. This, because of the medium in which the drug is carried, facilitates prolonged drug delivery.

However, using local delivery systems alone presents problems. It has been shown that the antibiotic is usually incapable of disrupting a biofilm. The biofilm has an exopolysaccharide matrix that is resistant to antibiotic penetration in the absence of mechanical disruption. Also, there has been little documentation to show that there is renewed attachment without disrupting the

biofilm and removal of calculus that may be present. The overall consensus is to always mechanically debride the area with scaling and root planning. This removes debris and breaks up the biofilm that harbors the pathogens.[13, 14]

Oral pathogens are associated with endogenous flora (normal flora). Normal oral flora has now been discovered to have many clonal types. Therefore, it is necessary to directly supervise their activity instead of trying to destroy them. To date, 32 clonal types of *P. gingivalis* and 10 clonal types of *A. actinomyctemcomitans* have been identified. Current literature does not reveal if *P. ginivalis* and *A. acitinomycetemcomitans* are endogenous or exogenous. Some of the clones may be either exogenous or endogenous, and it is also difficult to assess whether the clonal types are virulent or not. Merely culturing the bacterial type does not specifically identify it as a clone but generally only as a species. This difference may explain why in some patients a certain bacterial strain is pathogenic and not in other patients. In order to treat an endogenous pathogen, you cannot eradicate it from its normal environment. In other words, you manipulate their existence into a normal balanced community in the mouth.[15, 16]

Current Sequencing of Antibiotic Therapy

Antibiotics should only be an adjunct to scaling and root planning. Debridement must generally accompany antibiotic therapy, but antibiotics are rarely used alone to treat periodontal disease. The following represents a practical approach to periodontal antibiotic therapy.

1. First perform a thorough mechanical root debridement.
2. Prescribe antibiotics based on the need for further treatment, results of cultures, and the medical condition of the patient.

3. In two or three months, evaluate the patient's response. If there is no improvement and no resolution of inflammation, do a microbiological exam of the subgingival flora. This will help determine the amount and presence of putative pathogens.
4. One to three months after antibiotic therapy, do a clinical exam. Based upon the findings, another microbiological test might be needed. This will screen for super-infecting organisms and verify the elimination of target organisms. The finding of high levels of *Streptococcus viridans, Actimomyces*, and *Veillonella* species are suggestive of periodontal health or minimal disease.
5. Place the patient on an individually tailored maintenance program. Plaque control supragingivally will help deter the recolonization of putative periodontal pathogens. Any recurrence of progressive disease may necessitate repeated testing and antibiotic therapy targeted against specific microorganisms that are detected.[17]

In summary, keep in mind that the science of periodontal infections is continually changing. Periodontal disease greatly affects the systemic health of many patients. Resistance is causing us to curtail the indiscriminate use of antibiotics. A good clinician should refer to current literature often and stay abreast of this dynamically changing situation.

Periodontal disease is usually plaque-oriented—starting with gingivitis. If left unattended, it starts a series of qualitative shifts in the subgingival flora. Adult periodontitis is composed of 90 percent anaerobes, with the gram-negative anaerobes making up 70 to 75 percent, and motile forms (spirochetes) making up about 25 to 30 percent. About plus or minus 5 percent are attributed to aerobic bacteria, but these are probably not responsible for the destructive aspect of the disease.[11]

In summary, because of the complex nature of periodontitis and the fact that there are new forms or clonal types of bacteria identified constantly, it is not an exact science. We can, however, follow the regimen of teaching proper oral hygiene and nutrition along with performing scaling, root planning, and surgical procedures when warranted. The use of the correct antibiotic can be used in those cases that need the help. In all situations, when antibiotics are used they are only effective when many of the pathogens are mechanically removed or disturbed by the dental health professional. Using antibiotics and leaving impenetrable biofilms and colonies of bacteria behind is almost always ineffective and is furthering bacterial resistance. Studies have shown that regular scaling and root planning can be as effective as incorporating various surgical techniques. Severe pocket depth does have to be corrected to benefit from a patient's effective hygiene practices. The control of supragingival plaque is vital to the prevention of subgingival pathogenic flora in previously treated pockets. [18, 19]

Tissue-Invading Pathogens

Patients that are not responding to scaling and root planning may be infected with bacteria that actually invade the cells of the infected tissue.[20] This harboring of the bacteria makes **local** delivery of the antibiotic ineffective. *A. actinomycetemcomitans* and *P. gingivalis* have been detected in the cell walls of gingival tissues and are responsive to a systemic therapy of amoxicillin/clavulanate and metronitazol.

Antibiotics useful in the treatment of mostly gram-negative periodontal pathogens are metronidazol, tetracycline, clindamycin, and to some extent penicillin and amoxicillin/clavulanic acid. Metronidazol and tetracycline (Doxycycline) are the drugs of choice in the majority of periodontal infections.

Antibiotics

Following is a brief discussion of the most commonly used systemic antibiotics in dentistry. It is necessary for further understanding of their action and appropriate application.

THE PENICILLINS

When penicillin became widely available during the Second World War, it was a medical miracle, rapidly vanquishing the biggest wartime killer—infected wounds. Discovered initially by a French medical student, Ernest Duchesne, in 1896, and then rediscovered by Scottish physician Alexander Fleming in 1928, the product of the soil mold Penicillium crippled many types of disease-causing bacteria. But just four years after drug companies began mass-producing penicillin in 1943, microbes began appearing that could resist it.

The penicillins constitute one of the most important groups of antibiotics. Although numerous other antimicrobial agents have been produced since the first penicillin became available, penicillin is still widely used, and new derivatives of the basic penicillin nucleus still are being produced. Many of these have unique advantages, such that members of this group of antibiotics are presently the drugs of choice for a large number of infectious diseases.

Penicillin V and amoxicillin are the most commonly used penicillins in dentistry. They have a spectrum that is effective with many oral infections and in prophylactic administration. Their spectrum is similar, but amoxicillin is absorbed faster, and blood levels are higher at shorter intervals, making it more popular than penicillin V. This, however, is not without its problems. Amoxicillin has a greater effect on the flora of the gut. This causes more gastrointestinal upset. Penicillin V is often a better choice for long-term antibiotic administration when immediate

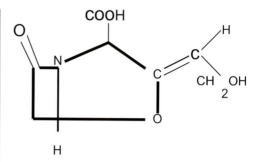

Figure 9-8. Clavulanic acid.

blood levels are not necessary. Penicillin V will reach an adequate blood saturation level quickly enough, especially with a significant loading dose. When you combine amoxicillin with clavulanic acid, the resulting drug is Augmentin. This combination binds the bacteria's beta lactamase (penicillinase) so the β-lactamase will not break down (lyse) the penicillin. Clavulanic acid is produced by the fermentation of *Streptomyces clavuligerus*. It is a β-lactam structurally related to the penicillins and possesses the ability to inactivate a wide variety of β-lactamases by blocking the active sites of these enzymes.

Odontogenic Infections

In noncompromised patients, penicillin still remains the empirical antibiotic of choice for mouth infections. If the infection is not localized but is manifest by cellulitis, penicillin will attack the *Streptococcus viridans* group bacteria that are a significant part of the infection. It is still the drug of choice in mild to moderate odontogenic infections because of its efficacy across the board. For more severe or recalcitrant infections, a culture and antibiotic sensitivity study may become necessary; however, empirically we know that gram-negative anaerobes are present, and the addition of metronidazol can be added to penicillin to increase effectiveness.

ABSCESSED TEETH

An abscessed tooth accompanied by long-term pathology at the apex is one of the more common scenarios in dentistry. A study of 98 isolates by Lewis et al.[21] in Great Britain determined that 23 percent of the isolates were resistant to penicillin. In this study, 15/98 isolates (15 percent) were resistant to penicillin V and 9/98 (9 percent) were resistant to amoxicillin. When clindamycin was administered, 94/98 (96 percent) of the bacteria were eliminated. The effect of amoxicillin/clavulanic acid destroyed 98/98 (100 percent) of the cultured bacterial strains. Metronidazol, an antibiotic effective against gram-negative anaerobes, killed 44/98 (45 percent). In combination with penicillin V, metronidazol was effective against 91/98 (93 percent), and in combination with amoxicillin it was effective against 97/98 or 99 percent of the bacteria.

Because amoxicillin/clavulanic acid (Augmentin) is so expensive, many patients will not purchase it unless they are covered by insurance. The use of penicillin first, then with the addition of metronidazol after two or three days (if there is no effect from the penicillin), is a good medication combination for infection in the mouth. The use of penicillin V is still a good antibiotic of choice over amoxicillin in the treatment of long-term polymicrobial mouth infections because of its low cost and narrow spectrum. It causes less GI upset long term.

Amoxicillin, clindamycin, and amoxicillin/clavulanic acid did show a slightly greater activity in this study than penicillin V but have a wider spectrum against species outside the oral cavity. This would make them more likely to cause complications by killing normal flora and upsetting the balance in the gut and elsewhere. Clarithromycin is a good alternative for erythromycin for mild infections when a patient is penicillin allergic. It cannot be used in combination with metronidazol because it is bacteriostatic and metronidazol is bactericidal.

The antibiotic table that follows (Table 9.6) is for adult or pediatric patients and is used primarily for periodontal infections. It may also be used for infections that invade periodontal tissues from an abscessed tooth. When the table is used for periodontal infections, the clinician should be familiar with the bacteria responsible for this disease as discussed earlier in the chapter.

Deep Fascial Plane Infections

Deep fascial plane infections can be one of most serious infections to the human body. They must be treated aggressively and without delay. The recognition of this type of serious infection is imperative, and the patient must be referred to an oral and maxillofacial

Table 9-6. Antibiotics Used in the Treatment of Periodontitis

Metronidazol	500 mg tid 8 days
Clindamycin	300 mg tid 8 days
Doxycycline	100–200 mg qd 21 days
Minocycline	100–200 mg qd 21 days
Azithromycin	500 mg qd 4–7 days
Metronidazole + amoxicillin	250 mg tid 8 days each drug
Metronidazole and ciprofloxacin	500 mg bid 8 days each drug

Source: Table modified from Systemic Antibiotics in Periodontics position paper. *J Periodont.*; 75; 1553–1565. 2004.[21] Information is suggestive only; comprehensive microbiological studies may be necessary.

surgeon or physician who may have to manage the patient with incision and drainage in a hospital setting. The drainage of the infection and administration of large amounts of IV antibiotics is the usual treatment. The welfare of the patient must be the main consideration. There are about 21,000 hospital admissions and 150 deaths annually from dentoalveolar infections.

Immediate attention with antibiotics and/or surgery is indicated in the following situations:

- Cellulitis of dental origin
- Pericoronitis with elevated temperature and trismus
- Infections that penetrate into deep fascial spaces
- Open fractures of the mandible or maxilla
- Deep wounds more that six hours old
- Dental infection in the medically compromised patient
- Prophylaxis for dental surgery in a patient with valvular heart disease or prosthetic valves

Antibiotic Prophylaxis

Antibiotic premedication is recommended for certain heart defects and some medically compromised joint replacement patients.

The current recommendations from the American Dental Association (ADA) and the American Academy of Orthopaedic Surgeons (AAOS) for joint replacement patients have been revised since 1997. The most recent statement concludes that antibiotic prophylaxis regimens are not recommended for patients with pins, plates, or screws, nor is it routinely indicated for most dental patients with total joint replacements. It is, however, advisable to consider premedication for a limited number of patients. These are patients that, for the most part, have experienced some complication with previous joint infection or have certain compromising medical comorbidities. These include but are not limited to those in Table 9.7.

The recommended dose of antibiotics for medically compromised patients with joint replacement is shown in Table 9.8.[22]

Table 9-7. Medical Conditions Requiring Antibiotic Prophylaxis for Joint Replacement Patients

1. Previous prosthetic joint infections
2. Immunocompromised/immunosuppresed patients
3. Malnourishment
4. Hemophilia
5. HIV infection
6. Insulin-dependant (type 1) diabetes
7. Malignancy

Table 9-8. Antibiotic Regimens for Joint Replacement Patients

Patient Type	Antibiotic	Prescribed Dose
Patients not allergic to penicillin	Cephalexin, cephradine, or amoxicillin	2 g orally 1 hour prior to dental procedure
Patients not allergic to penicillin but unable to take oral medications	Cefazolin or ampicillin Cefazolin 1g or ampicillin	2 g IM or IV 1 hour prior to the dental procedure
Patients allergic to penicillin	Clindamycin	600 mg orally 1 hour prior to the dental procedure
Patients allergic to penicillin and unable to take oral medications	Clindamycin	600 mg IM 1 hour prior to the dental procedure

The regimes in this table are one dose only, as no follow-up doses are recommended.

Table 9-9. Heart Problems Requiring Pre-Medication

1. Artificial (prosthetic) heart valve
2. History of previous endocarditis
3. Heart valves damaged (scarred) by conditions such as rheumatic fever
4. Congenital heart or heart valve defects
5. Hypertrophic cardiomyopathy
6. Prolapsed mitral valve with regurgitation

Antibiotic Regimens for Heart Patients

Patients with certain heart problems have need for a prophylaxis of penicillin, amoxicillin, or clindamycin.[23] This is the standard of care for all patients with the defects shown in Table 9.9.

What Is Bacterial Endocarditis?

Subacute Bacterial Endocarditis (SBE) is an infection of the heart's inner lining (endocardium) or the heart valves. It can damage or even destroy heart valves.

Endocarditis rarely occurs in patients with a normal heart. However, in patients with certain pre-existing heart conditions, care must be taken to prevent a bacterial colonization of the damaged heart. Table 9.10 is a list of possible risk factors that predispose a bacterial endocarditis complication.[24]

There is some controversy regarding the patient with a prolapsed mitral valve (MVP). Regurgitation or an audible heart sound is not always a true determining factor. Some experts feel that an audible nonejection click, even without a murmur, may identify patients with a potential for intermittent regurgitation, and therefore, there may be a risk of developing endocarditis. Although there are insufficient data on this issue, an isolated click may be an indication for more thorough evaluation of valve morphology and function, including Doppler-echocardiographic imaging or auscultation during maneuvers that elicit or augment mitral regurgitation. Men older than 45 years with MVP, without a consistent systolic murmur, might warrant prophylaxis even in the absence of resting regurgitation. Normal mitral valves with normal motion often have minimal leaks detectable by Doppler examination. This does not appear to increase the risk of endocarditis. In contrast, the regurgi-

Table 9-10. Prophylaxis Dosage for Bacterial Endocarditis Prevention

Situation	Antibiotic	Regime
Standard general prophylaxis	**Amoxicillin**	**Adults**: 2.0g; 1 hr before procedure **children**: 50mg/kg orally 1 h before procedure
Unable to take oral medications	**Ampicillin**	**Adults**: 2.0g IM or IV; **children**: 50mg/kg IM or IV within 30 min before procedure
Allergic to penicillin	**Clindamycin or**	**Adults**: 600mg; **children**: 20mg/kg orally 1 h before procedure
Allergic to penicillin	**Cephalexin or Cefadroxil**	**Adults**: 2.0g; **children**; 50mg/kg orally 1 h before procedure
	Azithromycin or Clarithromycin	**Adults**: 500mg; **children**: 15mg/kg orally 1 h before procedure
Allergic to penicillin and unable to take oral medications	**Clindamycin or Cefazolin**	**Adults**: 600mg; **children**: 20mg/kg IV within 30 min before
		Adults: 1.0g; **children:** 25mg/kg IM or IV within 30 min before procedure

tation that occurs with structurally normal but prolapsing valves originates from larger regurgitant orifices and creates broader areas of turbulent flow. Patients with prolapsing and leaking mitral valves, evidenced by audible clicks and murmurs of mitral regurgitation or by Doppler-demonstrated mitral insufficiency, should receive prophylactic antibiotics. These guidelines are meant to aid practitioners but are not intended as the standard of care or as a substitute for clinical judgment.[23, 24] The most common responsible pathogen is *Streptococcus viridans* spp. (a-hemolytic streptococci). This is the most prevalent bacteria in the oral cavity. Antibiotic prophylaxis to prevent SBE is recommended as shown in Table 9.11.

Table 9-11. Antibiotics for Oral and Fascial Infections

Antibiotic	With Food	Adult dosage	Childs dosage	Gm + Aerobes	Gm + Anaerobes	Gram − Anaerobes
Penicillin	Yes	250/500mg qid	25 to 50 mg/kg/day in 3 divided doses	Yes	Yes	Yes/No
Amoxicillin	Yes	250/500mg tid	25 to 50 mg/kg/day in 3 divided doses	Yes	Yes	Yes/No
Augmentin	Yes	875 mg bid or 500mg tid	90 mg/kg/day in 2 divided doses	Yes	Yes	Yes
Cefaclor	Yes	250 mg tid	20 to 40 mg/kg/day in 3 divided doses	Yes	No	Yes/No
Cefuroxime	Yes	250–500 mg bid	20 to 30 mg/kg/day in 2 divided doses	Yes	Yes	Yes
Erythromycin sterate	No	400 mg qid	20 to 40 mg/kg/day in 4 divided doses	Yes	No	No
Azithromycin	Yes	500 mg followed by 250-mg single daily doses on days 2 to 5	10 mg/kg followed by 5 mg/kg on days 2 to 5	Yes	Yes/No	No
Clindamycin	Yes	150 to 450 mg q 6 h in adults	10 to 30 mg/kg/day in 3 to 4 divided doses	Yes	Yes	Yes
Metronidazole	Yes	250 to 500 mg tid	35 to 50 mg/kg/day divided tid for children	No	Yes	Yes
Doxycycline	Yes	200 mg in 2 divided doses on the first day then 100 mg/day	Over 8 yr, 4 mg/kg/day divided in 2 doses given orally first day then 2 mg/kg/day	No	Yes	Yes
Minocycline	No	200 mg followed by 100 mg q 12 h in adults.	Over 8 yr, the oral or IV dosage is 4 mg/kg followed by 2 mg/kg q 12 h	No	Yes	Yes
Vancomycin	Yes	125 mg q 6 h in adults	40 mg/kg/day in 4 equally divided doses	Yes	Yes	Yes
Clarithromycin	Yes	250–500 mg q 8 to 12 hr	7.5 mg/kg every 12 h	Yes	Yes/No	Yes/No
Cefalexin	**Yes**	250–500 mg qid		**Yes**	**No**	**No**

Occasionally, a patient may already be taking an antibiotic before coming to the physician or dentist. If the patient is taking an antibiotic normally used for endocarditis prophylaxis, it is prudent to select a drug from a different class rather than to increase the dose of the current antibiotic. In particular, antibiotic regimens used to prevent the recurrence of acute rheumatic fever are inadequate for the prevention of bacterial endocarditis. Individuals who take oral penicillin for secondary prevention of rheumatic fever or for other purposes may have viridans streptococci in their oral cavities that are relatively resistant to penicillin, amoxicillin, or ampicillin. In such cases, the dentist should select clindamycin, azithromycin, or clarithromycin for endocarditis prophylaxis. Because of possible cross-resistance with the cephalosporins, this class of antibiotics should be avoided. If possible, one could delay the procedure until at least 9 to 14 days after completion of the antibiotic. This will allow the usual oral flora to be reestablished.[25] This has to be approved by the prescribing doctor, if other than the treating dentist, and it is assumed that the infection being treated is under control.

Choosing the Right Antibiotic

PENICILLIN

Penicillin V or amoxicillin remain the antibiotics of choice in the treatment of dentoalveolar infections in a noncompromised patient. Even though many gram-negative organisms have developed resistance, the antibiotics are still effective against the majority of them. Penicillin is the first of the β-lactams, and with the combination of metronidazol, it is effective against almost 100 percent of the pathogens in oral infections. Amoxicillin combined with clavulanate is almost 100 percent effective, but the cost of amoxicillin/clavulanate is a factor.

Penicillin has been one of the most over-used drugs since it was developed but continues to be effective and to be the standard for treating millions of people each year. It is also safe to give large doses because the therapeutic index is high.

CEPHALOSPORINS

Cephalosporins are also β-lactams. They attack the cell wall much like penicillin. They have a less-effective spectrum than penicillin, and there is a risk of allergic reaction if used on a penicillin-allergic patient. The second- (Cefuroxime) and third-generation (Cefpodoxime) cephalosporins are broader spectrum than first-generation Cephalexin. It can also be used with clindamycin or metronitazol in the compromised host. It is not the first drug of choice because as many (60 percent) of the gram-negative anaerobes are resistant—especially to the first-generation drugs.

ERYTHROMYCIN

Erythromycin is not as effective as penicillin, because it is poorly absorbed and does not have much effect against anaerobic bacteria. **Azithromicin** is a newer macrolide and is effective against more gram-negative anaerobes but still lacks the spectrum necessary for it to be useful in all but milder cases. Erythromycin is effective against the streptococcus viridans group of bacteria and can be substituted for clindamycin with SBE prophylaxis in penicillin allergic patients. Azithromycin generally is less active than erythromycin against gram-positive organisms (*Streptococcus* spp. and enterococci) and is slightly more active than either erythromycin or clarithromycin against *H. influenzae*. Azithromycin is very active against *Chlamydia* spp., *M. pneumoniae*, *L. pneumophila*, *Fusobacterium* spp., and *N. gonorrhoeae*. The mechanism of action is to bind to the 50S ribosomal subunits disrupting protein synthesis and replication.

TETRACYCLINE

Tetracycline antibiotics were discovered by systematic screening of soil specimens collected from many parts of the world for antibiotic-producing microorganisms. The first of these compounds, chlortetracycline, was introduced in 1948. Tetracyclines are effective against a few gram-positive bacteria, but in the oral environment they work well against the common oral anaerobes. The lipophillic drugs doxycycline and minocycline usually are the most active by weight and are taken with more compliance because of their once/day regimen. They are absorbed much more slowly with half-lives of up to 16 hours and stay in the tissues long after their administration has stopped. Tetracycline has to be taken one hour before meals and two hours after, but doxycycline and minocycline are not affected by food. The tetracyclines are active against many anaerobic and facultative micro-organisms, and their activity against a-*actinomyces, bacteriodes,* and spirochetes is particularly useful in periodontal disease.

Differences in clinical efficacy are minor and attributable largely to features of absorption, distribution, and excretion of individual drugs. Tetracyclines enter microorganisms in part by passive diffusion and in part by an energy-dependent process of active transport. This provides an intracellular concentration of the drug. Once inside the cell, tetracyclines bind reversibly to the 30 S subunit of the bacterial ribosome, blocking the binding of aminoacyl-tRNA to the acceptor site on the mRNA-ribosome complex.

CLINDAMYCIN

Clindamycin is active against most anaerobes, including *bacteroides, prevotella, clostridium, peptococcus, peptostreptococcus,* and *fusobacterium* organisms. However, 10–20 percent of *bacteroides* isolates are re-

sistant. It is frequently used to treat moderately severe infection in which anaerobes are significant pathogens, often in combination with other drugs (aminoglycosides, cephalosporins, and fluoroquinolones). Common side effects are diarrhea, nausea, and skin rashes. Bloody diarrhea with pseudo-membranous colitis has been associated with the administration of clindamycin and other antibiotics.

METRONIDAZOLE

Metronidazole is an antiprotozoal drug that also has striking antibacterial effects against most anaerobic gram-negative bacilli (*bacteroides, prevotella,* and *fusobacterium* and *clostridium* species). It has some activity against other anaerobic gram-positive and microaerophilic organisms. It is well absorbed after oral administration and is widely distributed in tissues. It penetrates well into the cerebrospinal fluid, yielding levels similar to those in serum. The drug is metabolized in the liver, and dosage reduction is required in severe hepatic insufficiency or biliary dysfunction. Metronidazole is less expensive and equally as efficacious as oral vancomycin for the therapy of *C. difficile* colitis and is the drug of choice for the disease. A dosage of 500 mg orally three times daily is recommended. If oral medication cannot be tolerated, intravenous metronidazole can be tried at the same dose; however, this route is unproved and usually less effective than the oral one. Because of the emergence of vancomycin-resistant enterococci as a major pathogen and the role of oral vancomycin in selecting for these resistant organisms, metronidazole is now used as first-line therapy for *C. difficile* disease (colitis).[26]

ANTIBIOTIC-INDUCED COLITIS

Antibiotic-associated colitis (AAC) is a significant clinical problem almost always caused by *C. difficile*. Hospitalized patients are most susceptible, especially those who are severely ill or malnourished or who are receiving chemotherapy. This anaerobic bacterium colonizes the colon of 5 percent of healthy adults. In hospitalized patients, however, it is present in more than 20 percent of patients, most of whom have received antibiotics that disrupt the normal bowel flora and, thus, allow the bacterium to flourish. Most of these patients are asymptomatic. Recently, patients receiving enteral tube feedings have been found to have a higher risk for acquisition of *C. difficile* and the development of *C. difficile*–associated diarrhea. The organism is spread in a fecal-oral fashion. It is found throughout hospitals in patient rooms and bathrooms and can be transmitted from patient to patient by hospital personnel. Fastidious hand washing and use of disposable gloves are essential in minimizing transmission. Clindamycin is the antibiotic that has been tagged as the responsible agent because of the normal flora susceptibility to it. However, many other antibiotics can cause the onset if the *Clostridia difficile* is present. The clostridia bacterium gives off toxins that damage the walls of the intestine in severe cases.

Conclusion

When a clinician is treating infection, each of the previously considered factors must be evaluated. Then a decision about of the appropriate antibiotic can be made. In any case, where drainage or debridement can be performed, it should be done. The infection, whenever possible, must be removed in order to render the antibiotic more effective. This would include debridement, plaque and biofilm removal, and the incising and drainage of abscesses. Protection of the antibiotics we have is essential, and as health care providers, we must do our part to preserve their effectiveness.

Bibliography

1. R. Lewis. The Rise of Antibiotic Resistant Infections. US Food and Drug Admin. *Consumer Magazine.* September, 1995.
2. K. U. Todar. Wisconsin Dept of Bacteriology. Bacterial Resistance to Antibiotics lecture. 2002.
3. G. Greenstein. Changing periodontal concepts. *Compendium* Feb. p. 81. 2005.
4. Peterson, Ellis, Hupp, Tucker. *Contemporary Oral and Maxillofacial Surgery*, 4th edition. p. 345. 2002.
5. Topazian Goldberg Hupp Oral and Maxillofacial Infections 4th edition.
6. A. S. Dajani, K. A. Taubert, W. Wilson, et al. Prevention of bacterial endocarditis. Recommendations by The American Heart Association.
7. J. Slots, C. Chen. The oral microflora and human periodontal disease. In G. W. Tannock, ed. *Medical Importance of the Normal Microflora.* London: Kluwer Academic Publishers, p. 101–127. 1999.
8. A. Asujaubeb, C. Cgeb. Oral ecology and person-to-person transmission of *A actinomycetemcomitans* and *Porphyromonas gingivalis. Periodontol.* 2000.
9. Peterson, Ellis, Hupp, Tucker. Contemporary Oral and Maxillofacial Surgery. 4th edition. p. 346**.** 2002.
10. Systemic Antibiotics in Periodontics position paper; Academy of Periodontology. November, 2004.
11. M. H. Goldberg. The changing nature of acute dental infection. *J Am Dent Assoc.* 80: 1048. 1970.
12. M. K. Jeffcoat, K. S. Bray, S. G. Ciancio, et al. Adjunctive use of a subgingival controlled-release chlorhexidine chip reduces probing depth and improves attachmentlevel compared with scaling and root planing alone. *J. Periodontol.* 69: 989–997. 1998.
13. J. M. Goodson, M. A. Cugini, R. L. Kent, et al. Multicenter evaluation of tetracycline fiber therapy: II. Clinical response. *J Periodont Res.* 26: 371–379. 1991.
14. G. Greenstein. Changing periodontal concepts. *Compendium.* Feb. p. 82–84. 2005.
15. J. Slots, M. Ting. *Actinobacilus actinomycetemcomitans* and *Porphyromonas gingivalis* in human periodontal disease: occurrentce and treatment. *Periodonto* 2000. 20: 82–121. 1999.

16. G. Greenstein, I. Lanster. Bacterial transmission in periodontal diseases: a critical review. *J Periodontol.* 68: 421–431. 1997.

17. Systemic Antibiotics in Periodontics position paper. Academy of Periodontology. November, 2004.

18. J. W. Knowles, F. G. Burgett, R. R. Nissle, et al. Results of periodontal treatment related to pocket depth and attachment level: eight years. *J Periodontol.* 50: 225. 1979.

19. K. S. Kornman. The role of supragingival plaque in the prevention and treatment of of periodontal disease: a review of concepts. *J Periodontol Res.* 15: 111. 1980.

20. G. Greenstein. Changing periodontal concepts. *Compendium* Feb. p. 82. 2005.

21. J. Baumgartner, T. Xia. Antibiotic susceptibility of bacteria associated with endodontic abcesses. *J. of Endodontics.* Vol 29, No 1, p. 44–47. Jan., 2003.

22. Antibiotic Prophylaxis for Dental Patients with Total Joint Replacements Advisory statement. *JADA.* July p. 895–897. 2003.

23. American Heart Association Circulation Prevention of Endocarditis. 96: 338. 1997.

24. B. A. Carabello. Mitral valve disease. *Curr Probl Cardiol.* 7: 423–478. 1993.

25. A. S. Bayer, R. J. Nelson, T. G. Slama. Current concepts in prevention of prosthetic valve endocarditis. *Chest.* 97: 1203–1207. 1990.

26. L. M. Tierney, Jr., S. J. McPhee, M. A. Papadakis, eds. R. Gonzales, R. Zeiger. Current Medical Diagnosis & Treatment. 2005.

ADDITIONAL REFERENCES

J. Slots, D. Moenbo, J. Langback, et al. Microbiota of gingivitis I man. *Scand J Dent Res.* 86: 174. 1978.

R. B. Devereux, C. J. Frary, R. Kramer-Fox, R. B. Roberts, H. S. Ruchlin. Cost-effectiveness of infective endocarditis prophylaxis for mitral valve prolapse with or without a mitral regurgitant murmur. *Am J Cardiol.* 74: 1024–1029. 1994.

Chapter 10

Management of Perioperative Bleeding

Dr. Karl R. Koerner and Dr. William L. McBee

Introduction

Most general dentists extract teeth. However, they are usually discriminatory in their case selection—choosing teeth that present within their ability and comfort zone. Even with this precaution, unexpected situations can arise. Bleeding is one of the complications that frequently occurs, leading to intraoperative and even postoperative problems. There are several factors that can cause or exacerbate a troublesome bleeding episode from an oral surgery procedure.[1] Tissues of the mouth are highly vascular; many wounds are left open (as with most extractions); pressure dressings don't work very well; talking and eating can irritate surgery sites; negative pressures in the mouth from the tongue and eating can dislodge clots; and salivary enzymes may lyse clots before they have a chance to organize.

This chapter identifies and discusses those things that the general dentist should consider in terms of both prevention and management options. With an understanding of the material that follows, oral surgery can be approached with greater confidence and

skill. It will also help expedite surgery procedures and make them more routine and predictable. Unfortunately, dental school does not always provide the graduate with an adequate understanding of how to control excessive bleeding during or after surgery. The pages that follow will serve to fill in the gaps and help generalists increase competency in this extremely important area.

Primary Reasons for Coagulation Failure

What are reasons that blood fails to clot normally? Some of the most serious ones are listed here.[2]

THROMBOCYTOPENIA

The concentration of platelets in the blood is too low.

Usually blood contains about 150,000 to 350,000 platelets per mm^3. However, when this count decreases below 50,000, there can be abnormal bleeding, with spontaneous bleeding occuring if the platelet count falls below 10,000. Signs may include gingival bleeding, frequent epistaxis (bloody nose), ecchymosis, blood in the stool or urine, or menstrual periods that are unusually heavy. Oral surgery or trauma may also lead to bleeding that is difficult to control.

There are five main reasons why platelet deficiency occurs:

1. Bone marrow doesn't produce enough platelets (heavy alcohol consumption, bone marrow disorders, vitamin deficiencies, aplastic anemia, certain drugs or infections, and so on).
2. Platelets become entrapped in an enlarged speen (for example, portal hypertension with congestive splenomegaly).
3. Platelets become diluted (major blood or fluid replacement, heart bypass surgery, and so on).
4. The use or destruction of platelets increases. (Viral infections such as Epstein-Barr [EB] or human immunodeficiency virus [HIV]; drugs such as heparin; oral diabetes drugs; sulfa-containing antibiotics, quinidine and rifampin; systemic lupus; some cancers; septicemia; and so on).
5. Increased use of platelets. Patients with disseminated intravascular coagulation (DIC) will have thrombocytopenia, as well as other disorders of coagulation.

VON WILLEBRAND'S DISEASE (VWD)

Platelets don't clump together to adequately plug a tear in a vessel wall.

This is a hereditary deficiency of the von Willebrand factor in the blood—a protein that affects platelets. It is the most common hereditary disorder of platelet function. This factor is found in plasma, platelets, and blood vessel walls. When missing or abnormal, the first step in plugging a blood vessel injury (platelets adhering to one another at the site of vessel wall injury) doesn't happen. Consequently, bleeding temporarily continues, and coagulation is delayed.

Generally, a person with this disease has a parent or other close relative with a history of bleeding problems. It is often manifest when a person bruises easily or has excessive bleeding after a minor skin laceration, tooth extraction, or other surgery. It may be confusing to the patient, since there are some situations that can stimulate the body to temporarily increase the production of the factor, such as stress, pregnancy, inflammation, infection, and hormonal changes.

The four types of VWD are types I, IIa, IIb, and III, progressively more rare and serious from I through III. The definitive diagnosis can be difficult, requiring multiple labs, a physical exam, and a thorough understanding of the patient's bleeding history.

Many people with this disease do not require preoperative treatment. Yet, if there is a question of excessive bleeding in the patient's history or in the family's medical history, a consultation from a hematologist should be obtained.

The patient may require preoperative Desmopressin (DDAVP) or replacement therapy with von Willebrand Factor (VWF) concentrate (Humate-P), or the dentist may be advised to use just local measures during surgery (reviewed later in this chapter).

HEMOPHILIA

This is characterized by decreased amounts of coagulation factors VIII or IX.

Classic hemophilia (A) makes up about 80 percent of cases and is a deficiency of factor VIII. Hemophilia B (Christmas disease) is a deficiency in clotting factor IX. Both are inherited through the mother but almost always affect male children. The severity of the symptoms depends on how the gene abnormality affects the activity of factors VIII and IX. A patient's clotting condition may involve any of the following (according to the amount of the clotting factor present):

- 1% of normal: severe bleeding and/or recurrence of spontaneous bleeding.
- 1–5% of normal: moderate hemophilia—surgery or injury can cause significant or uncontrolled bleeding from even minor trauma.
- 5–25% of normal: mild hemophilia—still dangerous.
- Greater than 25% of normal: May not be diagnosed. Still potentially dangerous.

DISSEMINATED INTRAVASCULAR COAGULATION (DIC)

Clotting factors are depleted from excessive clotting.

With this condition, small clots form throughout the blood stream. They block smaller blood vessels and use up the clotting factors required to control bleeding. This condition usually arises from a toxic substance in the blood, such as uterine tissue from complicated obstetric surgery or endotoxins from a severe bacterial infection. In addition, it can be from certain leukemias or cancer of the stomach, pancreas, or prostate. Generally, the problem is resolved when the cause is properly addressed.

Systemic Disease Conditions That Can Cause Bleeding During Surgery

Most systemic diseases will produce some alteration in the blood. Blood dyscrasia may accompany the disease, or it may be the presenting feature of a general systemic disease. Examples include the following.[3]

DISSEMINATED MALIGNANCY

This finding is commonly accompanied by the presence of tumor cells in the bone marrow. Some bleeding disorders related to cancer appear to be caused by the selective impairment of coagulation from pathological inhibitors of different parts of the coagulation system or from isolated factor deficiencies.

ANEMIA

There are three forms of anemia that can contribute to bleeding problems:

1. Anemia as a complication of chronic renal failure. The management of bleeding in these patients is through dialysis and appropriate replacement therapy. Management has been revolutionized by the availability of recombinant erythropoietin.
2. Less common forms of anemia associated with cancer. Autoimmune hemolytic anemia is sometimes a feature in patients with lymphoma and ovarian tumors. Autoimmune hemolysis can also occur in patients with tumors of the lung, stomach, breast, kidney, colon, and testis.
3. Anemia from pituitary deficiency, thyroid disease, adrenal disease, or parathyroid disease.

ACUTE AND CHRONIC BACTERIAL INFECTIONS

Most bacterial infections can be associated with a hypervascular tissue called granulomatous tissue. The vessels themselves are not only dilated, but there is usually a greater number of vessels that have proliferated within the area of the infection. Functionally, this allows for a greater response by the body's own defense mechanisms, while trying to fend off the unwanted organisms.

Toxins produced and released by microorganisms within the area of infection can damage tissues (including the endothelium associated with vascular walls) and also cause impairment of liver function and hemostasis. Therefore, in the presence of damaged hypervascular tissue and an impaired hemostatic response, undesired surgical or spontaneous bleeding may occur.

Viral Infections

This includes rubella, cytomegalovirus (CMV), and AIDS.

HIV-Associated Coagulapathies

Besides the immunological changes related to HIV infections, there are also several hematological problems. Lymphopenia (an abnormally small number of lymphocytes in the circulating blood) is common, as is neutropenia (an abnormal decrease in the number of neutrophils in the blood). Neutropenia reportedly varies between 0 and 30 percent in HIV antibody-positive asymptomatic patients and in 20–65 percent of patients with AIDS. Thrombocytopenia is present in 5–20 percent of asymptomatic HIV-infected persons but rises to 25–50 percent in patients with AIDS. In addition to these complications there is also a risk of drug-induced marrow hypoplasia related to treatment with zidovudine (AZT).

Rheumatiod Arthritis

Anemia in these patients is common but usually follows the pattern of anemia from chronic disorders. It can be exacerbated by iron deficiency resulting from poor diet, chronic blood loss, or because of the effects of treatment with aspirin, other NSAIDS, or corticosteroids.

Systemic Lupus Erythematosus

In this autoimmune disease, rogue immune cells attack body tissues. Antibodies may be produced that can react against blood cells, organs, and other tissues. It affects nine times as many women than men. Blood disorders occur in up to 85 percent of those with the disease. Both arterial and venous blood clots can form and may be associated with pulmonary embolism, strokes, hemoptysis (coughing up blood), miscarriages and other disorders. Clots and/or bleeding occur because of antibodies against lipids that are involved in clotting. It is known as antiphospholipid antibody syndrome (APS). Commonly platelets are decreased thus causing bleeding or clotting problems. There can also be anemia in the course of Systemic Lupus Erythematosus (SLE).

Parasitic Disease

This includes malaria, leishmaniasis, hookworm, visceral larva migrans, schistosomiasis, and various other trematode infestations.

Inflammatory Diseases of the Bowel

These are often made worse by drugs used in managing the diseases.

Liver Disease

Liver disease causes a reduction of certain clotting factors required in the coagulation cascade. There is usually anemia in patients with chronic liver failure. Especially with alcoholics, anemia may be from a deficient diet, chronic blood loss, hepatic dysfunction, or the direct toxic effects of alcohol on the bone marrow.

Pneumonia

Particularly with pneumonia caused by *Legionella pneumophilia*, there can be severe thrombocytopenia and lymphopenia. Some cases have also been reported to be complicated by disseminated intravascular coagulation.

Primary Sources of Serious Bleeding around the Oral Cavity

There are four vascular sources that provide blood to the oral cavity that can cause serious and sometimes life-threatening bleeding if disrupted during oral surgery procedures.

MANAGEMENT OF PERIOPERATIVE BLEEDING

These are the lingual, facial, inferior alveolar, and the greater palatine arteries.

The **lingual artery** branches directly from the external carotid. Upper airway obstruction from bleeding has occurred from puncture wounds of the tongue, biopsies of the tongue or floor of the mouth, and implant perforation out the lingual cortex of the mandible.

The **facial artery** also branches directly from the external carotid. It is accompanied by the anterior facial vein, and they pass in the cheek lateral to the lower molars. A long incision for a vertical release into the mucobuccal fold, buccal to the mandibular posterior teeth, could cut one of these vessels causing profuse bleeding.

The **inferior alveolar artery** branches from the maxillary artery, which is the larger of the two terminal branches of the external carotid. As it descends, it splits off the mylohyoid artery before entering the mandibular foramen and mandibular canal. A mental branch emerges from the mental foramen to supply the chin and lower lip. The mylohyoid artery traverses along the medial surface of the mandible in the mylohyoid groove and supplies the muscle of the same name. Sometimes a small lingual branch can arise from the inferior alveolar artery and descend with the lingual nerve to supply the mucosa of the floor of the mouth.

The inferior alveolar artery is usually above the inferior alveolar nerve in the mandibular canal in the molar area. An inadvertent cut with the bur into the canal would likely injure the artery before injuring the nerve. The nerve would continue intact after such an injury but could still result in a neuropathy from a disruption of the nerve's blood supply.[4]

The **greater palatine artery** is found emerging from a foramen on the palate superior to the second molar where the horizontal and vertical aspects of the palate converge. Unlike the vessels emerging from the incisive canal, the greater palatine artery is significant in size and will result in difficult-to-control spurting if cut. This can occur when removing a palatal torus or obtaining donor tissue for a free gingival or connective tissue graft. It can also happen with periodontal surgery, especially if there is loss of the alveolus from periodontal disease and a significant portion of the vertical palatal bone is diseased—causing the artery to be closer than anticipated. Tears of the posterior palatal tissues involving the greater palatine artery are common when the gingival tissues have not been completely separated from the tooth during a maxillary posterior extraction.

A previous calculation[4] reported that these arteries are 1–2 mm in lumen diameter. If so, with 0.2 mL per beat at 70 beats per minute, it would be possible for 14 mL of blood to escape in 60 seconds. In 30 minutes, this could represent approximately 420 mL of blood loss. The authors, however, find this to be a significant underestimation. In our experience, the previously mentioned vessels can produce a significantly greater amount of bleeding in a shorter time period if not controlled immediately. This being said, they are also usually relatively easy to temporarily tamponade, preventing excessive blood loss until definitive treatment can occur.

Preventing Bleeding Problems

Preventing bleeding problems prior to surgery is preferable to having to treat them intra- or postoperatively. The sections that follow review considerations and procedures that help dentists avoid excessive hemorrhage during oral surgery.

PATIENT HISTORY

Every new patient fills out a dental/medical history, which is reviewed by the dentist in the presence of the patient. This history should be updated on an annual basis. This screening of prospective patients will usually reveal bleeding disorders serious enough to be of consequence (see Table 10.1). Depending on the severity, consultation with the patient's physician or a hematologist may be advised. Following is a list of questions that can be reviewed with the patient:

Is there a history of bleeding problems?

The dentist should ask whether at any time in the past with a previous surgery or even an accident where bleeding took place, has there been persistent bleeding? What about previous oral surgery, a tonsillectomy, or any other surgical procedure? The question should be asked: "Did bleeding last more that 24 hours, or did you require special attention from a dentist or physician?"

Do they have a history of nosebleeds? Do they bleed easily? Do they have heavy menstrual bleeding? Do they bleed spontanteously? If the patient answers positively to any of these questions, then they should probably be referred to an oral and maxillofacial surgeon for treatment or to a hematologist for coagulation screening.

Does the patient bruise easily?

If the answer to this question is in the affirmative and if the patient is not taking any over-the-counter prescription or homeopathic medications that might be responsible for it, then it might suggest the need for a bleeding time test. This problem could be indicative of a disease involving decreased platelet formation or possibly increased capillary fragility.

Is there a history of bleeding problems in the family?

Most people will know whether they have an inherited bleeding disorder. However, with some, prolonged bleeding after an oral surgery procedure may be their first indication that they have a bleeding problem. von Willebrand disease affects 1–2 percent of the U.S. population.[5] If this condition is suspected, the patient should

Table 10-1. Bleeding Assessment Prior to Surgery: Serious Concerns

Risk Factors

1. Bleeding with prior surgical procedures
    a. dental, other
2. Heavy menstrual bleeding
3. Liver disease
    a. Hepatitis B or C
    b. Cirrhosis
    c. Chronic alcohol abuse
4. Renal disease
5. Congenital diseases
    a. Hemophilia
    b. von Willebrand's disease
    c. Other inherited coagulopathies
6. History of abnormal blood count
    a. Leukemia
    b. Throbocyopenia
        (Either decreased production of platelets or increased destruction of platelets.)
    c. AIDS
7. Medications
    a. Aspirin
    b. Other NSAIDs
    c. Anticoagulants
    d. Antibiotics
    e. Chemotherapeutic agents

Source: Adapted from Figure 5-1 and 5-2, p. 55. Dym, H and Ogle, OE. *Atlas of Minor Oral Surgery.* Philadelphia: W.B. Saunders Co. 2001.

be referred to a hematologist or a hemophilia treatment center.

The patient may have signs indicating a platelet defect, such as easy bruising. It could be quantitative or qualitative, in either case suggesting the possible need for a platelet transfusion. Factor replacement may be required if they have von Willebrand's disease, hemophilia A or B, or another clotting factor deficiency.

Has the patient ever had a history of liver dysfunction?

How about a history of hepatitis, hepatic carcinoma or jaundice? Is there a history of excessive alcohol intake that might affect hepatic health? All of the blood clotting factors except Factor XIII are produced in the liver.

What are the patient's baseline vital signs, particularly blood pressure?

A high systolic blood pressure alone (over 180) can be a cause of excessive bleeding during surgery. In this event, they should be treated by their physician for hypertension prior to performing an oral surgery procedure.

What medications are being taken by the patient?

This question relates to both prescription and nonprescription drugs. Drug usage is the most common undocumented cause of bleeding in the oral surgery patient.[6] The patient may not know whether a given medication contributes to increased bleeding.

Medications That Influence Bleeding

We know that there are many medications that can interfere with coagulation. With some patients, these medications are therapeutically necessary and are part of a treatment regimen for a medical condition. Prior to surgery, it is prudent to consult the patient's physician regarding the situation (see Table 10.2). One way to remember these medications is to know that seven of them start with the letter A. These are listed here:

1. **Aspirin.** One 325-mg aspirin or low-dose (81-mg) aspirin can irreversibly inhibit platelet function for the life of the platelet. If the surgery is significant and the patient's physician is in agreement, then it should be discontinued 7–10 days prior to the procedure (life span of a platelet is nine days). If the health risks of discontinuing are too high and the surgical procedure is relatively minor, then usually intraoperative bleeding concerns may be managed with "local meas-

ures" (to be discussed further later in the chapter).

2. **Anti-inflammatories.** Other NSAIDs operate in the body by a similar mechanism as aspirin but are qualitatively less serious—only reversibly inhibiting platelet function. They should be stopped 2–3 days prior to oral surgery.

3. **Anticoagulants**, such as warfarin (Coumadin), heparin, or low molecular weight heparin (Ardeparin, Dalteparin, Enoxaparin).

    These medications are prescribed for the treatment of atrial fibrillation, dilated cardiomyopathy, systolic congestive heart failure, valvular heart disease, valve replacement, deep vein thrombosis and pulmonary emboli, post myocardial infarction or cerebral vascular accident, or a need for extracorporeal blood flow, such as hemodialysis.

    Coumadin inhibits the synthesis of vitamin K–dependent coagulation factors, altering the extrinsic pathway of the coagulation cascade. It is usually taken orally by dental patients. Unless vitamin K is administered, it requires several days for coagulation to normalize after its continuous use. Its anticoagulant effects are monitored every few weeks by hematologic laboratory tests. More recently, the most commonly used test is the International Normalized Ratio (INR), but Prothrombin Time (PT) is also used. The INR considers both the patient's prothrombin time (PT) and the control and is more standardized than a PT. It is becoming the standard test for monitoring the anticoagulant effects of warfarin (or the function of the extrinsic pathway), and the prothrombin time ratio (PTR) is becoming more obsolete.

    Heparin, on the other hand, requires IV access for administration. It binds to antithrombin III, giving assistance in the inhibition of thrombin formation and prolonging the intrinsic pathway. Its

284 CHAPTER 10

Table 10-2. Managing Therapeutically Anticoagulated Patients and the Laboratory Values Commonly Used to Monitor Anticoagulation

Drug	Lab Value
Aspirin/NSAIDs/Antiplatelet 1. Consult with physician on safety of stopping the medication for several days. 2. Defer surgery for at least five days, depending on the type of antiplatelet medication they are taking. 3. Use extra measures during and after surgery to help promote clot formation and retention.	Bleeding time

Warfarin (Coumadin)
1. Consult with physician on:
  a. Treating the patient with no alteration in anticoagulation therapy.
  b. Safety of discontinuing warfarin and allowing INR to fall to 1.5 for a few days prior to performing surgery, or
  c. Having the patient start on IM heparin that would cease for at least a 12 hour window during which surgery could be performed.
2. Use extra measures during and after surgery to help promote clot formation and retention.
	PT and INR

Heparin
1. Consult the physician on:
  a. Safety of stopping heparin therapy during the perioperative period.
  b. Restarting heparin once a stable clot has formed.
2. Use extra measures during and after surgery to help promote clot formation and retention.
	PTT

Low Molecular Weight Heparin (Lovenox)	No tests

blood thinning effects can be gone in a few hours or sooner if reversed by Protamine. Monitoring is with a PTR value.

Low molecular weight heparin (LMWH or SQ heparin) is typically used for deep vein thrombosis (DVT) treatment or prevention and is administered subcutaneously. Similar to heparin, it binds to antithrombin III. However, it inhibits factor Xa more than thrombin formation. Its antithrombotic effect is extremely predictable, requiring no laboratory values for its monitoring.

4. **Antibiotics (broad-spectrum).** These medications can alter the nature of the body's intestinal flora, which can de-

crease the production of vitamin K. Many of the clotting factors require vitamin K for their synthesis.

5. **Alcoholism.** Alcohol can cause enough liver dysfunction to decrease production of the clotting factors.

6. **Anticancer drugs.** Patients may be on chemotherapy drugs that reduce the number of circulating platelets.

7. **Antiplatelet drugs.** Medications such as thienopyridines (Ticlid and Plavix) and glycoprotein IIb/IIIa inhibitors (Reopro and Integrilin).

In addition to the previously mentioned types of drugs, many herbal medications have anticoagulant properties. A significant

MANAGEMENT OF PERIOPERATIVE BLEEDING   **285**

portion of the population self-medicates with these nonregulated formulations. Commonly, they inhibit platelet aggregation and prolong bleeding times. If a difficult surgery is planned, it would be wise to ask about these things (along with other more conventional medications) as the patient health history is reviewed. Examples of some of the herbal products that affect clotting are as follows:

- **Ginko biloba.** Taken for depression, macular degeneration, vertigo, and increased mental acuity.
- **Garlic.** For lowering cholesterol and triglycerides, to prevent colds, and so on.
- **Feverfew.** For treatment of migranes, asthma, arthritis, and so on.
- **Ginseng.** For increasing energy and libido. It is also said to stimulate immune function and normalize glucose levels after meals in diabetics.
- **Chamomile.** For stress and muscle (including menstrual) cramps. It is reported to have antiseptic and anti-inflammatory properties.

If the patient does happen to be taking a substance that compromises the body's clotting ability, then the dentist needs to be prepared to implement local measures to enhance hemostasis. For example, the patient may be on warfarin. Their INR will usually be less than three. For most anticoagulated patients, their INR will be 2.0 to 3.0 (therapeutic range). It has become acceptable, even recommended, to perform oral surgery on patients in this range without altering their anticoagulation regimen.[7] The authors recommend that the INR be less than 2.5 for surgical dental procedures performed by general dentists and that the practitioner have local measures (substances) on hand, as they will probably be needed. Persistent bleeding in a patient on warfarin can be difficult to manage. Furthermore, the administration of vitamin K to aid hemostasis is not only un-

predictable but can increase the chance of an embolic phenomenon.

In some cases, to discontinue wafarin, even temporarily puts the patient at extreme risk. In this scenario, a physician will most likely choose to stop the warfarin 2–3 days before surgery but start the patient on low molecular weight heparin (Enoxaparin/ Lovenox) that the patient self-administers. Lovenox was the first injectable, low molecular weight heparin approved for at-home use and has a 12-hour duration. As warfarin stops, the heparin begins. It is given every 12 hours and then usually discontinued 12 hours before the oral surgical procedure. If there are no bleeding problems, then another subcutaneous heparin may be administered the night of surgery, followed by warfarin beginning again the next morning. This treatment method narrows the window of risk and vulnerability while allowing the surgery to be performed in the safest manner.

Frequently, a physician will recommend discontinuing warfarin 2–3 days prior to the oral surgery, allowing the INR to temporarily drop from 2.5 or 3 to as low as 1.5, and then resume warfarin the day following surgery. There is greater potential risk with this method, but it is the physician's call.

Similarly, the patient may have a known or suspected coagulopathy. With a known bleeding problem, it is appropriate to confer with the patient's physician or enlist the assistance of a hematologist. If the problem is only suspected because of a past history of bleeding irregularities, then the dentist may want to order coagulation studies prior to treatment such as a complete blood count (CBC) including platelets, partial thromboplastin time (PTT), INR, and/or bleeding time. If the patient needs multiple extractions or other more extensive oral surgery, or if the general dentist is not familiar with the interpretation of lab values, it may be better for him or her to defer treatment to someone with more experience treating these situations.

Preventing Bleeding Problems with Careful Surgery

Quite often, bleeding problems during surgery are made worse by poor surgical technique. Much bleeding can be avoided by careful management of the soft tissues. The operator needs to make clean incisions and not tear flaps. One should be careful not to lacerate or abrade soft tissue with a bur, crush it with a forcep, or puncture it with elevators or other instruments since these are some things that increase and prolong bleeding. Sometimes we get so focused on **hard tissue** that we may tend to not pay attention to the handling of **soft tissue**. In addition, areas of sharp bone should be smoothed and diseased, and/or cyanotic tissue should be excised from the gumline after extractions. Periapical granulomatous lesions should also be removed from extraction sites.

One fault of many general dentists is having a flap that is too small. Enlarging the flap to give better visibility and access will, at the same time, prevent stretching, pulling, and tearing of the mucosa. This may involve doing something many generalists are reluctant to do—making a releasing incision. A releasing incision is generally made one tooth mesial or distal to the tooth being removed, thus helping to ensure that the incision is over bone for better healing. It doesn't need to be long. Five to ten millimeters is often sufficient, just into the unattached tissue. The incision is usually angled slightly to give a wider base to the flap and provide a more adequate blood supply. Making this triangular flap also prevents tension on the flap or the need to apply excessive retraction pressure.

Sometimes, despite our best effort during surgery, troublesome bleeding occurs. In this event, we must do our best to control it. The first question we need to ask is, "Where is it coming from?" Is it from soft tissue or bleeding diffusely from a bony socket? Is it from a nutrient canal (artery) in the bone that was cut by a bur, or could it be from a severed vessel in the mandibular canal? The treatment modality will depend on the bleeding source. Identification requires good lighting, suction, and competent retraction assistance.

Soft Tissue Bleeding

In a patient with normal clotting, any bleeding from soft tissue incisions or periosteal reflections will generally subside within a few minutes. An exception might be if an artery or vein within the soft tissue is severed. For example, when making a releasing incision for a triangular flap in the mandibular second molar area, the incision could inadvertently extend too far apically. If it goes beyond the mucobuccal fold into the cheek, the facial artery or anterior facial vein could be nicked or even severed. This would cause major bleeding and would need to be treated before proceeding with the surgery. In this case, a mosquito hemostat could be used to clamp the bleeder, after which suture material could be used to tie off the vessel. Soft tissue bleeders (larger blood vessels) can also be packed, although hemostasis is more frequently obtained with careful suturing or electro/chemical cauterization.

The following are local measures that can be used to help stop soft tissue bleeding:

- Electrocautery
- Hemostatic liquid
  Examples are Hemodent (aluminum chloride), Viscostat (20% ferric sulfate coagulative gel), Astringedent (15.5% aqueous ferric sulfate), Astringedent-X (12.7% equivalent ferric sulfate and ferric subsulfate). The latter is the most potent of those listed.
- Local anesthetic with 1:50,000 epinephrine
- Sutures
- Pressure

Socket bleeding

Occasionally, bleeding from a **tooth socket** following tooth extraction can be persistent and annoying. This often occurs when there has been drilling in the socket to help remove a root. The operator may have drilled with a bur to help create a purchase area adjacent to a root, or an interradicular bone may have been removed to lessen the body's hold on a root. If bleeding fails to subside prior to the patient leaving the office, then the socket should be packed with something to help with hemostasis.

The following are local measures that can be used to help stop socket bleeding:

- Hemostatic gauze (such as ActCel or HemoStyp Hemostatic Gauze™) (See Figure 10.1)
- Gelfoam (see Figure 10.2)
- Collagen (Colla-Plug or Colla-Tape) (see Figure 10.3)
- Surgicel (see Figure 10.4)
- Gelfoam with bovine thrombin
- Bone wax (see Figure 10.5)

Hemostatic gauze looks like a cotton fabric (originating from cotton) but has been chemically treated with a proprietary process to dissolve into glucose and saline within 1–2 weeks. When one or more small (1 × 1 inch) pieces are placed in a socket, it enhances hemostasis and serves to stabilize the clot. This material is the authors' choice for obtaining hemostasis within extraction sites. Gelfoam works in a similar manner. Both are held in place with a figure-eight suture over the socket.

Colla-Plug and Colla-Tape are highly cross-linked collagen products that also promote hemostasis. They help coagulation by

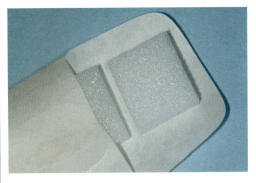

Figure 10-2. Gelfoam.

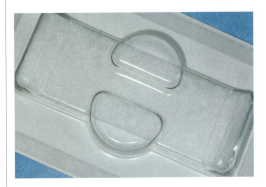

Figure 10-3. CollaTape.

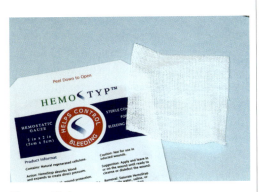

Figure 10-1. Hemostatic gauze.

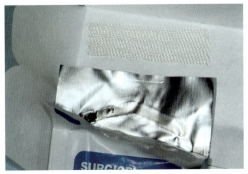

Figure 10-4. Surgicel.

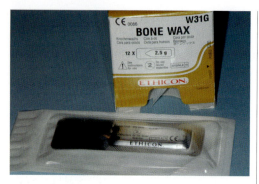

Figure 10-5. Bone wax.

enhancing platelet aggregation. Another form of collagen that can be placed in a socket is the microfibular type (for example, Avitene). This material is more fluffy and loose-knit.

Surgicel is oxidized regenerated cellulose. It can be more effective at hemostasis than Gelfoam because it has more strength and can be packed under pressure; however, it commonly causes delayed healing of the socket. For this reason, it is usually only used for persistent bleeding.[1]

In difficult situations, a liquid preparation of bovine thrombin can be applied to Gelfoam and placed in a socket. By using thrombin, all the steps in the coagulation cascade are bypassed, and fibrinogen is converted to fibrin enzymatically. Since this product is of animal origin, it might occasionally lead to allergic reactions.

NUTRIENT CANAL BLEEDING

When removing bone with a bur for a surgical extraction, a nutrient blood vessel (branch of the inferior alveolar artery) can sometimes be cut in the process, causing profuse bleeding. If this happens, several actions can help remedy the situation. One is to localize the bleeding orifice with suction. Second, bone should be crushed into the lumen with a periosteal elevator or other similar instrument. Third, a small amount of bone wax can be burnished into the bleeding orifice. It should be noted that the mechanical effect of bone wax may not be very long-lasting.

With nutrient canal bleeding, if the tooth is still present and can quickly be extracted, then control the bleeding with suction and remove the tooth. If bleeding is too great to allow visibility, and it will take more than a few minutes to remove the tooth, then the extraction should be postponed to another time, and all efforts can be expended on hemostasis. In addition to bone burnishing and bone wax, one or more of the methods (local measures) listed previously may be implemented, followed by closure of the soft tissue with sutures over the socket. The patient can then bite on conventional gauze. This type of bleeding can, at times, become life-threatening.

In a study with 175 adult patients who had extractions averaging 18 teeth, it was reported that the blood loss varied from 35 to 912 mL, with a mean of 223 mL.[8] Another study[9] using radioactively labeled I131, found that the blood loss during multiple extractions ranged from 148 to 912 mL. Sinclair found that blood loss during extractions was greater when teeth were removed from the upper than the lower jaw and that the amount was related to tooth type.[10] There was a mean loss of 1.9 mL from lower canine sockets and a mean of 14.05 mL from upper molars. Sinclair suggested that blood loss was related to the surface area of the roots.

Some operators, in the midst of an episode of profuse bleeding, count the number of 2 × 2 gauze sponges saturated with blood to determine the magnitude of blood loss. This method has inherent problems unless pre- and postoperative weight measurements are performed with the brand of gauze used in the office. For example, two different brands of 2 × 2s were saturated with venous blood to determine how many milliliters they would hold. Figures 10.6A and 10.6B show that a Sullivan-Schein brand holds 4.5 mL, and a Johnson &

MANAGEMENT OF PERIOPERATIVE BLEEDING   289

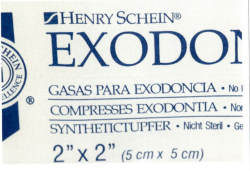

Figure 10-6A. Two-by-two inch, lightly filled cotton-filled gauze commonly used in dental offices.

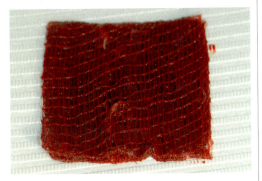

Figure 10-6B. The same gauze saturated with venous blood holds 4.0 mL.

Johnson brand holds 9.0 mL. See Figures 10.7A and 10.7B.

There are multiple reports of external carotid ligation or selective vessel embolization during oral surgical procedures in order to save the patient. If blood loss is estimated to approach 500 mL, the emergency medical system (EMS) should be activated, or the patient quickly transferred to the emergency room since there may be signs of shock at 800–1000 mL of blood loss.[1]

Signs of shock can include the following:

- systolic BP 70–80 mm Hg
- rapid but weak pulse
- increased rate but shallow respirations
- limited consciousness
- cyanosis of lips and nail beds
- cold sweat

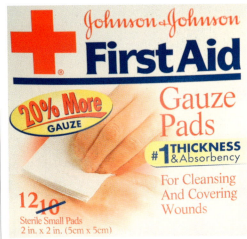

Figure 10-7A. Two-by-two inch, densely filled cotton-filled gauze.

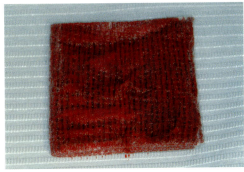

Figure 10-7B. The same gauze saturated with venous blood holds 9.5 mL.

- thirst
- restlessness
- subnormal temperature

An example of a patient with heavy bleeding is shown in Figures 10.8A–C. The radiograph (see Figure 10.8A) shows tooth #32, which is a partial bony impaction. As bone was being removed with a bur on the distobuccal of the tooth in this 30-year-old man (see arrow), a nutrient canal was cut, causing immediate spurting of blood into the socket. Adjacent bone was burnished into the bleeding vessel; bone wax was applied; and suction used to maintain visibility for the brief

290 CHAPTER 10

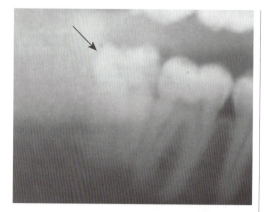

Figure 10-8A. Radiograph of tooth #32, which is a partial bony impaction in a healthy 30-year-old man.

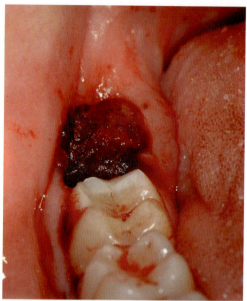

Figure 10-8C. As the previously mentioned measures were not successful, about 10 1×1 inch pieces of HemoStype hemostatic gauze were placed in the socket, after which hemostasis was achieved. The socket was then sutured and the patient observed for about 30 minutes before being allowed to leave the office.

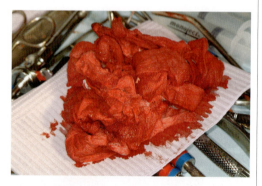

Figure 10-8B. After cutting a nutrient canal (artery) adjacent to the tooth during bone removal, emergency measures were implemented including burnishing of bone into the bleeding orifice and the use of bone wax. Additionally, 15 4×4 gauze sponges were used one after another to exert pressure and control bleeding.

time it took to remove the tooth. Then conventional gauze (4 × 4 inch) was used as packing to control bleeding. (*Note*: Gauze should not be used to just soak up the blood, but to pack the site, causing a higher pressure outside the vessel than inside. This is a temporary measure, but the goal is for the vessel to clot or at least for the gauze to prevent significant blood loss while other preparations are being made to stop the bleeding.)

Despite these measures, heavy bleeding continued. Approximately 15 gauze sponges were used, one after the other, as pressure dressings in the socket (see Figure 10.8B). Each one equaled four 2 × 2s. As they became saturated and ineffective, they were removed. Since this was not working, about 10 1 × 1 inch pieces of resorbable hemostatic gauze (HemoStyp™) were placed in the socket with conventional gauze placed on top of it to provide pressure. The bleeding stopped within a few minutes (see Figure 10.8C). At the end of the procedure, it was estimated that the pieces of 4 × 4 gauze likely contained roughly 270 mL of blood. This does not include blood aspirated into the high-speed evacuation system.

Mandibular Canal Bleeding

If, in the process of removing roots of a mandibular molar, it is suspected that a

MANAGEMENT OF PERIOPERATIVE BLEEDING **291**

blood vessel in the mandibular canal has been cut, causing serious bleeding from the depth of the socket, then treatment cannot be as aggressive as with nutrient canal bleeding. This is because of proximity to the inferior alveolar nerve (IAN). In this situation, either Gelfoam or hemostatic gauze (both resorbable) should be placed in the depth of the socket. Then moistened strung-out gauze (as with several 2 × 2 gauze sponges) can be packed on top of the bleeding vessel. Again, this is to allow for a fibrin clot to form and/or prevent significant hemorrhaging while gathering thoughts and necessary materials. Typically, this is left in place for 5–10 minutes. The more superficial gauze is then removed and the situation evaluated. If the site continues to bleed, a packing of Iodoform or Vaseline-impregnated gauze should be inserted over the resorable material for 10–15 minutes. The packing should be tight enough to prevent any bleeding although carefully placed to avoid damaging the IAN. If persistent bleeding continues, additional resorbable hemostatic material can be laid over the vessel and the socket packed again with moistened gauze. If unable to control the hemorrhaging with these methods, tight closure of the soft tissues over the gauze should be performed, and the patient should be immediately transported to an oral and maxillofacial surgeon or nearest medical facility.

Postoperative Bleeding

At this point, the surgery is over. It was successfully completed and bleeding was controlled during the procedure. We can assume that soft tissue was managed properly and sufficient sutures have been placed. Any bony bleeders have been controlled. The patient is about to leave the office with bleeding within normal limits and under control. Of course, there may be some oozing of blood from the area for 24–36 hours after the surgery, but it will not be excessive.

IMMEDIATELY POSTOPERATIVELY

The following instructions verbally or preferably in writing can be used to help ensure that postoperative bleeding problems do not occur:

- Bite on a piece of damp gauze for 20–30 minutes.
- Keep head elevated and rest so as to not raise the blood pressure.
- Rest for 2–3 hours.
- Do not rinse for 24 hours.
- Do not smoke for at least the first 12 hours. The smoke is an irritant. Additionally, suction from smoking causes negative pressure and may make bleeding worse.
- Avoid talking.
- Don't spit.
- Avoid strenuous exercise for the first 24 hours.
- Avoid touching the surgery site with the tongue.
- Avoid hot liquids, carbonation, or hydrogen peroxide rinses because they can promote clot lysis.
- Avoid aspirin or other nonsteroidal anti-inflammatory medications.
- Maintain a liquid diet for 24–48 hours.
- Don't chew near the surgery site for three days.
- If bleeding continues or restarts, bite again for 20–30 minutes (repacking and resuturing by the dentist may be required).
- Use a moist tea bag instead of the gauze for a few times. (The tannic acid in tea has vasoconstrictor properties.)

The dentist must be available in case of an emergency. Reasons for a return visit by the patient would be prolonged bleeding, large clots in the cheek or floor of the mouth, or profuse bright red bleeding. Over the phone, review the list provided previously. If, after a reasonable time, it is still actively bleeding, the dentist should see the patient.

If the dentist does see the patient back in the office, make sure there is good light, retraction, and suction. This may mean calling in help after hours for the needed assistance. For medico-legal and safety reasons, it is not advisable to be alone with the patient when providing this treatment.

Try to identify the source. Remove all sutures, gauze, and so on. If the patient is uncomfortable, anesthetize the area with a local anesthetic without a vasoconstrictor. The vasoconstrictor may fool the practitioner into thinking that hemostasis is obtained, when in fact only temporary vasoconstriction has occurred. Rebleeding may occur as soon as the vasoconstrictor has worn off (usually as soon as the patient arrives back home). Packing the site may be required to differentiate the source (soft tissue versus bone, or specific vessel versus diffuse oozing). Diffuse oozing is more likely to occur in a patient with a systemic disorder (hypertension, medically anticoagulated, bleeding disorder, and so on) as opposed to a vessel injury from surgery. Evaluating the type and discovering the site of bleeding can direct treatment.

If bone is the source of the bleeding, then follow the preceding steps for packing the site with resorbable hemostatic material, such as hemostactic gauze or Gel foam, and overpacking with Iodoform or Vaseline-impregnated gauze. A figure-eight suture over the socket should always be performed to assist in stabilizing the clot.

If generalized oozing (from bone, soft tissue, adjacent sulci) is difficult to manage, and especially if it is felt to be from a systemic disorder or anticoagulation, systemic management needs to be performed by the patient's primary physician or emergency personnel. Laboratory values will be obtained with ensuing fluid resuscitation, correction of abnormalities, and persistent monitoring.

Especially when treating patients on anticoagulants, the use of tranexamic acid mouthwash is an adjunctive hemostatic agent to consider for inhibiting the breakdown of fibrin clots. It is used to irrigate the socket before suturing, after which it is used as a mouthwash for two minutes, four times a day for one week. It is effective but very expensive (about $230 for seven days). However, when compared to other local hemostatic measures, it may not be that much more useful. It is more a tool of the oral and maxillofacial surgeon in a hospital environment.

SECONDARY BLEEDING

Secondary bleeding is after the fact. Some describe it as bleeding that takes place 24 hours after a surgical procedure. One should first consider the least invasive method of bleeding control.

1. Initially, it is good to have the patient at home rinse gently with cold water and bite on gauze for 20–30 minutes. If bleeding persists, the patient can substitute a moist tea bag for the gauze—trying this several times for 20–30 minutes each time. If unsuccessful, then the patient should see the dentist.
2. When in the office, the dentist should rinse and clean the mouth of any clots or bleeding. With good lighting, examine the surgical site to determine the source. Again, pressure should be applied by biting on gauze or by having the dentist press gauze on the area for five minutes or so. Many times, the cause of secondary bleeding is from the patient sucking, spitting, chewing, or engaging in some type of physical activity that irritates the wound and exacerbates the problem.
3. Finally, if these two measures don't work, it is time for a more aggressive approach. Anesthetize the area (a block is preferable to infiltration because an infiltration may provide a false positive of hemostasis) and curette the socket to establish fresh healing. Identify sources of bleeding and deal

with them appropriately according to their location (soft tissue or bone). One or more of the previously listed hemostatic agents can be applied. This time, one should be more thorough in instructing the patient how and where to place the gauze pack. Wait a sufficiently long time to make sure that bleeding has stopped before dismissing the patient. If bleeding continues to be a problem, there may be a coagulation disorder that should be evaluated by laboratory tests—generally under the direction of a hemoatologist.

In Figure 10.9, a lower third molar was removed and hemostasis achieved prior to the patient leaving the office. When the patient was called that night, he said there was still oozing from this one site. Instructions were given on what the patient should do to control the situation, and he was asked to call back if bleeding didn't subside. The next morning the patient called the dentist to say that it had been bleeding all night. The patient had been up changing gauze and biting on gauze continually. The dentist saw the patient within a short time. Several pieces of resorbable hemostatic agent (in this case Gelfoam) were placed, and the patient asked to bite firmly on gauze placed directly over the socket. After about five minutes, the bleeding stopped and did not start up again. More invasive methods were not needed.

Surgical Contraindications from Hematologic Conditions

There are two situations that present absolute contraindications to extraction of teeth. They are arteriovenous or sinusoidal aneurysms and central hemangiomas. Removal of teeth with root structures that are involved with one of these lesions can cause death from three different means: the patient may exsanguinate, go into shock, or aspirate blood.

Arteriovenous aneurysms or fistulas are

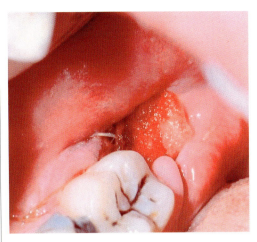

Figure 10-9. Control of secondary bleeding with Gelfoam and pressure from 2 × 2 inch gauze.

uncommon vascular abnormalities that may either be congenital or traumatic in origin. Those due to trauma are generally singular fistular channels resulting from injury to an artery and adjacent vein. Congenital arteriovenous aneurysms are hemangiomas with large-bore, high-flow channels. The latter have also been described as pulsating, central, and central cavernous hemangiomas. They have a tendency to develop in the head and neck but seldom affect the mandible or maxilla. When in the jaws, however, they are more common in the mandible than the maxilla by a ratio of 2:1. Also, there is a higher incidence in females than males by 3:1. They are most common in the molar region during the second decade of life. In the mandible, signs and symptoms include tooth mobility, pain, and pulsation or throbbing. Other reports include paresthesia, derangement of normal arch and occlusion, premature exfoliation of deciduous teeth, congenitally missing teeth, root resorption (30 percent), and referred pain to the ear. Radiographically, lesions range from diffuse destruction to multiloculation with a soap-bubble appearance and well-defined borders. Congenital lesions arise most often within bone from marrow spaces near the mandibular canal, where they can resorb and/or expand the mandible, demonstrating radiographically as a lucency.

This type of vascular lesion should always be kept in mind when performing surgery. Extraction or deep periodontal surgery of an involved tooth or a biopsy of this lesion could result in life-threatening exsanguinations. This situation may even resist carotid ligation, radiation therapy, injection of sclerosing agents, or other forms of treatment. Radiolucencies should be aspirated with a 20-gauge needle prior to surgical intervention. If blood is readily withdrawn, surgery should not be performed until a vascular lesion has been ruled out. That will usually require referring to an oral and maxillofacial surgeon to set up the patient with an interventional radiologist for angiographic studies and then treatment—first limited to observation and then possibly with single or multiple treatments of selective embolization followed by surgical excision.

Bibliography

1. L. J. Peterson, Sr. Ed. *Contemporary Oral and Maxillofac. Surg.,* 4th ed. St. Louis: Mosby. 2004.

2. *Merck Manual of Medical Information.* Mark H. Beer, ed. Section 14. Blood disorders. Whitehouse Station: NJ: Merck and Co. 1999.

3. D. J. Weatherall. The blood in systemic disease. In: *Oxford Textbook of Medicine,* 4th ed. Oxford, England: Oxford University Press. 1999.

4. D. Flanagan. Important arterial supply of the mandible, control of an arterial hemorrhage, and report of a hemorrhagic incident. *J Oral Implant.* 29(4): 165–173. 2003.

5. Centers for Disease Control, National Center on Birth Defects and Developmental Disabilities. Heriditary Blood disorders. *http://www.cdc.gov/ncbddd/hemophilia.htm.*

6. H. Dym, O. E. Ogle. *Atlas of Minor Oral Surgery.* Philadelphia, PA: W.B. Saunders Co. 2001.

7. M. J. Wahl. Myths of dental surgery in patients receiving anticoagulant therapy. *JADA.* 131: 77–81. 2000.

8. R. L. Johnson. Blood loss in oral surgery. *J Dent Research.* 35: 175–184. 1956.

9. M. Spengos. Determination of blood loss during full-mouth extraction and alveoplasty by plasma volume studies with I 131 tagged human albumin. *Oral Surg, Oral Med, Oral Path.* 16: 16–17. 1963.

10. J. H. Sinclair. Loss of blood following the removal of teeth in normal and hemophilia patients. *Oral Surg, Oral Med, Oral Path.* 23: 415–420. 1967.

Chapter 11

Third World Volunteer Dentistry

Dr. Richard C. Smith

Introduction

The majority of people in developing countries live with daily pain, and the word dentist is not in their vocabulary. The fortunate ones may have access to a local medicine man or paraprofessional who may be able to extract one or all of their teeth under a tree or by the kitchen table. Some may even travel a great distance to find a trained practitioner with expertise but very little in the way of instruments or equipment. Because of deep poverty and little income, few patients can afford more than basic palliative measures. This kills incentive for people to go into dentistry as a profession since the income-producing prospects are so meager. Even with some government and international aid trying to solve such widespread problems, most of these disadvantaged populations will never see a change in their lifetimes. Volunteer dentists, hygienists, and other team members that travel to treat and teach these people in this "other world" literally bring light and hope with them.

The purpose of this chapter is to encourage more of such altruistic humanitarian service. See Figures 11.1–11.3. This chapter is divided into four sections:

- I. Dental Conditions in the Third World
- II. Levels of Assistance (including preparation)
- III. Planning and Preparing for Volunteer Service
- IV. Gaining a New Perspective

I. Dental Conditions in the Third World

We live in a time when the "Golden Age of Dentistry" with its innovations, inventions, research, and scientific methods, has given us preventive programs in oral hygiene and diet, water fluoridation, and topical fluorides that have reduced the impact of dental disease. Dental manpower has increased, and organized dentistry has done a big part by elevating the profession and rewarding the practitioners. However, a visit to many foreign countries is a step back in time. As far as dentistry is concerned the term **underdeveloped country** means no preventive programs. **Unindustrialized** means most of the population cannot afford dental treatment. Regrettably, we live in a world of the very rich and the very poor. See Figures 11.4 and 11.5.

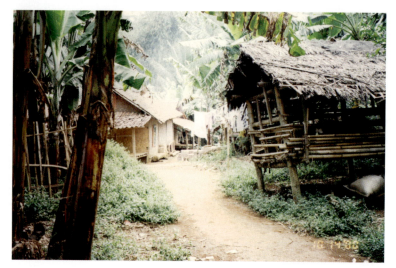

Figure 11-1. Village in Indonesia.

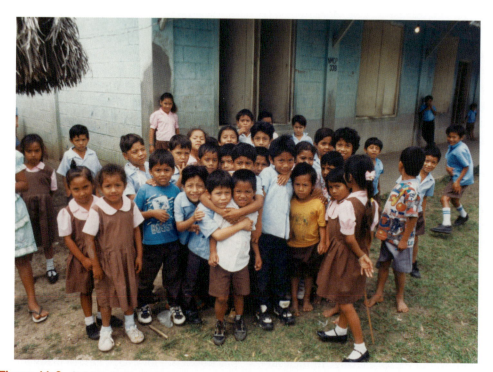

Figure 11-2. Children in Mexico.

For example, the GDP (gross domestic product) per capita or the production of goods per person in a year, in Norway is US$34,310.00, contrasted with US$90.00 in Ethiopia. Table 11.1 illustrates the differences in these nations with regard to the possibility of a patient receiving dental care. Norway has a ratio of 1,100 patients per dentist, Ethiopia has a ratio of 1,200,000 people per dentist.

One country may graduate 5,600 dentists each year from 122 dental schools as op-

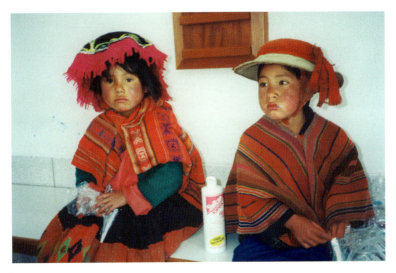

Figure 11-3. Patients in Peru.

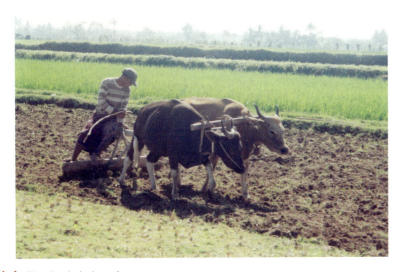

Figure 11-4. Plowing in Indonesia.

posed to another country that graduates 25 students from one school to serve their population of 11.5 million. It is statistics like these that are causing organizations like the Federation Dentaire Internationale (FDI), World Dental Federation (WDF), and World Health Organization (WHO) to formulate programs and push for results. In the words of Dr. Sam Thorpe from Sierra Leone, who is the former Regional Advisor for Oral Health of the Regional Office of the World Health Organization, "Previous approaches to improving oral health in Africa have been modeled on those of affluent countries and have, therefore, failed to recognize the epidemiological priorities of the region. The main problems can be traced to the following: (a) lack of national oral health policies and plans; (b) inappropriately trained dentists (c) services that benefit only affluent and urban communities; (d) services that are almost entirely curative; (e) and lack of

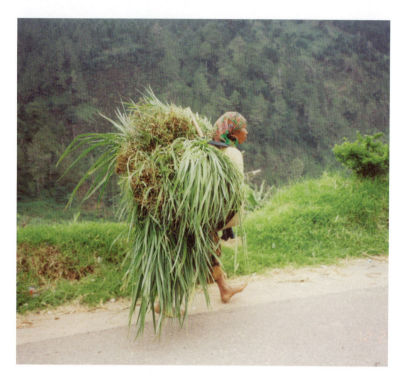

Figure 11-5. Produce going to market.

Table 11-1. Ratio of Dentists to Population

Country	Number of Dentists	Population per Dentist	Number of Dental Schools
Ethiopia	52	1,200,000 to 1	0
Malia	47	225,000 to 1	0
Nepal	100	220,000 to 1	1
Guinea	53	138,000 to 1	1
Cameroon	120	119,000 to 1	2
Maldives	3	100,000 to 1	0
Kiribati	2	40,000 to 1	0
Cambodia	296	38,850 to 1	1
India	26,000	36,538 to 1	122
Gabon	42	28,500 to 1	0
Namibia	60	28,000 to 1	0
Indonesia	8,128	24,852 to 1	11
Sri Lanka	1,353	14,000 to 1	1
United Kingdom	27,957	2,100 to 1	15
Israel*	8,500	1,700 to 1	2
France*	40,000	1,503 to 1	16
United States*	169,894	1,471 to 1	56
Japan*	92,874	1,358 to 1	29
Argentina	28,000	1,200 to 1	10
Norway	4,000	1,100 to 1	2

Statistics from FDI World Dental Federation for Year 2000, *2004.

equipment and materials, supplies and maintenance."[1]

At the annual FDI World Dental Congress in New Delhi, India, in 2004, 189 delegates from 48 African and other countries met. One result of their planning meetings was the Nairobi Declaration on Oral Health in Africa, which confirmed the commitment to increase the number of countries with functioning oral health policies in the region. They emphasized that the integration of oral health into general health activities and primary health care is essential.[2]

It is very important for those going to a developing country to provide humanitarian service to know what problems they are dealing with as well as the resources that are already being used. It behooves those anxious to serve in these countries to have a good understanding of the overall plan that is already in place with its priorities, goals, and methods to accomplish them.

The World Health Organization has a very detailed plan called the Basic Package of Oral Care (BPOC), which addresses the urgent need for change among disadvantaged populations that are without adequate community oriented preventive services. It has three components or goals: 1) Oral Urgent Treatment (OUT), 2) Affordable Fluoride Toothpaste (AFT), and 3) Atraumatic Restorative Treatment (ART). Its objectives are to address nonestablished market economy (non-EME) countries that often have little access to basic emergency treatment and no organized system for the prevention of oral diseases.

ORAL URGENT TREATMENT

This is the first step in primary health care (PHC) providing basic emergency care to meet the needs and conditions of each local population. It involves:

- Extraction of teeth that cannot be saved
- Treatment of postextraction complications

- Drainage of abscesses
- Palliative drug therapy
- Trauma first aid

AFFORDABLE FLUORIDE TOOTHPASTE

It has been demonstrated that it was not until the acceptance of mass preventive measures using fluorides that the incidence of caries started to decline in market economy countries. The use of fluoride toothpaste is considered to be the most efficient means of controlling dental caries, especially in developing countries without the resources for water or salt fluoridation. The following recommendations have been proposed by WHO planners:

- Developing effective low-cost fluoride toothpaste
- Promotion campaign
- Supervised daily tooth brushing with flouride toothpaste (1,000 ppm F)
- Oral hygiene education

ATRAUMATIC RESTORATIVE TREATMENT

This is the concept of caries removal and cavity preparation **without a dental handpiece, water or electricity**. It uses hand instrumentation with a minimum of instruments, glassionomer restorative materials, and trained dental auxiliaries. It makes restorative treatment more affordable, more available, and more accessible, meeting the requirements for primary health care for large, needy populations. Field studies on the technique were done in Tanzania, Malawi, Syria, Thailand, Zimbabwe, and Pakistan. When compared to conventional amalgam restorations, no statistically significant differences in survival rates were reported.[3]

It will take methods "other than those of affluent countries" to have the greatest impact in taking care of dental problems in countries where up to 90 percent of the population is indigent. Murray Dickson in his book *Where There Is No Dentist* states, "Two things can greatly reduce the cost of adequate dental care: popular education about dental health, and the training of primary health workers as 'dental health promoters'. In addition numbers of 'community dental technicians' can be trained in 2 to 3 months (plus a period of apprenticeship) to care for up to 90 percent of the people who have problems of pain and infection." A university-trained dentist would be the secondary line of care. Simpler more commonplace procedures could be done in villages everywhere. Where a program such as this is in place already, these technicians have become quite skilled.[1]

What is also needed is the training of more auxiliary personel (local people) in simple inexpensive preventive methods. Oral health progress will not be made by the unmodified transfer of skills, equipment, or personnel. It should be adapted in each country, not just adopted from another country.[4]

In Dr. Thorpe's assessment, those out-of-country volunteers who come in to serve for a short time can combine with the BPOC (Basic Package of Oral Care) to increase the availability of needed services without imposing concepts "modeled on those of affluent countries." In Belize there is a two-year training program in a WHO facility for female students who will then return to treat primary teeth only. This is a two-tier system, but one that is very appropriate for the conditions and needs in that country. This two-tier system is accepted by Guatemala, Ecuador, Papua New Guinea, and Mozambique. In these countries dentists train technicians that then do cleanings, extractions, fillings, work in schools, and help with health education.[5] The third component of the BPOC plan, the ART technique, has been in use in New Zealand for several years and in Cambodia, where dental nurses are being trained in its use (see Figure 11.6). A single dental school like theirs cannot train enough people to ever treat the large rural population.

For example, oral health care is virtually nonexistent in rural areas in Pakistan, where more than 80 percent of the population live.

Dr. Ayyaz Ali Khan is Coordinator of the National Oral Health Programme at the Ministry of Health in Pakistan. He has stated, "over the last two decades, it has been seen that the existing traditional oral health systems, focusing on restorative approaches,

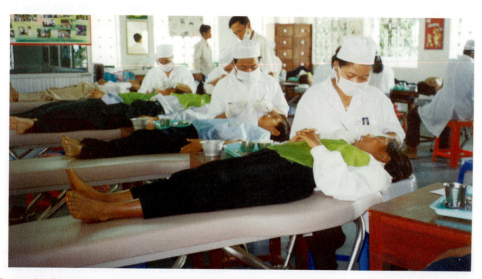

Figure 11-6. Regional training center for dental nurses in Kompong Cham, Cambodia.

staffed by highly qualified, highly paid personnel using sophisticated technology have been unsuccessful in controlling the deterioration of oral health in developing countries. It would be unrealistic to assume that adequate resources will ever be available for the dental surgeons to perform traditional high tech dentistry. In addition there will never be enough dentists in any developing country to provide these services to the whole population. Furthermore, auxiliaries provide services at locations where the dentist is not willing to go or live."[6]

II. Levels of Assistance

Without considering the preventative aspect of the second goal (Affordable Fluoride Toothpastes), there are basically two types of care that we (volunteer dentists) can deliver in third world countries: 1) relief of pain by extraction (Oral Urgent Treatment) and 2) filling carious teeth and perhaps even teaching the Atraumatic Restorative Treatment procedures. As volunteers step into third-world situations, these two types of care will be the primary emphasis for their expenditures and expertise. The sections that follow will elaborate on these and other elements of treatment. In fact, we will break down our treatment into three levels or approaches—from the most simple to the more sophisticated.

Level One: Bush dentistry. Treatment in the wild with forceps to remove diseased teeth, thereby alleviating pain and infection.

Level Two: Dental care with the benefit of power and water. This may involve mobile units, multiple dentists, and auxiliary personnel. There may even be portable suction and/or x-rays along with oral hygiene instruction for patients. The location could be a church or government building such as a school.

Level Three: Permanent and ongoing facilities in a community set up by volunteers.

This is obviously more desirable but more difficult to establish. When foreign dentists are not there, care can be provided by local dentists who rotate in and out of the clinic. Hopefully, patient scheduling would be done by someone to maximize use and efficiency.

At some point in their lives, many professionals consider the skills and experience they have attained and want to expand their horizon to help others. The act of serving others to relieve pain and suffering without monetary return fulfills a desire to make the world a better place. Dental professionals are fortunate in that their dental skills can be adapted for use in underserved areas. Even dental specialists can be integrated into a team that can effectively treat and teach populations that otherwise would not be reached.

When an individual or team of volunteer dentists begins to treat patients in a village or town, there are certain invisible barriers that need to be recognized and overcome. These involve cultural differences, local taboos, status issues, and prevailing attitudes about foreign visitors. This is usually accomplished quite easily if the volunteers know the language and talk to local leaders—asking questions and explaining what their purpose and methods will be. Of more importance are some general principles that need to be followed. There are certain guidelines that apply to all volunteer activities in third-world communities.

Dr. Jamie Robertson, who has vast experience working in Vietnam, gives these observations:

1. Volunteers are there to augment existing programs, to enthuse and perhaps establish local workers, to teach, to innovate and offer themselves as role models.
2. Volunteer projects cannot and should not be the sole delivery system of some dental activity as ends in themselves.

3. Local ownership is essential for sustainability.
4. Projects should work on the KISS principle (Keep It Simple Stupid). It is better to teach all health workers how to minimize cross-infection than to show one or two dentists advance techniques.
5. One objective of any project is to make it redundant. The ideal way to do this is to equip local workers with skills and resources.[7]

The American Dental Association's publication, *International Dental Volunteer Organizations: A Guide to Service and a Directory of Programs,* also offers good insights for those looking for opportunities to serve. It discusses "Why Volunteer?," "The Nature of Volunteer Work," "Types of Projects," and "Organizations" that have foreign projects. The ADA Directory currently lists 64 volunteer programs. The Academy of Dentistry International is the first organization listed with the stated purpose of elevating dental care standards worldwide through continuing education. The last one on the list is World Medical Relief Inc. Their volunteers collect supplies, equipment, and pharmaceuticals in response to requests from other organizations giving assistance. A group called World Concern is just one of many Christian organizations that is well known working in Africa, Asia, and Latin America.

Operation Smile is an organization providing reconstructive surgery and related dental treatment. Since Operation Smile's first mission to Bolivia in 1999, 789 children have been treated. In 2004 they were again in Bolivia for 10 days. Thirty-four volunteer team members including plastic surgeons, anesthesiologists, pediatricians, nurses, a dentist, and speech therapists worked with a Bolivian team that screened 258 patients and treated 110.[8]

Many other organizations, not on the ADA list, have programs using volunteers for projects with agriculture, home building, water development, health, and so on. By using local project directors, populations with the greatest needs are recognized, and then volunteeer groups with resources and volunteers are invited to help. Many times they will organize missions to their projects with just dental personal. They plan all details, arrange for patients, and provide other needed support. This type of dental treatment, especially in schools and churches where there is permanent water and power resources, allows more sophisticated dental procedures to be done. Also, it increases the possibility of return visits to that area to treat even more patients.

When dental groups and individual dentists partner with endowed humanitarian organizations or foundations, both of them are more successful, and their mission statements are more likely to be accomplished. Choice, Chasqui Humanitarian, and Eagle-Condor are just a few. Another partner in many foreign projects is Rotary Inernational. When a local Rotary club unites with a foreign one, it brings together the needed expertise, the volunteers, and the people to make the arrangements on site. This is real synergism with the whole accomplishing more than the individual parts. See Figure 11.7.

LEVEL ONE

There are many approaches to the successful treatment of third-world patients. Some have proven their worth over the years. On the most basic level of care, it can be bush dentistry in the jungle with forceps only to alleviate as much pain as possible. This fulfills the first goal of WHO's BPOC approach (OUT) for urgent care. There is also the opportunity for oral hygiene instruction (OHI) and the possibility of training local villagers to continue doing some procedures. This is a Level One classification of volunteer involvement.

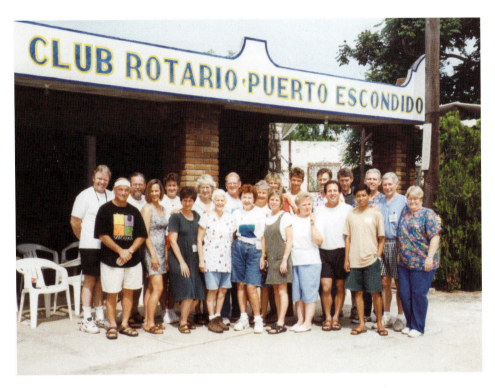

Figure 11-7. Rotary International–sponsored project in Puerto Escondido, Mexico.

There is an old saying "he that travels alone travels faster." Some feel that with large groups of people with inexperienced volunteers, accompanying baggage, and necessary dental equipment, problems are introduced that they would rather do without. In contrast, for those who want to travel light and do extractions in remote wilderness environments, there are plenty of countries where this can be done. See Figure 11.8.

There are also many opportunities for the "do it alone" dentist to tag along with humanitarian foundations, mentioned previously, where other volunteers are working on their own nondental projects. In this situation, a dentist and maybe a companion have the advantage of a location that not only needs their services but a support team to take care of travel arrangements and living accommodations without worry or responsibility for others. Many times, dental expedition leaders with large teams feel like travel agents with the extra duties, taking away from their enjoyment of doing dentistry.

One oral surgeon, Dr. Dan Bluth, exemplifies this spirit of individual service. Since 1993 he has serviced the poor in the northern section of the state of Chihuahua, Mexico. Once a month he is on a plane to El Paso, Texas. Picking up his car at the airport, he crosses the border and heads south to his first stop in Ascension at the DIF (Desarrollo Integral De La Familia.) This is an all-purpose facility set up and run by the wife of the state's President for Relief of the Poor. It provides food, education, and counseling by a small staff and, once a month, a visit by a dentist. The word is sent out over the local radio station that the doctor will be there on a certain morning. People are ready and waiting when he arrives. Patients pay a small amount (based on their ability to pay), which helps out with the maintenance and the running of other programs in the facility.

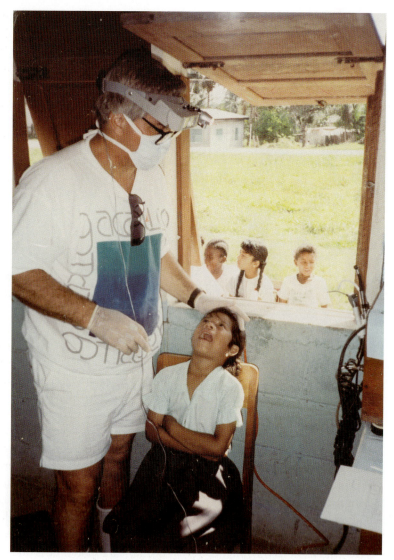

Figure 11-8. Dr. Harris Done treating a patient in Belize.

At the first stop, 15 to 30 patients may be seen for extractions on a given day. While waiting for the anesthetic to work, a discussion on oral hygiene may take place. Obviously, it helps if the dentist and/or his assistant speak the language. In this case, the dentist speaks fluent Spanish. After a while and with goodbyes all around, he is off to the next little community of Janos. It is not as well suited to delivering dental care, and sometimes the word has not been spread that he will be there. Not to worry, though, he will be back next month. If this is the case, then he will just spend more time in the next city of Buenaventura. This time it is a Red Cross building with two ambulances in the driveway, but the treatment protocol is the same as in the other locations. The radio has been announcing his arrival, and patients are there ready to be seen by the Spanish-speaking gringo doctor from the United States. Many have been in before, and friendships have been previously established. The patients are calm knowing that the treatment will be almost painless. The doctor knows his job well. With ease and speed, the tooth or teeth are slipped out. Some comforting words are offered by the doctor, and gratitude is expressed by his patients. Soon, it is time for the next town in line where similar procedures are done on many more patients. The last day on the circuit would be Florez Margon. This town is situated near a river, and it is not uncommon for the local treatment facility to have been flooded. If so, the doctor would not be able to see patients that trip.

When one looks at this schedule—once a month for 11 years: $12 \times 11 = 144$ trips with an average of 75 to 85 patients per trip. This equals approximately 11,520 people seen and treated with not only great skill but a lot of love and kindness. This dentist truly is someone who is showing compassion to less-fortunate fellow beings.

Rendering one-on-one basic care is often the best environment for teaching a local person the skills necessary to treat their own people at a future time when a need arises but no one more qualified is there. Teofilo Cafiero, a Nivacle Indian in Abundancia, Paraguay, is a good example. He had some experience working in Asuncion in a hospital. When visiting dentists came to treat tribe members in his village, he showed a lot of interest in what they were doing. He already was the village medic helping with pregnancies, calling for the ambulance, and dispensing some medications. In the course of the week-long clinic, he was trained in some basic fundamentals by a Spanish-speaking dentist (see Figure 11.9). (Teofilo was the only one that spoke Spanish, the native tongue being Nivacle.) In time and hopefully with some more training, he will be able to adequately treat dental emergencies for his people.

An approach that has proven successful for including native people in the oral health care of their villages includes several important steps:

1. Have communication with the government. Many times they will want the people to know that they approve and even are responsible for the good that is being done.
2. When there is an in-country project manager of a humanitarian group, volunteers can use his or her knowledge to select a

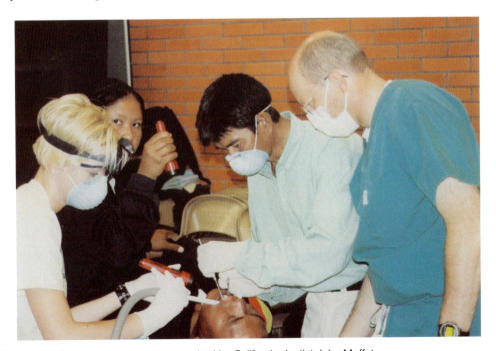

Figure 11-9. Teofilo Cafiero being coached by California dentist John Moffat.

local person who would have the interest to be trained. This person would likely have the trust of the people to possibly provide some simple care in the future or at least recognize danger signs of a life-threatening emergency.
3. In a week-long clinic, the new practitioner observes the dentist for a couple of days.
4. Then he or she does some treating, and the dentist observes.
5. Instruments are left in a kit to be used in a level of treatment that they feel they can handle (see Figure 11.10).
6. By observing the use of boiling water and rubbing alcohol for instruments infection control is learned.

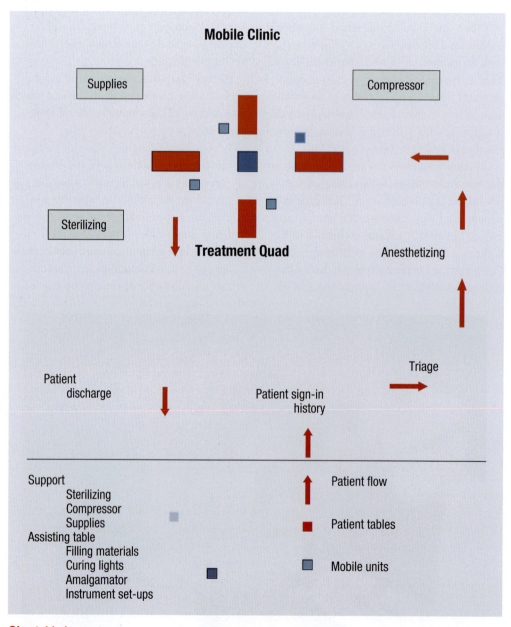

Chart 11–1

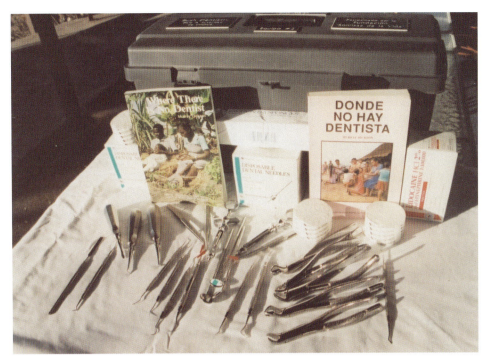

Figure 11-10. Emergency dental kit and manual left with a villager on missions by Dr. Roy Hammond.

7. Small payments for services are encouraged. This person's standard of living is raised as is his status in the community.
8. Replacement items are sent when possible.[9]

LEVEL TWO

Level Two treatment of the poor involves oral hygiene instruction, interceptive restorative care to prevent the otherwise inevitable loss of teeth, and, of course, extractions. Treatment is usually provided with the benefit of electricity and running water—generally using mobile/portable equipment. This level of treatment of necessity usually involves multiple doctors and auxiliary personnel for optimum production.

An organization that illustrates Level Two (giving more comprehensive operative treatment) is Ayuda Inc. See Figure 11.11. *Ayuda* means help in Spanish. This organization has a simple philosophy with the first premise being to "See as many patients and save as many teeth as possible." This is accomplished with a model of patient care for effectively utilizing equipment (see Table 11.2) and personnel. It is based on using a compressor and facility that can service modules of up to four operating stations. An example is the "Treatment Quad" using mobile A-dec units. It can be expanded to two modules (four units each) for a total of eight operating stations. Although mobile chairs can be used, a typical setup would utilize school or church tables with the patient lying supine (see Chart 11-1).

Ayuda's second premise is: "You can't do all things for all people." (See Table 11.3.) Primary teeth are not restored on children. By focusing on and treating first and second molars in children age 6–12, this age group will have fewer carious lesions in permanent teeth. More of the "at risk" teeth that are restored will enable that child to perhaps keep a more lasting dentition into adulthood. Amalgam is the restorative material of choice. Maxillary anterior teeth are almost universally decayed in the older age groups.

CHAPTER 11

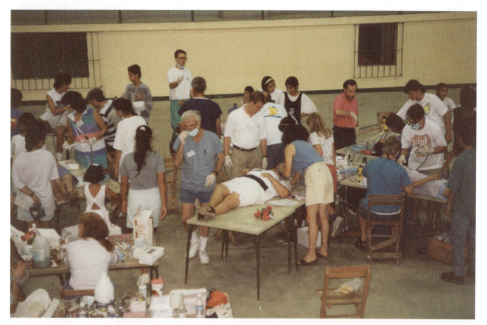

Figure 11-11. An Ayuda Inc. clinic in Mexico with eight mobile units set up with two treatment quads.

Table 11-2. Instruments and Supplies in Kit

1. Mouth mirrors (15)
2. Explorers (15)
3. Syringes, aspirating (3)
4. Scalers, Ivory c-1 (1)
5. Gracy curette 11–12 (1)
6. Filling instrument (1)
7. Cotton pliers (15)
8. Cement spatula (1)
9. Elevators, straight #34 (3)
10. Excavator, spoon (3)
11. Forceps, upper universal #150 (3)
12. Forceps, lower universal #75 (3)
13. Anesthetic, cement, needles, cotton rolls, and flashlight

Table 11-3. Statistics on Four Foreign Mission Trips

	#1	#2	#3	#4
Number of:				
Days	6	4	4	5
Dentists	8	4	7	6
Hygienists	1	2	0	0
Auxiliaries	4	17	5	5
Patients	1489	236	408	266
Fillings	1440	475	653	292
Extractions	1515	354	197	168

Note: #1 = Phnom Penh, Cambodia, 2002; #2 = Abundancia, Paraguay, 2004; #3 = Chiclayo, Peru, 2004; #4 = Puerto Escondido, Mexico, 1998.

In some situations, they can be restored with composite restorations. These people, on whom anterior composites are done, are generally also the same ones who will require some extractions in the posterior.

Using this philosophy and physical setup, an ideal team would consist of the following personnel: Dentists (4–6), Hygienists (1–2), and Auxiliaries (7) for a total of 12–15 members. If an additional treatment quad were used, the total would be 26–28. This philosophy and equipment setup is very efficient with many patients screened, treated, and instructed daily. See Figure 11.12.

LEVEL THREE

Progressing to Level Three would add the incorporation of local professionals that ob-

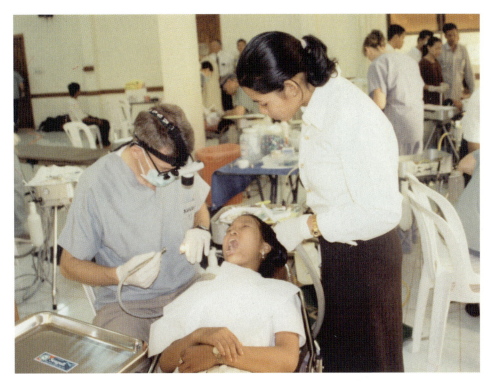

Figure 11-12. Dr. Paul Fillmore utilizing a local assistant.

serve and participate (treat) in clinics in poor areas (see Figures 11.13 and 11.14).

These local people can be instructed in preventive, advanced, and newer procedures and many times get the vision on their own to continue with an out-reach program to the poor in their country. With motivated individuals like this, there can be more long-term benefits for more people. Other projects can supplement these efforts as time goes on with the installation of new equipment or updating of existing dental chairs and units. There could be remodeling or building of new facilities or even establishing teaching programs in dental schools and clinics.

Each level, whether one, two, or three, contributes in its own way to the general goal of decreasing dental disease in these countries. Each has its limitations and will also have its successes and failures. The challenges can be overwhelming, but, at the same time, very rewarding for those going to developing nations to provide care. Many say that their first time was a life-changing experience. Their priorities and views of life and the world are changed.

To see some of the components that go into Level Three projects, we can start with the second organization on the ADA list, the Academy of LDS Dentists. This is not a church organization but just members of a church (The Church of Jesus-Christ of Latter-day Saints) who have organized to give service. One of their projects will serve as a good example of incorporating resources and volunteers within the country to be visited with resources and volunteers from the visiting country. They combine into one continuing project that expands much like the ripples on the water when a stone is dropped. Sometimes viable humanitarian programs often begin quite by chance. Such is the case with the project described in the following case study in Tegucigalpa and Choluteca, Honduras. The sequence

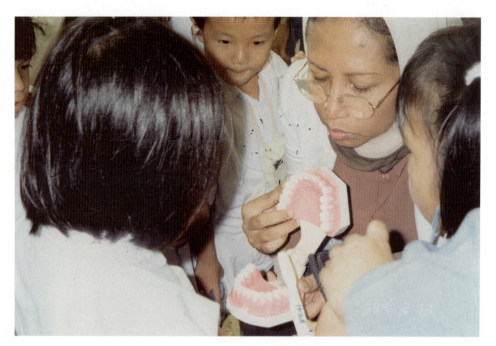

Figure 11-13. A professor at the University of Indonesia giving instructions during an outreach program.

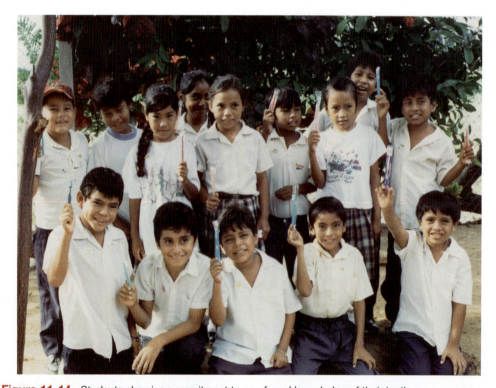

Figure 11-14. Students showing commitment to newfound knowledge of their teeth.

of events in conducting this program were as follows:

August 2003

Academy members met Dr. Ramon Arguelles, Vice Dean of a Dental School, in Tegucigalpa Honduras. Need for dental care was discussed. It was decided that four goals should be set:

1. Conduct a dental project in Choluteca in December for providing patient treatment.
2. Ship dental equipment and supplies to the dental school.
3. Send hospital equipment to the hospital.
4. Establish and maintain a permanent dental clinic at the dental school mainly for the purpose of treating the indigent but also for dentist/auxiliary education.

November 2003

A container of dental equipment, instruments, and supplies was shipped. Some hospital equipment was also included in the container.

December 2003

Forty-six volunteers including 5 general dentists, 1 oral surgeon, and 15 pre-dental students treated patients in the hospital in Choluteca. At this time, Academy members and Dr. Arguelles were the main people involved in the project, but it gave these foreign volunteers the opportunity to meet and become friends with many local dentists and community leaders.

After the school finished renovating existing rooms and installing the donated equipment, there would be a new dental clinic equipped with the following: seven new dental chairs, x-ray machines, compressors, and dental supplies. This new facility was to be used for the following:

1. A certified sixth-year residency program for 12 graduated dental students where they would fulfill their one-year government service requirement by treating the poor.
2. A dental assistant training program.
3. A center for advanced learning and specialty training.
4. A staging area for future service projects for the community with treatment provided by either local dentists or volunteers from abroad.
5. Additional opportunities to increase revenue for the school.
6. A program of continuing education by visiting dental educators (Academy of LDS Dentist or others).

January to April 2004

The dental equipment was installed. The renovations for the new clinic were completed.

May 3, 2004

Academy members returned again for a week-long dental service project for indigent patients utilizing the new clinic as well as other departments in the school. Thirteen dentists, 2 dental assistants, and 12 pre-dental students treated 675 patients doing 787 procedures. The visiting dentists presented three lectures on basic oral surgery, endodontics, and periodontal surgery. That same week inauguration ceremonies were held and the new clinic was officially opened.[6]

III. Planning and Preparing for Volunteer Service

Many circumstances dictate the where, when, why, how, who, and what of a foreign dental mission. This applies to a single practitioner or a large group of volunteers. The project illustrating Level III from the preceding section can accomplish a considerable amount over time, but this may not always be possible or desired.

Regardless of the Level (I, II, or III), if the kind of dentistry to be performed is not clearly understood by all team members with the proper preparation of equipment, instruments, and materials, the trip may not be as successful as anticipated. This being said, there should be contingent plans for not only emergencies but also for ample materials and supplies so that shortages don't arise. It should be made very clear what each team member should bring on the trip and what their duties will be.

"Where" is determined by the particular needs of a country and you finding out about those needs. Projects have been started because of a chance encounter with someone on vacation or by hearing about another humanitarian trip. Many times local officials asking through friends request that a certain non-government organization (NGO) or other humanitarian group help them. The question always becomes one of logistics and viability. Is this place right for the effort to be expended? Are the recipients truly in need?

"When," of course, is easy. A scheduled date needs to consider weather (not monsoon season), availability of locals (not a holiday), and so on.

"Why," is an easy and simple one, too. The underserved population of that country will not have dental treatment unless you and your colleagues provide it.

"Who" has already been answered. "Who" is probably a population of indigenous people that needs help in all too many countries.

"How" is the hardest one. How can volunteers from a foreign country best help them with the treatment of dental disease? This is where humanitarian partnering organizations, usually with a native project leader in-country, can be come into play. For example, there is one project in remote areas of the Dominican Republic that provides ex-

odontia, operative (amalgam and light-cured composites), prosthetic (transitional partial dentures to replace maxillary anterior teeth), and preventive (toothbrushes and sealants) services to approximately 2,700 people each summer. These services are provided using totally portable equipment. The dental teams travel to a different rural village each day establishing their clinic in a school, church, or other suitable building. Dominican Republic dentists have begun providing similar services to the poor during the rest of the year, which is the ultimate solution to these problems.[8]

Conditions, of course, in foreign clinics will be far less than ideal and many times difficult. The importance of correct diagnosis, correct cavity preparation, and proper surgical technique should be stressed. Infection control is important and needs to be emphasized. Certain things may have to be modified, however, and adapted to changing conditions. The most obvious deterrents for the best dentistry are as follows:

- **Lighting.** Head lamps are by far the most useful and dependable.
- **Communications between doctor and patient.** At the very least one member of the team needs to speak the language. Even then, dental-related facts or post-op instructions may not be understood by the patient, depending on local dialects.
- **Lack of medication.** Medications are usually brought by volunteers.
- **Equipment failure.** Repair kits for units and other tools need to be included when packing.
- In addition, some other potentially troublesome areas are as follows:
  1. Problem with dryness of field.
  2. Longer time needed to perform procedures.
  3. Less than ideal patient positioning.
  4. Less help from chairside assistant.
  5. Long work hours.

THIRD WORLD VOLUNTEER DENTISTRY   313

Table 11-4. Ayuda Foreign Clinic Armamentarium*

Equipment	#	Instruments exam/anesthetic	#
Dental units	4	Aspirating syringe	12
Compressor	1	Mirror (exam)	12
Sterilization unit	1	Explorer (exam)	12
Amalgamator	1		
Curing light	2		
Cavitron	1		
Handpieces	8		

Operative setup	#	Surgery setup	#
Nine Instruments			
Explorer	12	Forceps-upper-universals	3
Amalgam carrier	12	Forceps lower-universals	3
Excavator	12	Forceps-lower-cowhorns	3
Mirror	12	Forceps-upper-cowhorns	3
Cotton pliers	12	Elevator-large, and small straight, Potts	6
Plastic instrument	12	Root-tip pick	2
Burisher	12	Rongeurs	1
Carver	12	Periosteal elevator	3
Condenser	12	Scalpel and blades	3
		Needle holder	3
		Bone file	2
		Bite block	3
		Tissue scissors	2
		Curette	2

Team Members/Assignments		
Dentist	**Hygienist**	**Auxiliary**
Anesthetizing	Triage	Assisting
Triage	Anesthetizing	Patient education
Operative, surgery	Patient education	Sterilizing
	Prophy	Charting

Note: #, number of each item needed.

* Based on 4 mobile units, 4–5 dentists.

The equipment, instrument, and material list (see Tables 11.4 and 11.5.) will suffice as a checklist for anyone finding himself in charge of a foreign clinic.

Another important step is to check the web page of the Centers for Disease Control for the immunizations required for the country to be visited (see Table 11.6).

IV, Gaining a New Perspective

There is an almost universal consensus from people returning from third world volunteer missions that good things were accomplished. Comments like "I learned so much," "I want to go back," "I wish I could have done more," "I love those people." It is a wonderful learning experience. It is too

Table 11-5. Ayuda Foreign Clinic Material List*

Materials	Quantities
Alloy (double spill)	1,000 capsules
Composite kit (anterior)	100 applications
Sealant kit	100 patients
Anesthetic (with epi.)	1,000 cartridges
(without epi.)	200 cartridges
Anesthetic (topical)	2 jars
Needles (27 ga L)	500
(30 ga S)	500
Burs (557, #2, #4, #8 rd.#12 fluted)	
Flame-football	50 each
Gauze 2 × 2	1,600
Cotton rolls	1,600
Gloves (SML)	2,000
Masks	200
Prophy angles/paste	50
Evacuator tips	800
Cold sterilizing solution	1 gal
Distilled water (sterilizer)	5 gal
Surface disinfectants (wipes)	2 bottles
Alcohol	1 bottle
Wedges, matrix strips-bands	
Mixing pads, finishing strips	
Temporary cement, cotton pellets	
Base material, articulating paper	
Glass ionomer build-up mat	1 box each

* Quantities based on 4–5 days, 4 mobile units, 4–5 dentists (40 patients/Dr./day = 800 patients).

Table 11-6. Centers for Disease Control Immunization Guidelines for Traveling to South America 2004 (subject to change*)

- Hepatitis A or immune globulin (IG).
- Hepatitis B if you might be exposed to blood (for example, health care workers), stay > 6 months in the region.
- Rabies if you might be exposed to wild or domestic animals.
- Typhoid, particularly if you are visiting developing countries in this region.
- Yellow fever vaccination, if you will be traveling outside urban areas.
- As needed booster doses for tetanus-diphtheria and measles.

* See Centers for Disease Control Web site for vaccines required for the specific country to be visited.

bad that more people can't have the opportunity.

It is also a time of personal growth and perhaps a changing of attitudes. The first trip leaves a sense of satisfaction and appreciation for the people and culture. With a subsequent visit there is usually a desire to not only treat and teach as before but to get to know the people better. After a few trips one really looks forward to returning to see good friends again.

To share one of the author's surprising memories: A young girl was probably 11 or 12 years old and looked pretty much the same as the others waiting to be examined and receive dental treatment by a visiting dental team. It was very hot and would be a very long day before all the people were treated.

The people who had traveled some distance to be seen were wonderful, friendly, cooperative, and appreciated everything that was done for them. The village and countryside with their customs and way of life was a source of awe and admiration for the visitors. These foreigners appreciated the simple oneness with nature that they saw.

Typically, the adults would have few teeth left. Many had been extracted; others had roots that were slowly being avulsed due to infection. Some patients had acute pain; others did not. The children were the main focus. How many of their teeth could be saved and how many would need extraction?

At her age this girl would likely be the same as most of the others—never having seen a dentist, never having had any oral hygiene instruction, and with lower first molars decayed probably too deep to be saved.

"Abre la boca, por favor." (please open your mouth). "Grande" (wide) so that I can see." What a surprise. Her mouth wasn't typ-

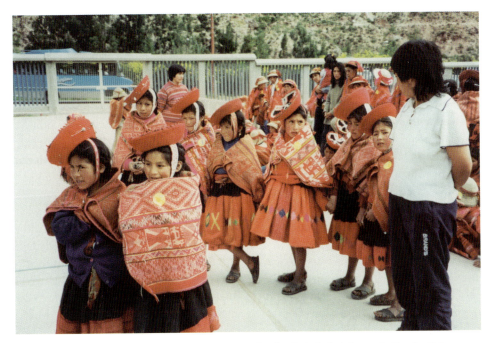

Figure 11-15. Children just arrived from the mountains for their first visit ever to the dentist.

ical. There had been some home care, and all four first molars stood out because of large silver fillings in each one. These restorations had saved those teeth until now and hopefully long into the future. Any dentist would be proud to have placed them under the circumstances. "¿Que es esta, de donde vinieron esos tapitas, cuando?" (What is this, where did these fillings come from, and when?) Her proud answer, "Una dentista, como tu de America" (A dentist like you from America). "Hace dos anos." (It has been two years.)[10]

Here is another example: We can read the remarks of Fredrick Meyers from his 2000 trip to Ollantaytambo in the Sacred Valley, Peru. This gives the reader not only an organizational and procedural overview of a working foreign clinic, but also the insights and feelings of a compassionate dentist.

"The clinic was set up in a church, and the children were transported in open trucks from the surrounding mountains (see Figure 11.15).

The first group of children would then either go into the diagnosis room or into a room to be taught dental and personal hygiene. In dental hygiene there were instructional pictures on the wall. Each person was taught about the causes of dental decay and prevention through brushing and flossing. Each patient was given a bag containing a toothbrush, toothpaste, and other useful items depending on their age group.

From there they went into another room for diagnosis where a doctor examined their teeth and an assistant held a flashlight and recorded a list of teeth needing treatment. I was touched to see many of them (children) try to calm the fears of others. As I started working in diagnosis, I was heartbroken to see the condition of their little mouths. Most had rampant decay, and many had teeth with abscesses. A feeling of complete hopelessness started to overcome my emotions, and I was at a loss on the best way to treat each patient with only minimal time allotted to each one. I was very unprepared for this.

The patient would then go into another room to receive injections of local anesthetic.

The patient would be placed into the next available spot and receive either fillings in permanent teeth or extractions of abscessed or painful teeth that were nonrestorable. Lastly, the younger patients without serious problems would go to an area to receive fluoride treatments and then be ushered outside to wait for the ride home.

In the center of the treatment room was a table set up with an amalgamator, curing light, and a variety of cements, liners, and materials for immediate use by the doctors. This helped because things they needed could be mixed and ready in an instant so the doctors and assistants didn't have to leave their workstations. Sterilization was set up in the kitchen area and was a marvel of efficiency. Like I said, the enthusiasm was incredible, and work proceeded at a rapid rate.

The first day we were able to see 208 patients, mostly children. By the end of the day volunteers had endured long hours and strenuous work. Our bodies cried out for rest and a good night's sleep, which came easily for most.

The conversation at the dinner table was filled with great stories and experiences of how all of us had been touched that day. I never saw a decline of enthusiasm for the work nor had I ever seen a happier group of volunteers.

The next day was a repeat of the first in intensity only this time we received a real treat. A whole village of pure Inca native people was brought down by Jamie and Terry Figueroa. Many of these villages survived the great conquest of the Spaniards and had preserved their cultures by living deep within the mountains at altitudes of 13–14,000 feet. They all showed up dressed in their beautiful native dress causing great excitement in all of us. It was incredible to treat these people. Most didn't understand Spanish and spoke only Quechua, the native Inca language.

The work was difficult for two reasons.

First, the language barrier made it hard to build their confidence. Second, we all felt intense sadness due to their poor health condition. One small child when asked how she felt and whether there was anything that bothered her answered, "At times my stomach hurts, and sometimes worms come out of my body."

I was excited to observe the behavior and actions of children as they came in and climbed onto the table. From the way they walked and carried themselves to the way they interacted with us showed vast cultural differences. All had severely chapped cheeks and dry skin due to windburn. On their feet, they wore sandals. Their feet looked like dried leather caked with dirt and dried clay, and by the appearance, you would think they had never been washed. Everything they wore was made by hand—nothing having been purchased in a store. Their world was completely different from mine; still, they put their total trust in us.

I don't remember a time in my life when I felt such an intense love and admiration for a people, all of whom were complete strangers. I was willing to do anything for them if given the chance. I was humbled to see the aura of contentment each had in spite of what appeared to us as poverty. These were happy people who suffered from physical hardships but loved life and their community and had a deep belief in their religion and moral codes. I am sure that we have more to learn from them than they do from us.

When we finished, we were honored with a presentation of native songs and dances prepared by the children. Once again, the emotion was intense, and I again marveled at the rich culture and pure joy emanating from these beautiful people. Experiences like this just don't exist in the Untied States.

It was hard leaving Cuzco because I was leaving a series of experiences that would change my life forever (see Figure 11.6). This place will always be a spot in the world

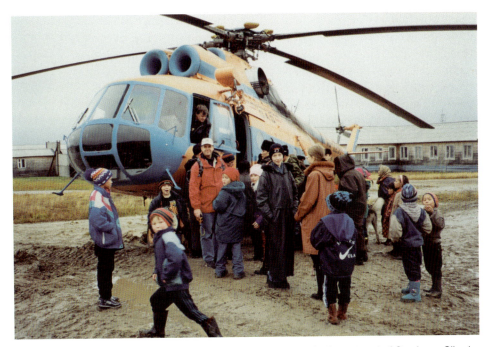

Figure 11-16. Craig Smith saying good-bye to grateful patients in the outpost of Samburg, Siberia.

where many of my deepest feelings of love for my fellowman were cultivated. For a long time, I will remember and relive in my thoughts the joy that comes from true acts of charity performed by these dental volunteers."[11]

Conclusion

Globalization has many facets—not the least of which should be recognition of the disparity that exists among nations. The world that has been described in this chapter waits for those who are willing to accept not only the challenges but also the innumerable rewards that come from sharing needed skills and talents with others.

Bibliography

1. S. Thope. Oral health in Africa. *Developing Dentistry* 5(1): 1. 2004.
2. C. Nackstad. *Ferney Communique.* March p. 3. 2004.
3. J. E. Frencken, C. J. Holmgren, W. Helderman, H. van Palenstein. Basic package of oral care. *WHO Collaborating Centre for Oral Health Care Planning and Future Scenarios.*
4. W. Mautsch. The Berlin Oral Health Declaration—10 Years Later: Where Are We Now? *Developing Dentistry.* 1/03 p. 2. 2003.
5. M. Dickson. *Where There Is No Dentist,* 8th ed. Berkeley, California: The Hesperian Foundation. Introduction by D. Werner. p. 169. 1983.
6. A. A. Khan. Oral Health Services in Developing Countries: A case for the Primary Health Care Approach. *Developing Dentistry* 5 (2). 2004.
7. J. A. Robertson. McL. Unpublished paper. *Volunteer Dental Projects.* pp. 1–4.
8. F. G. Serio, H. M. Cherrett. *International Dental Volunteer Organizations: A Guide to Service and a Directory Of Programs.* 2nd ed. Chicago, Illinois: American Dental Association. pp. 7, 18, 22, 44, 52. 1993.
9. R. A. Hammond. Author Interview. 2005.
10. R. C. Smith. *Ayuda-Inc.Newsletter.* 2002.
11. F. Meyers. *Diary Peru 2000.* 2004 *Honduras Project Report to the LDS Academy.* 2000.

Index

Academy of LDS Dentists, 309
Affordable Fluoride Toothpaste (AFT), 299
Alveoplasty, 85
Aneurysm, 293
Anxiety, 9, 10, 222, 224, 228, 236, 239
Antibiotics, 255, 268, 273
    Bactericidal, 262
    Bacteriostatic, 262
    Cephalosporin, 273
    Clindamycin, 274
    Erythromycin, 273
    Local delivery, 266
    Metronidazole, 274
    Penicillin, 268, 273
    Prophylaxis , 270
    Tetracycline, 274
Arteries,
    Inferior alveolar, 281
    Facial, 281
    Greater palatine, 281
    Lingual, 281
Atraumatic Restorative Treatment (ART), 299
Ayuda Organization, 307

Bacteria,
    Aerobic, 258
    Anatomy, 256
    Anaerobic , 258, 261
    Characteristics, 255
    Gram negative, 259, 260, 262
    Gram positive, 259, 260
    Resistance, 257
    Spontaneous mutation, 257
    Plasmid transfer resistance, 257
Basic Life Support (BLS), 13, 15
Benzodiazepines, 228, 236
    Halcion (triazolam), 237, 238, 240, 245
    Valium (diazepam), 225
    Versed (midazolam), 237
    Ativan (lorazepam), 238
Biologic width, 99, 121
Biopsy,
    Aspiration, 209

    Brush, 207
    Excisional, 212
    Form for submission, 217
    Incisional, 212
    Needle, 210
    Instrument list for, 213
    Oral CDx, 207
Bleeding, 12, 77, 133, 277
    History of, 282,
    Medications influencing, 283
    Nutrient canal, 288
    Post-operative, 291
    Prevention of, 281, 286
    Primary sources in oral cavity, 280
    Secondary, 292,
    Socket, 287
    Soft tissue, 286
Blood,
    Disseminated Intravascular Coagulation (DIC), 279
    Hemophilia, 278
    Hypertension, 278
    Thrombocytopenia, 277
    von Willebrand's Disease, 278
Bone removal, 19, 64, 73, 129,

Cardiovascular disease, 10
Chalazion forcep, 215
Chemiluminescent diagnosis, 210
Complications, 75, 133, 196
Consent forms, 7, 57, 108, 109

Dentist to population ratio, 298
Dentures, 84
Diabetes, 12
Dry socket (alveolar osteitis), 76

Emergency kit, 16
Epilepsy, 12
Epinephrine, 17, 163
Epulis fissuratum, 90
Exodontia
    Indications, 20

319

320 CHAPTER 11

Exodontia (*continued*)
   Multiple teeth, 42,
   Technique, 32, 33, 42, 46

Federation Dentaire Internationale (FDI), 296
Flaps,
   Design, 26, 62, 71, 124, 167
   Envelope, 43, 63
   Scalloped, 169
   Trapezoidal (rectangular), 169
   Triangular (3-cornered) , 45, 64, 167, 168
Force (controlled), 31
Fractures (mandible, maxilla), 54, 79
Frenectomy, 93, 96

Gelfoam, 77
Grafting, 96
Gingivectomy, 114
Gram staining, 259

Health history, 201
Hemangioma, 293
Hemostatic gauze, 287
HIPPA, 18
Human Immunodeficiency Virus (HIV) , 280

Incisions, 26, 62, 85, 115, 126, 167, 213
Infection, 50, 76, 133, 255, 258, 259, 262, 264, 268, 269

Lesions, 201
   History, 202
   Decision tree, 206
Levels of Assistance (for 3rd world volunteers), 301
Liver dysfunction, 11, 282

Malignancy,
   Risk factors, 207
   Signs, 205
Maxillary sinus, 23, 149
Maxillary tuberosity, 86
Medical history form, 4, 5, 150, 158, 281
Microscope (surgical operating), 152
Microsurgical instruments, 153
Mineral Trioxide Aggregate (MTA), 191
Mucocele, 208

Nerve injury, 52, 55, 78,
Nitrous oxide, 227, 229, 231

Oral Urgent Treatment (OUT), 299

Pain, 54, 76, 133
Papillary hyperplasia, 92
Planning for volunteer service, 311
Patient Evaluation, 3, 5, 9, 81, 201
Pericoronitis, 50
Periotomes, 46
Pregnancy, 13
Pulse oximeter, 236

Retrograde filling, 189
Retropreparation, 184
Ridge augmentation, 90
Romazicon (flumazenil), 247
Root resection, 176
Root resorption, 51
Root tips, 36, 39, 159

SBE prophylaxis, 271
Sedation,
   Drugs , 225, 227
   Intravenous, 227
   Levels, 222
   Oral, 226
   Safety, 224
Sounding bone, 115, 124,
Speculoscopy, 210
Super EBA cement, 190
Surgical crown lengthening, 99,
Surgicel, 44, 77, 287
Suturing, 43, 46, 71, 130, 131, 133, 195

Third molar impactions, 49, 58, 71
Third world dental conditions, 295
Tori, 90
Treatment planning, 26, 83, 101

Ultrasonic instruments, 138, 153

ViziLite, 210
Vestibuloplasty, 92

World Dental Federation (WDF), 297
World Health Organization (WHO), 297